Urodynamic and Reconstructive Surgery of the Lower Urinary Tract

Published volumes in this series

Arterial Surgery of the Lower Limb
P. R. F. Bell

Operative Paediatric Urology
J. David Frank and J. H. Johnston

Stone Surgery
Michael Marberger, John M. Fitzpatrick,
Alan D. Jenkins, Charles Y. C. Pak

Operative Spinal Surgery
M. J. Torrens and R. A. Dickson

For Churchill Livingstone:

Publisher: Simon Fathers
Project Editor: Clare Wood-Allum
Copy Editor: Ruth Swan
Production Controller: Neil Dickson
Sales Promotion Executive: Louise Johnstone

PRACTICE OF SURGERY

Urodynamic and Reconstructive Surgery of the Lower Urinary Tract

A. R. MUNDY MS FRCS MRCP

Professor of Urology in the University of London at Guy's Hospital and the Institute of Urology, London, UK

ILLUSTRATIONS BY
PHILIP WILSON FMAA AIMI

Churchill Livingstone

EDINBURGH LONDON MADRID MELBOURNE NEW YORK AND TOKYO 1993

CHURCHILL LIVINGSTONE
Medical Division of Longman Group UK Limited

Distributed in the United States of America by
Churchill Livingstone Inc., 650 Avenue of the
Americas, New York, N.Y. 10011, and
throughout the world.

First published 1993

ISBN 0-443-03348-X

**British Library of Cataloguing in Publication
Data**
A catalogue record for this book is available from
the British Library.

**Library of Congress Cataloging in Publication
Data**
A catalog record for this book is available from
the Library of Congress.

The
publisher's
policy is to use
**paper manufactured
from sustainable forests**

Printed and bound in Great Britain by
William Clowes Limited, Beccles and London

This book is a personal view of urodynamic and reconstructive surgery of the lower urinary tract. It is by no means an encyclopaedic review of the subject; it describes the way I deal with the problems I see in clinical practice. If a clinical problem is not described it is either because it is so common that it does not seem necessary to discuss it in a book such as this (e.g. benign prostatic hyperplasia and meatal stenosis — both, being obstructions, are technically speaking urodynamic), or because it is more properly dealt with by someone else (e.g. urethral valves, hypospadias and exstrophy — by a paediatric urologist), or so rare that I have never had to deal with it. Everything here is tried and tested.

Equally I have made no attempt to describe all the ways a particular procedure might be performed but only the way I perform it. There seems little point in describing numerous trivial variations if I have never felt they were indicated. Given their current popularity, descriptions of the various gut pouches for continent diversion are the best example I can give of the sort of thing a reader might be surprised to find missing from this book.

Because the book is a personal view of the subject I have written it in the first person rather than in the third person as is more usual in 'scientific' writing. I hope that this might help readers to maintain a healthy degree of scepticism as they read the book so that they will not accept any statement as the last word on the subject. There are too many last words on the subject as it is. There are many ways of skinning a cat and each surgeon develops his own way of dealing with a problem that works best in his own hands. This book is not intended for those who already know how to skin a cat but for those who might like to learn. Equally, I have given only a few carefully selected references at the end of each chapter, chosen on the basis that they substantially expand on points made in the text and therefore make it worthwhile looking them up and reading them. In my opinion the prolific use of references in books such as this is to be deprecated on three counts — they clog up the text, they often refer to articles with a theme that is only peripheral to the main point at issue and they often merely serve to substantiate the author's own prejudices by quoting some other author with similar prejudices.

Preface

It would have been possible to write this book in one of two ways — either as a series of operations discussing the indications for each as a preliminary to a description of the technique itself; or as a series of clinical problems, discussing and describing the treatment in relation to the problem to be solved. I have chosen the latter approach although it produces more repetition and a greater amount of referral back to earlier chapters as one proceeds through the book. The reasons for choosing this approach are that patients usually present with clinical problems rather than with a request for a particular operation and because I feel that this approach makes it easier to understand the general principles and rationale of the proposed surgical procedure. As a general rule each operation is described in detail on the first occasion it is mentioned in the book and the reader is subsequently referred back to that description if it is mentioned again as a treatment option in a later chapter. Thus the book is best read from start to finish so that when the reader is referred back to a previous point or technique he or she will hopefully already be familiar with what is being referred to.

The order of chapters is loosely based on the idea of going from common to less common and from easier to more difficult problems. And, because I believe that an understanding of urodynamic problems is fundamental to the management of the more complex reconstructive problems, I have subdivided the book into 'urodynamic' and 'reconstructive' sections, recognising the rather artificial nature of such a distinction, with an introductory section on general perioperative considerations.

It has been said that research is taking ideas from lots of people whereas taking ideas from one person is plagiarism. I had no formal training in reconstructive urology because there was no such thing at the time, so most of the ideas I have had and most of the procedures I perform I have developed from what I have read and from what I have heard in conversations I have had over the years involving people too numerous to mention. Several very specific acknowledgements deserve to be recorded. To the others, if I am guilty of plagiarism, I apologise.

I always wanted to be a surgeon and Harry Naylor taught me how. Most of the basic surgical techniques I use I learnt from him and most of my surgical philosophy is derived from his. To him and to Eric Murray and Bill Hamer who also influenced my first steps in surgery at the South Essex group of hospitals I express my gratitude.

Urology was never what I intended for myself until that sudden numbing realisation whilst staring mournfully at some strangulated piles that there must be more to life than this and until I worked for Hugh Kinder. He 'reorientated' me to urology and he and Michael Joyce and James Flannery encouraged me to develop an interest in incontinence which ultimately led me to the wider field of reconstructive urology. They are now my friends and colleagues at Guy's and continue to support me, probably more than I am aware of. To Michael Joyce I owe a particular debt in this regard.

In reconstructive surgery the two most profound influences in my career have been two men I never worked with — Richard Turner Warwick from London, who I now know well, and Hardy Hendren from Boston, who I have only had the opportunity of meeting once. They taught me by their example that it is surgery, not politics, that is 'the art of the possible'.

Most influences in recent years have been from conversations with a small group of friends particularly Tim Stephenson from Cardiff, Paul Abrams from Bristol, David Thomas from Sheffield, Tony Rickwood from Liverpool, Peter Worth from London and Howard Snyder from Philadelphia, bouncing ideas off them and working problems out with them. To Tony Rickwood I am particularly grateful as he was kind enough to read the manuscript and make comments and criticisms of which I have duly taken note.

In everyday life the Guy's unit wouldn't run as efficiently as it does without the help of Hugh Saxton and his colleagues in radiology, Margaret Borzyskowski in paediatric neurology, Cyril Chantler and his colleagues in paediatric nephrology and especially John Paddle my anaesthetic friend and colleague, who regularly works late into the night keeping patients alive at one end whilst I create havoc at the other end. To them and to Sister Janice Horton of Martha Ward and the other nursing and medical staff who have helped me over the years by doing all the real work of looking after the patients, my thanks.

Preface

The book would never have been written at all but for the typing skills and hard work of Nikki Lewis, Emily Mundy, Jane Restorick and Debra Hendley and the Department of Medical Illustration and Photography at Guy's headed by David Bragg. Finally, I always wanted to play the piano and to draw like Philip Wilson — to him goes the last word of thanks and the most important for the splendid illustrations. (I still can't play the piano either.)

London 1993   A. R. Mundy

For
Samantha

GENERAL CONSIDERATIONS

Chapter 1

Introductory comments

INTRODUCTION

The scope of urodynamic and reconstructive urological surgery is wide and, for the purposes of this book, is taken to include all the surgical procedures applicable to the treatment of the various structural and functional abnormalities that affect the lower urinary tract. By structural abnormalities I mean those congenital and acquired conditions that alter the morphology of the lower urinary tract and may thereby impair its function; by functional abnormalities I mean those congenital and acquired conditions of the lower urinary tract that directly affect its function without necessarily altering its appearance. Urodynamic and reconstructive surgery of the upper urinary tract, such as it is, is not considered here except where it is related to a lower urinary tract problem or its surgical treatment. Some conditions, notably previous untreated exstrophy, male epispadias and hypospadias, are not discussed here as they are more properly the scope of the paediatric urologist at first presentation and other conditions, such as benign prostatic hyperplasia, are only discussed in outline because they are within the province of all urologists and are in any case discussed in great detail and very well in many other publications.

In essence the scope of this book is a description of all the surgical procedures that an interested surgeon might be called upon to undertake if he runs a reasonably sophisticated video-urodynamic investigational unit with all the appropriate back-up services. The value of these radiological, nuclear medical, adult and paediatric nephrological, neurological and anaesthetic support services cannot be overstated — without them many of the procedures described in this volume would be impossible.

In the main the procedures described here are intended to deal with disordered continence, although not necessarily incontinence. This is an extremely common problem with a wide spectrum of both presentation and treatment. Within these spectra, the attitudes of both the patient and the surgeon are influenced by secondary considerations. In general, obstructive problems are taken more seriously by the surgeon and less seriously by the patient because the surgeon has in mind the serious potential effects on renal function whereas the patient often feels only minor inconvenience until a comparatively advanced stage. By contrast, problems of incontinence are more serious to the patient because of the considerable social and sometimes occupational embarrassment, whereas the surgeon recognises that at least the urinary tract is 'safe', with notable exceptions, as far as renal function is concerned.

With treatment the situation is similar because obstructive problems are more clear cut and there is little else to offer except corrective surgery, which is itself fairly straightforward, whereas incontinence problems vary enormously from the trivial to the extreme and have a variety of treatment options the relative merits of which are often, at best, controversial and, at worst, unproven (again with some notable exceptions).

Thus with obstructive problems the assessment and treatment are straightforward, even if the surgical techniques used, as with the correction of pelvic fracture strictures, are sometimes difficult. On the other hand, with problems of incontinence there are several associated factors to be considered other than the problem of incontinence itself when assessing many patients, and there is much debate about the role of surgery when it comes to considering treatment.

There is a body of opinion that expresses the view that there are two types of incontinence — curable and incurable. Curable conditions would include most forms of stress incontinence in women, simple fistulae and some instances of urge incontinence in patients of either sex. Incurable conditions would include those types associated with irreversible brain failure, neurological disease or congenital malformations and more complex forms of stress and urge incontinence and fistulae. For the latter group, it is argued, containment of the incontinence by the use of catheters, appliances or appropriately designed pads and pants or, alternatively, urinary diversion, are more appropriate than the treatment of the underlying condition.

Although one can appreciate the point of view and its rationale, this does seem a rather pessimistic oversimplification. A more optimistic viewpoint, to which I subscribe, is that with currently available surgical techniques and associated non-surgical treatments, everybody is potentially curable and that incontinence is a disability which carries a morbidity factor which has to be weighed up against other morbidity factors when deciding whether or not that potential can be realised.

The disability of incontinence (or abnormal continence), on the one hand, may be associated with other similar and related disabilities such as bowel and sexual dysfunction and is commonly complicated by both emotional/psychological problems and occupational/social problems, usually but not always as a direct result of the incontinence or its previous treatment, particularly if the previous treatment was a urinary diversion. On the other hand, nobody ever died of wetting themselves, whereas they do die occasionally as a consequence of surgery and they do more commonly suffer morbidity and loss of income/education from time off work/school. Thus, when deciding on the best form of treatment for the patient, the nuisance value of the incontinence has to be weighed against the risk factors for that particular individual taking into account the nature of the disability, the patient's age, sex, occupation, motivation, intelligence, general health, mobility, manipulative skills, the associated genital, ano-rectal or other problems and the possible secondary effects of the disease on the one hand; and the mortality, morbidity and nuisance value of treatment on the other. As a result of applying this complicated equation, after patients responding to medical treatment have been excluded, some patients will indeed be regarded as incurable, just as in any other disease, but these will only be those whose general medical condition or intelligence and motivation are so restrictive as to make *any* form of surgical treatment unrealistic unless for a life-threatening condition.

A final word on this point concerns the attitude of the referring physician or surgeon and others concerned with the care of the patient. Whereas obstructive urodynamic problems require treatment by anybody's standards, non-obstructive urodynamic problems and reconstructive problems are often approached in a negative fashion according to the personal prejudice of the individual concerned. In general, nephrologists have not the least interest in what happens to the urine once it has passed the distal convoluted tubule. An ileal conduit seems to them to be a perfectly satisfactory solution to every urological problem. Equally, to many urologists an ileal conduit is an easy and effective solution to many severe congenital problems, to the problems of the neuropathic bladder and in the management of patients having a cystectomy for bladder cancer. This is important because it sometimes has the knock-on effect of putting the reconstructive surgeon on the defensive, seeking to justify his mode of practice. One has to accept that there is often a lot of sense in the non-reconstructive approach and one must always resist the urge to be over-enthusiastic about the reconstructive approach to a problem, particularly as many patients are easily swayed by a confident presentation of an apparently easy solution to their problem or problems. The patient whose ill-advised reconstructive procedure has failed is hardly likely to thank you for it when he or she ends up with the ileal conduit that some other surgeon suggested in the first place.

ASSESSMENT OF PATIENTS WITH A VIEW TO SURGERY

It should not be necessary to say that the essential prerequisite for effective treatment is adequate preoperative assessment and postoperative follow up. The best chance of surgical cure of almost all the conditions described in later chapters is at the first operation and this point cannot be overstated. Nor should it be necessary to say that surgical treatment should not be considered until all available non-surgical treatment methods have been tried or shown to be inappropriate.

This is not the place to describe the techniques and details of the various assessment modalities, but certain general points are worth highlighting.

Symptomatic assessment
It is always important to be sure what the patient's principal complaint is. This is rarely a problem with strictures and fistulae, but is often a problem in incontinent patients. Young professional women will often tolerate a bit of incontinence, but find frequency and urgency intolerable because it interrupts meetings and other such commitments. Older women who no longer have such occupational commitments usually have a directly opposite point of view because they can go and empty their bladders whenever they feel the need. Young adults may find daytime symptoms acceptable but bedwetting intolerable because of its adverse effect on their sex lives. Some patients with neuropathic dysfunction may adopt a philosophical approach to their incontinence, but find recurrent urinary infection a major disability. Given that one is operating on these patients' abnormalities for their 'nuisance' value in many instances, it is obviously important to be sure what the 'nuisance' actually is, because some symptoms are more readily cured than others. In general it is easier to resolve daytime symptoms than bedwetting, incontinence than frequency and urgency, and obstructive causes of residual urine (and therefore of recurrent urinary infection) than non-obstructive causes.

A specific point to be made is that bedwetting is rarely, if ever, due to a bladder abnormality alone, except in patients who lack bladder sensation. It is therefore inadvisable to offer major surgery to a patient for whom bedwetting is the only troublesome symptom. The patient will rarely be pleased, even if all the other less troublesome symptoms are cured, if he or she still fails to wake up with a full bladder.

With reconstructive problems and particularly in patients with a urinary diversion it is also important to try to find out what the patient expects from you. Many patients have unrealistic expectations of what surgery can offer them and these must be explored and discussed. The more problems the patient has, particularly when the genital tract or anorectum or both are also involved, the more important this is. It is interesting for example that the vast majority of patients presenting at their own instigation for undiversion have had little or no sexual experience. It is common in them to find that they see undiversion as their psychosexual salvation. It is rare with major abnormalities for a reconstructive procedure to return a patient's abnormality entirely to normal. One usually aims to improve an unacceptable abnormality to an acceptable level. One can, for example, straighten out the severe dorsal chordee of epispadias to give the patient a straight erection but one cannot make the erection six inches longer — an obvious point to the surgeon but the patient must realise it too.

Having discussed the patient's symptoms with him or her it is then important to find out whether he or she actually wants treatment or just advice. Many patients get caught up in the system once they have been referred to hospital and their doctors tend to assume that because they have a problem they necessarily want to have it treated. This is often not the case. A typical example is a menopausal lady with stress incontinence of recent onset who is worried that she may become an incontinent, smelly, senile old lady unless she is treated promptly, although her symptoms are not really a problem at the moment. If she can be reassured that she may not deteriorate significantly, that there is no association between incontinence and premature senility and that she can be treated just as easily when her symptoms *are* a problem, then she may be perfectly happy to leave it at that.

Physical examination

It is generally recognised that constipation and major gynaecological abnormalities can have a profound influence on lower tract dysfunction, particularly in the elderly, but it is surprising how often they are overlooked in practice. Equally, there are many women who are embarrassed to talk about their genitalia and may not volunteer their concern about prolapse, but will describe their stress incontinence with enthusiasm. If, for example, an enterocoele coexists with stress incontinence and a cystocoele, then the patient should be told of it so that it can be dealt with if the patient so wishes. A persistent enterocoele is a

common reason for dissatisfaction after an anti-stress incontinence operation.

Investigation

Urodynamic investigation and other non-urodynamic imaging techniques are discussed in detail elsewhere (Mundy et al 1984, Saxton 1987, respectively). Essentially, no patient should be operated on without objective proof of his or her diagnosis. For the assessment of a structural problem this will involve the appropriate radiological assessment of the lower urinary tract, a urinary flow study and endoscopic evaluation; for a functional problem, a video-urodynamic study, usually followed by endoscopy even if only immediately preoperatively. For a previously untreated middle-aged or elderly male patient with symptoms of bladder outflow obstruction, a flow rate study alone may be appropriate and for a previously untreated female patient with stress incontinence, but no frequency, urgency or other symptoms, the objective demonstration of incontinence on coughing will usually suffice, but with these exceptions the full diagnostic armamentarium should be brought to bear.

Equally, when the potential for secondary upper tract complications exists, the upper tracts must be screened by ultrasound at least or by intravenous urography if the facility for a first class ultrasound study does not exist. Further detailed functional evaluation of the upper tracts will be necessary if either of these investigations shows an abnormality.

It is worth noting that it is quite common to hear experts on a particular subject say that such-and-such an investigation is unnecessary and that a less invasive or less detailed study is all that they require before initiating treatment. As a general rule, in major urodynamic or reconstructive urology, it is better to 'over investigate' rather than run the risk of getting into trouble because an investigation was omitted or

inadequate until one is sufficiently confident of one's expertise to minimise one's investigatory pathways (bearing in mind that 'sufficiently confident' usually means 'over confident').

PLANNING AND STAGING OF SURGICAL PROCEDURES

Once the patient has been properly evaluated, non-surgical treatment options have been tried or excluded and the available surgical options have been determined, there will often be two alternative approaches available — the 'safer (or simpler)' approach and the 'ideal' approach. As a general rule both should be discussed frankly with the patient, pointing out the advantages and disadvantages of each, including the potential short-term and long-term complications and problems. With many patients the choice of approach can be left for the individual to choose. In some, poor general medical condition, disability, lack of intelligence or similar factors should sway the surgeon to suppress his or her natural enthusiasm for heroic surgery and recommend the 'simpler' approach more or less strongly. Equally importantly, all patients should be warned that the operative findings may dictate the 'simpler/safer' approach even when both surgeon and patient, after the preoperative evaluation, are inclined to go for the 'ideal' approach.

For example, a young, fit, healthy lady presents with a vesico-vaginal fistula following a Wertheim's hysterectomy and a radical course of radiotherapy for carcinoma of the cervix. Evaluation shows no evidence of residual tumour but a grossly fibrotic, small capacity bladder and vagina. The choice will be between a 'simple, safe' ileal conduit urinary diversion and a 'best option' substitution cytoplasty and vaginoplasty. On the one hand she may decide that she has had enough hospital treatment just recently and wants the quickest possible return to her family and job. On the other hand she may want to be a 'whole woman' again although this may entail a higher risk of further complications and may leave her with a life-long dependence on clean intermittent self catheterisation to empty her bladder completely. She should not be pushed in either direction but choose for herself with *all* the advantages and disadvantages of each given to her. Should she choose the reconstructive approach she should be warned that the operative findings may make reconstruction impossible (although this is rarely the case) so that if, for example, nodal metastases or an unusually severe radiotherapy reaction in the ileum and colon are found that make a conduit urinary diversion a more sensible option, then this option can be taken up without unduly surprising or worrying the patient when she comes round from the anaesthetic.

With most conditions there is no reason to delay treatment once the diagnosis has been confirmed and the appropriate procedure decided upon. In some situations however it is a good idea to wait a while. This particularly applies to post-prostatectomy incontinence (and other post-prostatectomy problems), strictures, and voiding dysfunctions or structural abnormalities after recent surgery. Post-prostatectomy incontinence and related problems will sometimes resolve spontaneously and completely, given time, and this may take up to a year. Untreated post-traumatic strictures may also take some time before the associated fibrosis becomes established and treated strictures may take 3 months or so after treatment before they stabilise; these factors may influence the timing and interpretation of radiological and endoscopic assessment even if they do not influence the surgical decision. Likewise, voiding dysfunction following pelvic surgery in general or urinary tract surgery in particular will often improve over a 3 month period and investigation and treatment should therefore be

delayed until that 3 month period, at least, has elapsed.

Having decided on the timing of the treatment, some consideration will have to be given to the staging of treatment, although this really only applies to complex problems. Even then, 'staging' will usually mean a series of steps within a single procedure rather than a series of separate procedures, although this may be the best way of handling certain complex problems. Staging is therefore more of a thought process than anything else and even the simplest problem will require the same thought process, if only to be sure that important factors are not overlooked.

To give an example in the field of incontinence surgery — three factors are important for continence: an adequate capacity, adequate emptying and voluntary control. When, in addition to incontinence, there are upper tract or other problems to consider, then the order of priority becomes:

1. Define the urodynamic problem(s) and decide how they are to be treated and, equally important, warn the patient of any possible eventualities, particularly if there is multiple urodynamic pathology.
2. Treat associated non-urodynamic problems of the upper urinary tract such as renal stones. These are usually dealt with as an entirely separate procedure.
3. Anticipate the means of voiding, e.g. if clean intermittent self catheterisation (CISC) is to be used ensure that the patient is willing and able to perform the technique beforehand.
4. Eliminate outflow obstruction unless CISC is to be used postoperatively. This may also be dealt with as a separate procedure, often at the time of an otherwise diagnostic endoscopy and EUA, e.g. resection of any residual prostate before implantation of an artificial sphincter for post-prostatectomy incontinence.

5. Ensure an adequate capacity, low-pressure bladder.
6. Provide control of continence. This may sometimes be dealt with as a separate procedure, e.g. delayed implantation of an artificial sphincter after a previous urinary tract reconstruction.

For example, in the relatively simple case of a woman with stress incontinence who also has urge symptoms, only criteria 1 and 6 apply; in other words prove the diagnosis and exclude detrusor instability urodynamically, treat the stress incontinence by an appropriate procedure and warn her beforehand that her urge symptoms may persist. On the other hand, with a patient who has a neuropathic bladder, all six criteria will often apply. These factors will be expanded upon where relevant in subsequent chapters.

REFERENCES

Mundy AR, Stephenson TP, Wein AJ 1984 Urodynamics: principles, practice and application. Churchill Livingstone, Edinburgh
This, in many respects, is a companion volume, hopefully to appear in a second edition in the near future. It is the only book currently available in English that describes in one volume the techniques of investigation, the basic scientific aspects of lower urinary tract structure and function, and the clinical problems in urodynamic practice.
Saxton HM 1987 Urological imaging. In: Mundy AR (ed) Scientific basis of urology. Churchill Livingstone, Edinburgh
This is a good, up-to-date review of all types of urological imaging.

Chapter 2

General perioperative considerations

For many of the procedures described in this volume there are no special preoperative, peroperative or postoperative measures that require discussion. For some procedures there are points that require special attention that vary from case to case. The point of this chapter is to give a brief general overview of the sorts of considerations that should be given to every patient so that they are not overlooked, perhaps with unfortunate consequences.

The factors considered in this chapter are not therefore applicable to all procedures nor are they all-embracing, but they do form a basis for a philosophy of surgical management that is applicable to all types of urodynamic and reconstructive procedures.

PREOPERATIVE PREPARATION

It is assumed that, before he or she reaches hospital, the patient has been deemed fit for whatever procedure he or she is about to undergo. That aside, the principal aim of preoperative preparation is to eliminate real or potential sources of the reconstructive surgeon's greatest enemy — infection. The main potential source of infection is the urinary tract itself.

Urinary tract infection
The patient should have had a mid-stream specimen of urine cultured within 24–48 hours of operation. For a routine procedure it is not essential to have the result before operation if the urine looks clear; for more major procedures it is mandatory. Furthermore any factors that may predispose to urinary tract infection should be dealt with. This specifically refers to indwelling catheters which should always be removed preoperatively, if at all possible.

It is my experience (but not based on concrete evidence) that a minimum of 24 hours of parenteral treatment with a sensitivity-proven antibiotic is required for the treatment of urinary infection before reconstructive surgery for the operation to be safe. If pseudomonas is the causative organism, or if a prosthesis is to be implanted then 24 hours may not be sufficient and the operation should be deferred until the urine has been proved to be sterile.

Bowel preparation
Bowel preparation is necessary before any operation which may involve opening the bowel (e.g. cystoplasty) or before a retropubic implantation of an artificial sphincter (AUS). I also recommend a limited bowel preparation prior to a transperineal operation such as urethroplasty or a bulbar urethral AUS implantation or any other reconstructive procedure that may involve omental mobilisation.

A full 'bowel prep' requires 3–4 days and involves:

Day 4/3 preoperatively — low residue diet, magnesium sulphate 10 ml t.d.s. until diarrhoea develops (then stop it).

Day 3 preoperatively — continue as above. A 4th day is generally only required in patients with particularly severe constipation (e.g. spina bifida).

Day 2 preoperatively — as above, and metronidazole 200–400 mg t.d.s., morning and evening enema.

Preoperative day — fluids only by mouth, magnesium sulphate if necessary, neomycin 1 g q.d.s., metronidazole 200–400 mg t.d.s., morning and evening enema.

Day of operation — parenteral gentamicin, ampicillin and metronidazole with premedication.

In adults, sorbitol or mannitol are alternatives to magnesium sulphate, but children tolerate them poorly and should therefore not be given them.

A limited 'bowel prep' requires only 24 hours and involves:

Preoperative day — fluids only, morning and evening rectal washout.

Day of operation — morning rectal washout, parenteral gentamicin, ampicillin and metronidazole with premedication.

Note that magnesium sulphate is not given with a limited bowel preparation. The aim is to empty the bowel but to avoid diarrhoea that may otherwise leak from the anus preoperatively or postoperatively and contaminate the wound.

It is important to remember, particularly in children, that a full bowel preparation may be dehydrating and the occasional patient may require parenteral fluid replacement prior to surgery or a larger than usual fluid replacement during the operation to counter this effect.

Skin preparation
It is my practice to get patients for major reconstructive surgery to have twice-daily baths with antiseptic soap and at least one hair wash before operation. For more minor procedures one bath is sufficient. It never seems to have done anybody any harm and it may do some good. They certainly smell better.

The patients are shaved at the time of operation. No surgeon would ever dry-shave his face with a razor blade (I can only speak for male surgeons), so it is sensible to adopt the same rationale to pubic shaving of patients — wet shaving using aqueous chlorhexidine produces fewer skin nicks. A depilatory cream is an alternative although allergic reactions limit their usefulness.

Antibiotic prophylaxis
Before any major urinary tract surgery I give at least a single dose of gentamicin with the premedication. Before major

reconstructive surgery, particularly involving cystoplasty or implantation of an artificial sphincter, gentamicin, ampicillin and metronidazole are used in combination and are continued for 3–5 days thereafter.

It is difficult, if not impossible, to provide good evidence to justify the measures outlined in the last four paragraphs beyond saying that infection of a reconstructed urinary tract, particularly in the presence of an artificial sphincter, may be disastrous and, in my practice, the postoperative infection rate (of all types except chest infection) is only 3%. Given these two facts and the observation that, although it may be excessive, no-one has ever suffered adversely from this regime, it is difficult to decide where to cut back on the various measures to determine which of them are essential and which are superfluous.

PEROPERATIVE AND TECHNICAL CONSIDERATIONS

Position
Many procedures may or do require access to the perineum, the pelvis and the abdomen. In such instances it is important that such access is readily available, even if it may prove unnecessary. For this purpose an appropriate operating table is obviously important and the best position for the patient is the low lithotomy position with the legs widely abducted and the hips slightly flexed on Lloyd-Davies leg supports (what one might call 'social' lithotomy!). Apart from providing free access to the perineum, this position ensures that the legs, and particularly the flexed thighs, do not provide an obstacle to the surgeon during intra-pelvic surgery. The low lithotomy position also gives room for two assistants to stand, whatever the site of operation, and allows flexibility for the surgeon to move around the patient to whatever position is most appropriate for the procedure in hand.

Skin preparation
There is no clear evidence to suggest which skin preparation is best but I prefer either an iodine-based fluid, such as Betadine, or chlorhexidine in spirit. Contact time is probably more important than the solution used. I clean the operative area with Betadine first and with chlorhexidine afterwards. This is because Betadine seems a more potent bactericidal agent, assuming that adequate contact time is allowed, but leaves the skin unsuitable for the use of an adhesive film such as Steridrape (3M) or Opsite (Smith & Nephew), which I use routinely. Chlorhexidine leaves the skin suitably prepared for a Steridrape/Opsite adhesive film, but care must be taken if it is used in spirit form to prevent the spirit from coming into contact with the diathermy apparatus, as this may lead to diathermy burns during the course of the procedure.

Drapes
Drapes must allow access to all potential operative sites and exclusion of the anal canal. In the latter respect, indeed in all situations, wet drapes are probably not much better than no drapes at all and this is one of the reasons why I routinely use an adhesive film. In this way the wound is isolated, the drapes are kept in place and contamination through wet drapes is reduced.

Light
Good light is essential. Mobility of the light is also important and this is best provided by having more than one light source. If a readily mobile satellite lamp is not available a headlamp is a useful but often cumbersome alternative.

Diathermy
The choice between standard or purpose-built diathermy instruments, and between hand or foot operated diathermy is an individual decision. I prefer hand-operated diathermy, for its convenience and flexibility in use.

Instruments
The essential requirement for good access is good retraction. Assistants take up room and get bored and tired if they are not doing something interesting; a good mechanical retractor is therefore necessary. I use the Turner Warwick ring retractor system and have a particular preference for malleable copper blades which are more flexible in their use than rigid blades and which are available in several sizes. It is difficult now to imagine operating without them.

As regards what might be called 'effector' instruments, the main requirement is for light, atraumatic instruments of the right length for the job in hand. There is rarely any need, in reconstructive surgery, for toothed dissecting forceps, for any artery forceps other than mosquito forceps (or Lahey forceps for larger or deeper vessels), or for heavy scissors and heavy needleholders. Leave those for the gynaecologists.

I manage almost all procedures with two lengths of deBakey dissecting forceps, two lengths of Babcock forceps, some mosquito clips, Lahey forceps, a pair of McIndoe and Nelson scissors and two lengths of the Turner Warwick needleholder. Needless to say, they should all be in good working order.

Suture material
The mainstay for reconstructive work is an absorbable suture. Traditionally catgut was used, but this has been superseded by polyglycolic acid and polyglactin 910, i.e. by Dexon (Davis and Geck) and Vicryl (Ethicon). I find Vicryl easier to tie and less harsh on the surgeon's own hands. It is also a prettier colour. As a general rule 2/0 gauge is used for the bladder, 3/0 for the urethra, 4/0 for the ureter, 0 for the abdominal wall, 2/0 for subcutaneous tissues and 3/0 for skin in adults and one gauge lower in each instance for children.

General points of operative technique

Most points of technique will be discussed under the appropriate sections, but certain general principles warrant emphasis:

1. Skin preparation and draping should be such that the risk of contamination is reduced to a minimum, taking into account the possibility that incisions may need to be extended or otherwise modified to improve exposure.
2. Incisions should be made so that exposure will be adequate, taking into account the possibility that unforeseen circumstances may arise requiring them to be extended. This means that for any complex procedure a full length midline, pubis to xiphisternum incision is likely to be necessary.
3. Only atraumatic instruments should be used, unless the tissue being handled is to be excised.
4. Haemostasis should be complete or as near complete as possible.
5. Anastomoses and other suture lines should always be entirely tension-free.
6. Always check that a reconstructed ureter or urethra is satisfactory by catheterising it after completing the reconstruction but before closing the incision.
7. Always ensure that there is mucosal apposition at any suture line or anastomosis. For this reason inverting sutures are generally best. If a suture gives mucosal apposition and inversion, one layer is almost always sufficient.
8. Free urine drainage and, where necessary, free drainage of any other exudates must be secured.
9. All mesenteric defects or cavities must be closed or filled.
10. As far as possible, all anastomoses should be supported or wrapped with omentum or some suitable alternative.
11. No anastomosis should be allowed to lie against another anastomosis.
12. No procedure should be undertaken unless the surgeon is sure that he or she is equipped to deal with any circumstance that may arise.
13. Don't take short cuts.

Catheters

The type and size of catheter used varies according to the site and the age of the patient. As a rule, however:

— Urine that does not have a significant blood content only requires a fine catheter (c. 12 or 14 F) to drain it, whereas blood-stained or mucus-containing urine requires something larger (c. 18 or 20 F) and to a large extent this governs the siting of the catheter.
— If the urethra does not require 'stenting', a suprapubic catheter is preferable.
— For short-term catheterisation, latex catheters are adequate.
— For longer-term catheterisation, siliconised catheters are preferable.
— After a urethroplasty a pure silicone catheter is preferable, particularly in a child.
— Large calibre Malecot catheters are painful to remove, so a Foley-type catheter is preferable if a large-sized suprapubic catheter is necessary.
— All catheters should be firmly anchored to the surrounding skin.
— Certain situations require specific types of catheter (e.g. cystoplasty catheters).

Stents/splints

All urethral and ureteric anastomoses are best stented (or splinted, depending on which terminology one prefers). This serves three purposes:

1. It maintains alignment across the anastomosis.
2. It provides proximal diversion of urine from above the level of the anastomosis to below or to the outside, thereby reducing the likelihood of leakage through the anastomosis.
3. It prevents cross-adhesions at the anastomosis.

In addition, ureteric splinting prevents obstruction of the upper tract due to oedema at the anastomosis and urethral splinting allows internal drainage of

blood or other exudates along the catheter (as long as it is not too large), thereby preventing their accumulation.

Ureteric stents/splints. Although purpose-made stents of silicone rubber are available, they are expensive. For the 7–10 days they are needed, long infant feeding tubes are perfectly adequate. They should not be a tight fit, but should lie comfortably within the ureter. This usually requires a 4–6 F in a child and an 8 F tube in an adult, assuming a normal ureteric calibre. If the ureteric calibre is larger, a proportionally larger tube may be used. If a tube with a calibre of 10 F or more is used, there is an advantage in using a Ryle's tube as the radiopaque markers at the tip of the Ryle's tube provide a useful way for checking the position of the tube radiologically during the postoperative period, if necessary.

Urethral stents/splints. A 12–16 F urethral catheter is adequate in an adult, proportionally smaller in a child. Some surgeons like to cut holes in the shaft where the catheter will lie alongside a urethral suture line, to encourage drainage of blood and exudates but this often leads to bypassing of urine from the bladder, down the catheter, out through the holes, into the distal urethra and out around the catheter, which is exceedingly tiresome for the patient and the nursing staff. The important point is not to obstruct the urethra with a large calibre catheter, so that exudates can freely drain out of the urethra alongside the catheter.

Drains

These are used to allow the escape of extravasated urine and blood, or to drain pockets of actual or potential infection. With the exception of the perineum, tube drains are preferable, as they allow extravasated fluids to be collected in a drainage bag, rather than soaking into wound dressings, which is unpleasant for the patient and unhelpful for the nursing and medical staff because the dressings have to be changed more often and because the volume of drainage cannot accurately be assessed. Multiple side holes (e.g. the Robinson's drain) are a distinct advantage. Suction drains are not however an advantage, in general, as they tend to suck tissue into the side holes thereby occluding them, particularly when used near the omentum.

Drains, like catheters, not only let fluids out but are also a potential site for letting infection in. Closed drainage systems are therefore preferable to reduce this risk.

Peroperative antibiotics
Given that the aim of the preoperative preparation is to eradicate foci of infection as far as possible, there should be little need for peroperative antibiotics. When infection exists, drainage is more important than antibiotic treatment. On the other hand, when implanting an artificial sphincter or some other inert material, sterility is particularly important and in such a situation I use either an antibiotic solution (such as bacitracin/neomycin/polymyxin) or more usually an iodine-based solution or spray such as Betadine (Napp Laboratories) or a povidone—iodine spray (Stuart Pharmaceuticals).

Wound closure
The final legacy of any operation is the wound, and for this reason I always use subcuticular closure.

Dressings
Wound dressing should help keep infection out and should stay in place until the risk is past. Clear adhesive dressings for abdominal wounds serve both of these purposes and have the additional advantage of allowing inspection of the wound in the early postoperative period, particularly if the patient develops a fever and wound infection is high on the list of possible explanations.

The use of these dressings is less satisfactory for the perineum, where most types of dressings tend to fall off. These wounds also tend to ooze more and so a standard gauze dressing is sometimes preferable. In such instances, a flexible adhesive tape is necessary to keep the gauze in place and Mefix (Mölnlycke) is particularly good in this respect.

POSTOPERATIVE CARE
Again, a few general comments are appropriate.

Fluid balance and gastric drainage
For the first few days after any major procedure, a patient will obviously require parenteral fluid replacement until a normal oral intake and intestinal function are re-established. After complex procedures the effects of the usual paralytic ileus are compounded by:

— the dehydrating effects of the preoperative preparation,
— the effects of extensive intra-abdominal and particularly of retroperitoneal dissection,
— the disruption and restoration of intestinal continuity in some instances.

Fluid requirements are therefore sometimes high and this makes the monitoring of central venous pressure mandatory after major intra-abdominal surgery. Another effect of extensive intra-abdominal and retroperitoneal surgery is to delay the resolution of paralytic ileus. Commonly, intestinal activity begins to recover after 2 or 3 days, only to be followed by a further period of depressed activity at 5–10 days. This recurrent paralytic ileus should not be confused with mechanical bowel obstruction but, equally, a mechanical bowel obstruction should not be overlooked because of complacency.

Parenteral nutrition is not usually required in patients undergoing urodynamic or reconstructive surgery,

but it is sometimes necessary in older patients and after more than usually extensive surgery and its use should always be considered in the early postoperative period, so that when it is necessary its institution is not unduly delayed. In fact, nowadays, the intensive therapy specialists recommend that enteral feeding is preferable to intravenous feeding and suggest that early enteral feeding should be used routinely. They feel that this not only helps nutritionally but also to reduce the risk of multiple organ failure in seriously ill patients.

Bowel function
Although patients are not as obsessive about bowel function as they used to be, bowel action is nonetheless a generally accepted external sign that all is well internally.

Unfortunately, after preoperative bowel preparation, the return of bowel activity is usually heralded by an impressive degree of diarrhoea. In most patients this is not a problem but it may be so after perineal surgery when it may be a source of contamination. For this reason a bath is advisable after a bowel action if this occurs within 5 days. If it occurs within 3 days or very frequently a wipe with aqueous chlorhexidine is a more reasonable alternative.

Removing drains, splints and catheters
Drains are removed when they stop draining, usually within a few days, although extravasation of urine sometimes takes longer to cease. There is little or no place for shortening of drains prior to their removal in this type of work.

If the patient has ureteric splints, there will almost always be a suprapubic catheter as well. The splints are removed after about 7 days and always before removing the suprapubic bladder catheter (unless indwelling commercially-manufactured, purpose-built 'stents' are used). It is my general practice to remove ureteric splints on about day 7 and then to clamp the suprapubic catheter on day 8 and then, if voiding is promptly re-established, to remove the suprapubic catheter on day 9. If urethral voiding is not satisfactory, the suprapubic catheter is kept in place until it is. If, after urethral surgery, there are both urethral and suprapubic catheters, as is usual, the urethral catheter is removed first (often under X-ray control — see below) for a trial of voiding before the suprapubic catheter is removed. This is usually at 10–15 days with the female urethra, or at 15–20 days with the male urethra, rather than the 7–10 days with ureteric splints.

The importance of relying primarily on suprapubic catheters for most urodynamic and reconstructive procedures (the main exception being endoscopic procedures) cannot be overstated. For the patient they are more comfortable and avoid the need for recatheterisation should problems occur when one tries to re-establish spontaneous urethral voiding. For the surgeon there is the further advantage of allowing radiological assessment of such voiding difficulties without having to remove the catheter.

Thus, whenever a urethral catheter is used in reconstructive urology it should be used in conjunction with a suprapubic catheter and should be regarded primarily as a splint, just like a ureteric splint, rather than as a conduit for urinary drainage, although obviously drainage can and does occur. It should not be regarded as an alternative to a suprapubic catheter, making the latter unnecessary.

In certain groups of patients it is wise to have a radiological assessment of the lower urinary tract before removing the catheters. Thus a ureteric 'stentogram' is advised after transureteroureterostomy (as in undiversion), a cystourethrogram after a urethroplasty, and a cystogram after fistula surgery or after a cystoplasty in a patient who has had previous radiotherapy. Radiology is not routinely used otherwise.

Postoperative antibiotics
With all but the simplest procedures, there is a small but significant incidence of urinary tract infection during the first six weeks. For this reason I usually prescribe a prophylactic antibiotic, usually trimethoprim 100 mg nocte, to cover this period after major surgery.

Follow-up investigation
The success of the procedure can only be determined by repeating the definitive preoperative diagnostic investigation. For the relief of bladder neck or prostatic obstruction, this is a flow rate; for stricture surgery, it is an ascending urethrogram and micturating cystogram; for problems of continence, it is a urodynamic study. In addition, when the upper tracts have been operated on, as in undiversion or substitution cystoplasty, an IVU will be necessary and possibly a renal scan as well. Without such re-investigations it will be impossible to assess objectively the results of surgery and it will also be difficult to decide, in a patient who presents again months or years later, whether she or he has a new problem or a recurrence of the old problem. A surgeon therefore does his patient no service by avoiding the postoperative re-investigation, even if the patient has had a symptomatic cure. Furthermore certain procedures carry their own potential problems, such as voiding dysfunction after cystoplasty, and these are only defined by the appropriate investigations. Follow-up investigations are therefore important; their timing is also important.

As a general rule, it takes 3 months, sometimes longer, for the functional effects of urodynamic and reconstructive surgery to stabilise. During that time voiding efficiency improves, local inflammatory causes of frequency and urgency resolve and periureteric oedema, as a cause of dilated upper tracts, settles down. Pre-existing and coexisting abnormalities, such as upper tract obstructive changes or detrusor instability in outflow obstruction, may also take at least as long as this to improve or resolve. For this reason, I generally restudy my patients at 3–6 months after operation (assuming there is no problem before that time), although certain patients, as mentioned above, will have had radiological evaluation at the time of removal of their various tubes.

Chapter 3

Incisions and exposure

The point of this chapter is to describe the technical and anatomical factors that allow the surgeon to gain the access needed to perform most open urodynamic and reconstructive procedures. The various incisions will be described first, followed by a consideration of some aspects of surgical anatomy.

INCISIONS

The exposure of the pelvis

The Pfannenstiel incision. It is unnecessary to describe this in detail, as it is a routinely and widely used incision, but three points are worth mentioning.

Firstly, the incision should be made close to the pubis because otherwise the inferior margin of the incised rectus sheath will obstruct the view into the pelvis.

Secondly, care should be taken to avoid damage to the inferior epigastric vessels on each side, particularly if the vascularity of the abdominal wall has already been impaired, for instance by radiotherapy.

Thirdly, it is important to remember that pelvic access may be restricted inferiorly by the attachments of the rectus tendons to the pubis and that these attachments are to the anterior aspects of the pubis (not the superior border) where they are obscured in some patients by the overlying pyramidalis muscles. Thus, when access is restricted with this incision, it may be improved by splitting the rectus tendons down onto the anterior aspect of the pubic symphysis, reflecting the pyramidales off the rectus tendons, and then incising the insertion of each rectus tendon for 1 cm or so from medial to lateral.

The main use for this incision is for a colposuspension type of procedure, for a simple fistula repair and for similar straightforward procedures in which the rather restricted access will always be adequate and when extension of the exposure will not be necessary.

The Cherney incision. This provides an alternative to the Pfannenstiel incision, when a wider exposure of the anterior pelvis is necessary, for example for augmentation cystoplasty in a patient with detrusor instability, or for implantation of an artificial sphincter,

and particularly when a previous Pfannenstiel incision is being reopened.

The advantages of the Cherney incision are that it eliminates the restrictive effects of the rectus attachments at the lower margin of the incision and of the recti themselves at the lateral edges of the incision, and that it is readily extended.

The skin incision is made over the upper margin of the pubic symphysis, curving upwards on each side above the line of the inguinal ligaments, as for the Pfannenstiel incision. The rectus sheath is then incised transversely, low over the pubis in the middle of the incision, but higher laterally, to split the external and internal obliques and the transversus abdominis above the level of the inguinal canal on each side.

The pyramidales are then reflected off the rectus tendons (Fig. 3.1), which are then incised, leaving sufficient inferiorly to allow the tendons to be reconstituted at the end of the procedure (Fig. 3.2). Having incised the rectus tendons, the recti are then retracted superiorly with a ring retractor. As with the Pfannenstiel incision, care should be taken not to damage the inferior epigastric vessels.

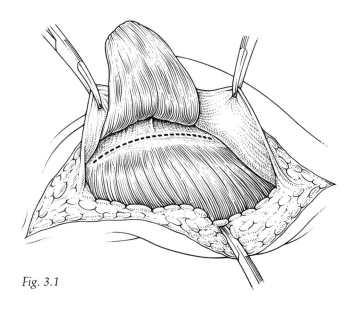

Fig. 3.1

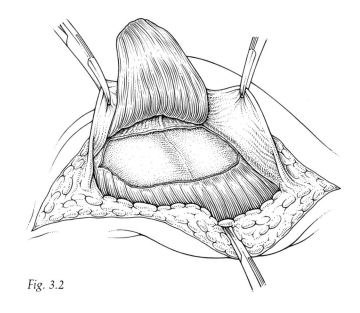

Fig. 3.2

This incision gives distinctly better exposure of the pelvis than is possible with the Pfannenstiel incision and also, by lateral extension of the incision on each side up to the level of the anterior superior iliac spine, affords reasonably good access to the lower abdomen. The incision is therefore a halfway stage between the Pfannenstiel incision, which is sometimes restrictive for the surgeon but nicer for the patient, and the midline incision, which provides the widest access for the surgeon, but is less satisfactory for the patient.

For exposure of the abdomen and pelvis

Midline incision. This is mainly used for substitution cystoplasty (or when there is doubt preoperatively as to whether augmentation or substitution cystoplasty may be required, as in patients with neuropathic detrusor hyperreflexia), for undiversion or for any other major reconstructive procedure, in other words, when access to the upper abdomen will be or may be required. Although it provides extensive exposure, the exposure of the pelvis is somewhat less satisfactory than with the Cherney incision, making the latter preferable if the height of the exposure of the midline incision is not going to be necessary. For all major reconstructive surgery the midline incision is the only incision worth considering except in very unusual circumstances.

For exposure of the male urethra

A midline perineal incision is used almost invariably. Like the midline abdominal incision, it is easily extended — if necessary to the tip of the penis — giving it flexibility.

For exposure of the female urethra

The anterior aspect of the female urethra is best exposed from above, the posterior aspect from below. A transverse incision is made about 0·5–1 cm below the external meatus, between it and the opening of the vagina. This is then deepened to separate the urethra from the anterior vaginal wall and can be extended with ease up to the level of the bladder neck and trigone.

SURGICAL ANATOMY

Pelvis

Having incised the abdominal wall and underlying fascia, the first step of any operation is to get good exposure, and good exposure requires a thorough knowledge of pelvic anatomy and particularly of the fascial layers within the pelvis.

It is probably more useful, rather than to describe the anatomy as such, to describe it as one would encounter it during a full mobilisation of the bladder and proximal urethra (including the prostate in the male patient) prior to a cystectomy or cystoprostatectomy, with comments where relevant on related subjects.

Apart from the attachments to the structures with which the bladder is in continuity (the ureters and urethra) the bladder is held in position by the fascial layers that surround it, and which, on the one hand, fix it to adjacent structures and, on the other hand, separate it from them.

It is difficult to overstate the importance of these fascial layers. In a healthy patient (or relatively healthy) it is possible to perform most if not all surgical procedures within the pelvis without taking any real notice of fascial layers and planes. But the worse the problem, the more important it is to be able to identify these planes and layers as they are the guide to the vessels and nerves one most needs to identify. The classic example is a cystoprostatectomy after radiotherapy. Here a 'wrench out' and ileal conduit may be possible with no more anatomical knowledge than that of a slaughterhouseman but a reconstructive substitution procedure may be impossible unless there is good control of the bleeding, no damage to adjacent structures and preservation of the relevant muscles, vessels and nerves. Repair of complex fistulae and reconstruction after previous surgery or trauma are other examples where a good working knowledge of the fascial layers and planes may make all the difference.

Two separate layers of fascia cover the bladder — one covers the anterior and lateral aspects (what one might call the retropubic surface of the bladder), the other covers the dome and the posterior aspect of the bladder between the two lateral pedicles (what one might call the pelvic or peritoneal surface of the bladder). The two layers converge at two sites, as shown in the sagittal section of the male pelvis in Figure 3.3:

— at the lateral vascular pedicles of the bladder to ensheath them as they run between the posterolateral side wall of the pelvis (in the region of the internal iliac vessels) and the bladder;
— at the junction of the dome of the bladder with the 'retropubic' surface of the bladder. From here the two layers, together with the overlying peritoneum, run upwards and outwards to the brim of the pelvis along the line of the external iliac vessels and round over the anterior abdominal wall to the urachus in the midline, where they become continuous with the fascia of the other side.

These two fascial conjunctions were described by the American anatomist Uhlenhuth, who called the fascia that runs from the dome of the bladder to the pelvic brim the superior hypogastric wing, and the fascia that surrounds the lateral pedicles, the inferior hypogastric wing or sheath.

Within the superior hypogastric wing, just lateral to the line where the retropubic and pelvic layers of fascia

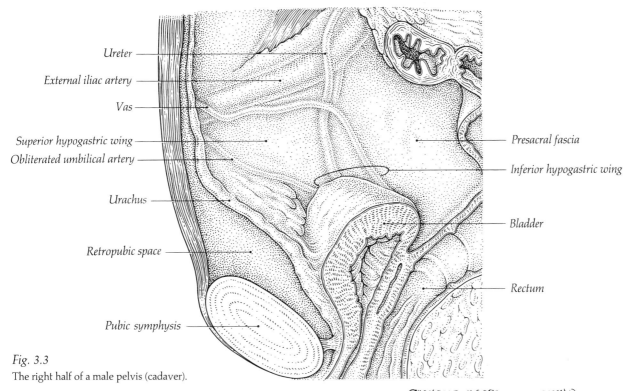

Fig. 3.3
The right half of a male pelvis (cadaver).

fuse to run together to the brim of the pelvis, lies the obliterated umbilical artery. Lateral to the obliterated umbilical artery, at the front of the pelvis and crossing it in the mid-pelvis, lies the vas or round ligament.

Within the inferior hypogastric wing or sheath are the superior and inferior vesical arteries and veins, the ureter and the pelvic autonomic nerve plexus.

The superior and inferior hypogastric wings meet at a right angle at the bifurcation of the common iliac vessels (Fig. 3.4) close to where the ureter runs over the vessels into the pelvis and where the vas runs horizontally, over the ureter, and then medially towards the ampulla and seminal vesicle on that side.

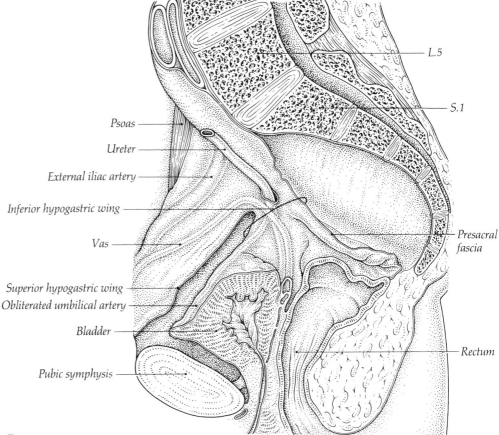

Fig. 3.4
The superior hypogastric wing has been incised and the presacral fascia mobilised off the sacrum.

Posterior to the lateral pedicle of the bladder these fascial layers are continuous with a third fascial layer that runs from the common iliac vessels above (and across both sides of the midline), to the inferior hypogastric wings (below and laterally) and to the rectum (below and medially) where it splits to form a sheath around the rectum. Uhlenhuth called this fascial layer the presacral fascia (Fig. 3.5).

The fascial sheath that surrounds each lateral pedicle of the bladder is therefore formed by the inferior hypogastric wing or sheath which is continuous posteriorly with the presacral fascia (Figs 3.4, 3.5). It is within the presacral fascia that the pelvic parasympathetic nerves run forward to enter the lateral pedicle (see below) and, in the reverse direction,

that the middle rectal vessels run back to supply the rectum (Fig. 3.6).

The retropubic space (Fig. 3.7) has the superior hypogastric wing as its roof and a fourth fascial sheet, the endopelvic fascia, as its floor. The medial wall is the bladder anteriorly, and the inferior hypogastric wing surrounding the lateral pedicle posteriorly. The lateral wall is the parietal pelvic fascia covering the obturator fossa. The anterior part of the retropubic space is continuous with the space on the other side and the posterior limit is where the inferior hypogastric wing, that is the fascia covering the lateral aspect of the lateral pedicle, fuses or becomes continuous with the superior hypogastric wing above, the obturator fascia laterally and the endopelvic fascia of the pelvic floor

below, along the vertical line of the internal iliac vessels and their anterior branches.

The endopelvic fascia of the pelvic floor runs from the obturator fascia, just superficial to the so-called 'white line' of origin of levator ani, across to the bladder, in the region of the lateral border of the trigone, and to the anterolateral border of the male prostate and the female urethra. At the anterior end of the endopelvic fascia on each side is the puboprostatic ligament in males and the pubourethral ligament in females. Between the two ligaments in the anterior midline the superficial branch of the dorsal vein complex of the penis/clitoris runs into the pelvis on the surface of the prostate/urethra within a pad of fat.

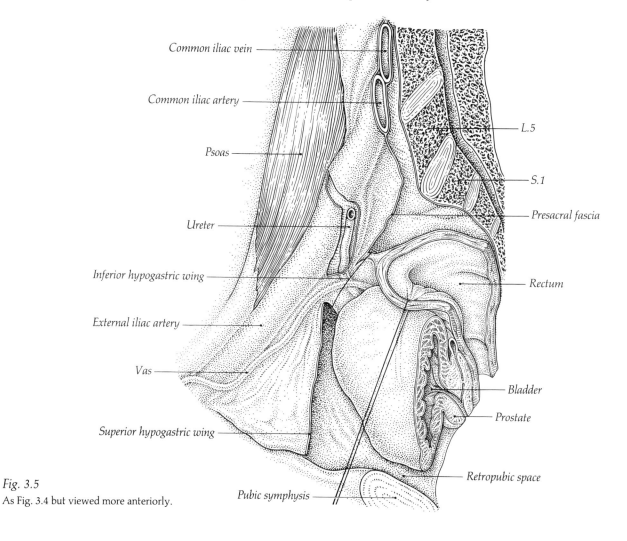

Fig. 3.5
As Fig. 3.4 but viewed more anteriorly.

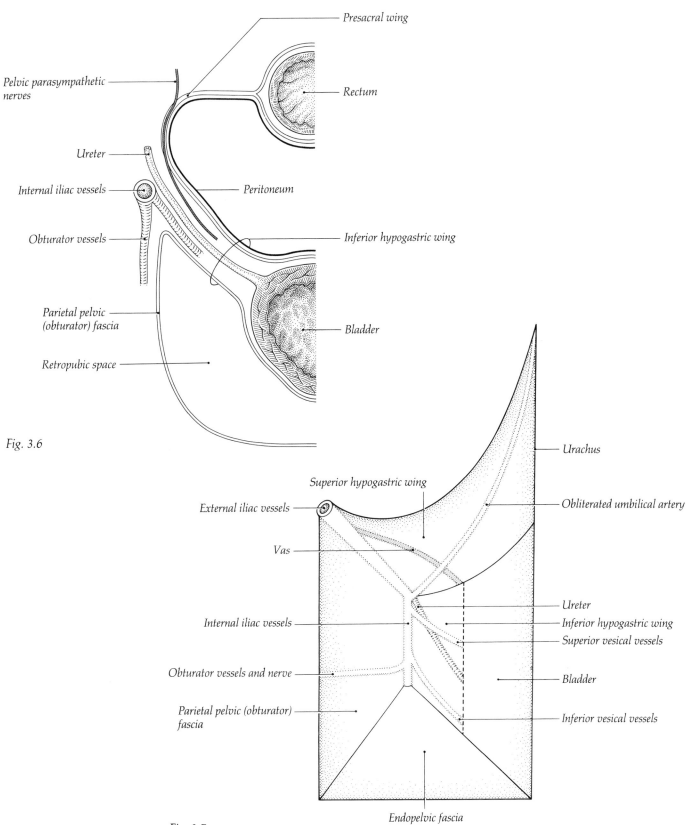

Fig. 3.6

Fig. 3.7
Diagram of the retropubic space viewed from in front.

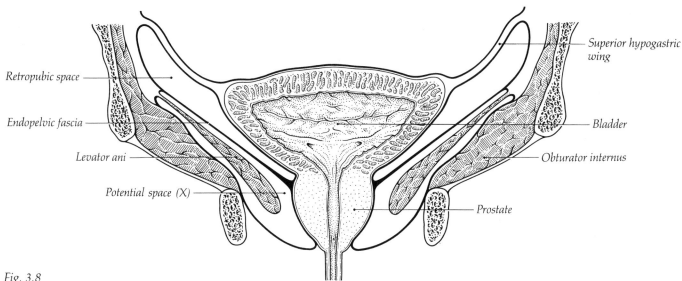

Fig. 3.8

There is a potential space (X) beneath the endopelvic fascia on each side between it and the underlying levator ani (Fig. 3.8) which can be opened up to expose the lateral aspect of the prostate. The other important point to note is that it is possible to get under the lateral pedicle of the bladder and prostate, and therefore all the major vessels to the pelvic viscera, by incising the endopelvic fascia of the pelvic floor at the posterior end of the retropubic space. Having previously exposed the posterior aspect of the lateral pedicle (see below), this incision in the endopelvic fascia allows the surgeon to put a sling under and around the lateral pedicle or to cross clamp the pedicle when performing a difficult cystectomy or similar procedure, particularly with massive pelvic tumours or in other situations where access is grossly restricted.

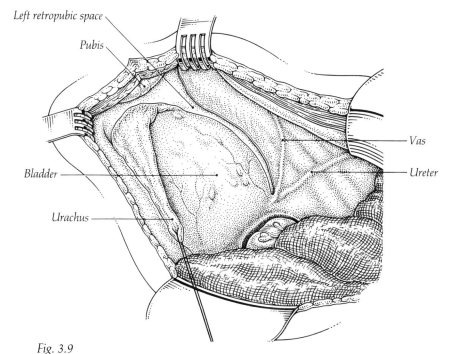

Fig. 3.9
View of the pelvis through a lower midline incision from the left hand side.

Having opened up the retropubic space on each side, so that the walls and the floor are clearly demonstrated, the first step in mobilising the bladder is to divide the urachus and obliterated umbilical arteries together, just below the umbilicus, and then to divide the superior hypogastric wing and the overlying peritoneum on each side, just lateral to the obliterated umbilical artery and between it and the vas, back to the point where the vas runs across, from lateral to medial, over the lateral pedicle (and ureter) to the ampulla and seminal vesicle of that side (Fig. 3.9). This manoeuvre mobilises the dome and the anterior and lateral aspects of the bladder.

If opening the retropubic space is difficult, usually because of previous radiotherapy or surgery, it is best to start at the front and work back or from the external iliac vessels and then downwards. 'Blind' sharp dissection in the region of the obturator fossae is likely to lead to bleeding, either from the obturator vessels laterally or from the prostatic/vaginal veins medially, both of which are difficult to control without good exposure. It is also liable to damage the origin of levator ani from the obturator fascia, making it difficult to know on which side of the levators one is and thereby risking damage to the pudendal vessels.

After previous radiotherapy, opening the retropubic space usually proceeds smoothly once the surgeon is in the correct plane because although the fascial layers may be grossly thickened and stiff, the planes are not usually obliterated. After previous surgery or trauma the planes are often obliterated anteriorly and it may be easier to start at the posterior end of the retropubic space and work forward.

The next step is to expose the posterior aspect of the bladder and the posteromedial aspects of the lateral pedicles.

The horizontal, pelvic part of the vas, as it crosses over the ureter, is surrounded by a fascial sheath which is continuous proximally with the fascia around the ampulla and seminal vesicle and thereby with the same fascia of the other side. This fascia is attached in front of the lower end of the vesicles to the posterior surface of the prostate, just above the level of the ejaculatory ducts, and behind the vesicles to the prostatic apex, in the area of attachment of the rectourethralis (Fig. 3.10). In fetal life this posterior fascial layer is covered by peritoneum, which runs down to the pelvic floor, at the posterior apex of the prostate, and then up on the anterior surface of the rectum, but during later fetal life the adjacent surfaces of peritoneum between the prostate and rectum (and to varying degrees upward on each side) fuse to form what is commonly known as the fascia of Denonvilliers, which is densest inferiorly.

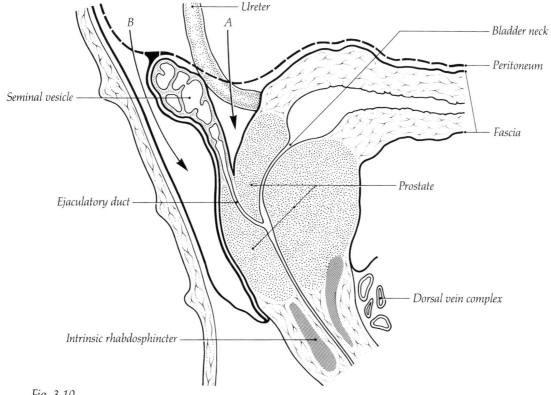

Fig. 3.10

Thus, to expose just the back of the bladder between the lateral pedicles (as, for example, for a subtotal cystectomy and substitution cystoplasty) the peritoneum is incised in front of the vas and across the midline to the other side (Figs 3.10 — plane A, 3.11), but to expose the posterior aspects of both the bladder and prostate (as, for example, for a total cystoprostatectomy) one must extend the peritoneal incision over the vas and then across the midline behind it (Figs 3.10 — plane B, 3.12). Deepening this incision behind the vasa and vesicles allows one to separate the vesicles and the prostate in front from the anterior aspect of the rectum behind, which is the crucial step to avoid damaging the rectum later on. When the rectum is damaged it is usually because the surgeon gets inside the fascial capsule of the seminal vesicles, rather than between it and the anterior fascial capsule of the rectum, and then has to dissect sharply backwards and downwards through the tough layer of Denonvilliers fascia to get down to the posterior aspect of prostate, and in so doing, goes too deep, damaging the rectum. To avoid this it is a simple matter to check that you are in the right plane by checking that you can palpate a catheter in the urethra at the apex of the prostate. If you can feel it you are in the right plane (B in Fig. 3.10) and the rectum is safe. If you cannot but can only feel the prostate then you are inside the fascia of the seminal vesicles, one layer too anterior (A in Fig. 3.10). Rather than persist and risk damaging the rectum you should make a fresh peritoneal incision further posteriorly and try again.

In female patients, the corresponding peritoneal incisions would be in front of the round ligament (for a simple or subtotal cystectomy) or behind the round and broad ligaments (for an anterior exenteration).

Attention to detail in these peritoneal incisions and their subsequent deepening, to separate the various fascial planes, should allow the midline exposure of the posterior aspect of the bladder, or bladder and prostate together, which simultaneously exposes the posteromedial aspects of the lateral pedicles. It should be stressed that if the exposure of the seminal vesicles and prostate from the posterior aspect and the separation of these structures from the rectum, right the way down to the apex of the prostate, is not easy then you are in the wrong plane and you risk damaging the rectum later on. All efforts should be made to get into the correct plane from the outset.

At this stage, the lateral pedicles will have been clearly defined on both their anterolateral aspects (in the retropubic space) where the covering layer of fascia is thick, and on their posteromedial aspects (in front of the rectum) where the fascial covering is much thinner. For this reason, ligation of the various parts of the lateral pedicle is likely to be less bloody if artery forceps are passed through the pedicle from posteromedial to anterolateral, rather than the other way round (Fig. 3.13).

Loosely speaking, there are four parts to each lateral pedicle from above down — the obliterated umbilical artery, the rest of the superior vesical pedicle, the ureter, and the inferior vesical pedicle. These are fairly easily recognised as distinct parts in children and young thin adults, less so in the elderly, the obese and after radiotherapy. Obviously there is some overlap between the four parts and the inferior vesical vessels in particular may be extensive.

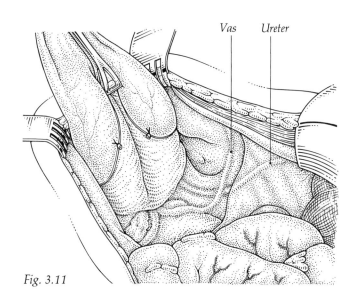

Fig. 3.11

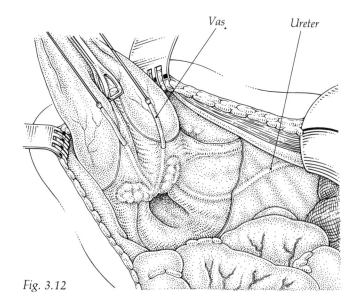

Fig. 3.12

At this stage only the upper three parts should be individually ligated and divided (Figs 3.14, 3.15), leaving the inferior vesical vessels until later because these are closely related to the pelvic parasympathetic nerves and it is obviously desirable to preserve these as far as possible.

Attention is then directed to the anterior aspect of the prostate in males and the urethra in females. In the male the anatomy is rather more complicated.

The fascia on the anterior aspect of the bladder is continuous below with the fascia covering the anterior aspect of the prostate. On the lateral aspect of the prostate on each side this fascia merges with the endopelvic fascia which forms the floor of the retropubic space. Laterally, the endopelvic fascia is thinner where it merges with the fascia covering the obturator fossa and the so-called 'white line' of origin of levator ani. Anteriorly there is usually a hiatus on each side (Fig. 3.16), just before the endopelvic fascia fuses with the puboprostatic ligaments. This hiatus is

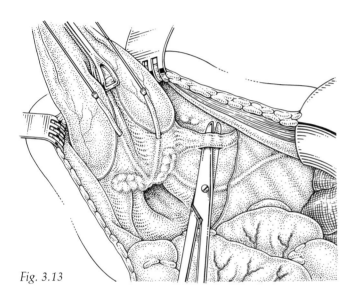

Fig. 3.13

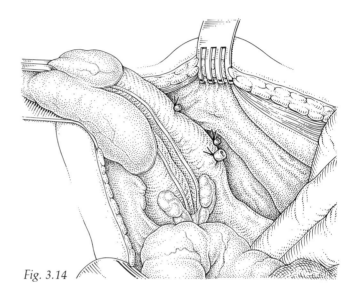

Fig. 3.14

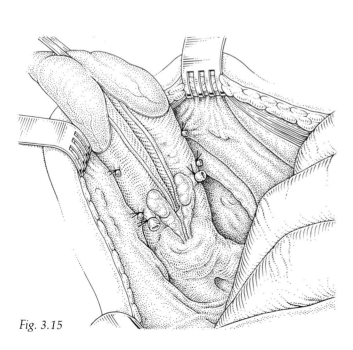

Fig. 3.15

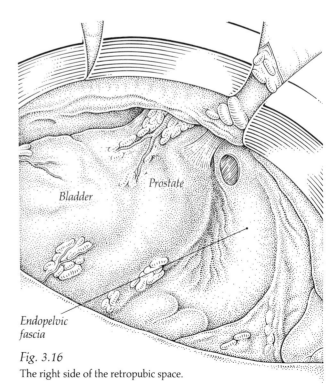

Bladder

Prostate

Endopelvic fascia

Fig. 3.16
The right side of the retropubic space.

usually obscured from view by the pad of fatty tissue which lies over the puboprostatic ligaments and the midline gap between them which transmits the friable superficial branch of the dorsal vein of the penis. (After radiotherapy this hiatus is usually plugged by a fatty hernia from the fascia on the anterolateral aspect of the bladder.) Deep to the lateral, thin part of the endopelvic fascia lies the anterior part of the levator ani. Deep to the thicker medial part of the endopelvic fascia lies the lateral aspect of the prostate and the overlying venous complex that drains the lateral branch of the dorsal vein of the penis.

Deep to the two puboprostatic ligaments is the point where the superficial branch and the two lateral branches of the dorsal vein complex arise from the deep dorsal vein of the penis, and deep to this is the subprostatic or membranous urethra (Fig. 3.17). Alongside the membranous urethra, on each posterolateral aspect, are the neurovascular bundles which (according to the English anatomist Gosling) supply this region of the urethra and more distally provide the innervation of the corpora cavernosa that is important for potency. More

proximally, the neurovascular bundles lie along the posterolateral margin of the prostate and within its fascial sheath, in the gutter of the levator ani. More proximally still the vessels of the neurovascular bundles are continuous with the inferior vesical vessels and the nerves are continuous with the pelvic plexuses — hence the reason for not dissecting below the ureters when dividing the lateral pedicles, until the neurovascular bundles have been defined distally.

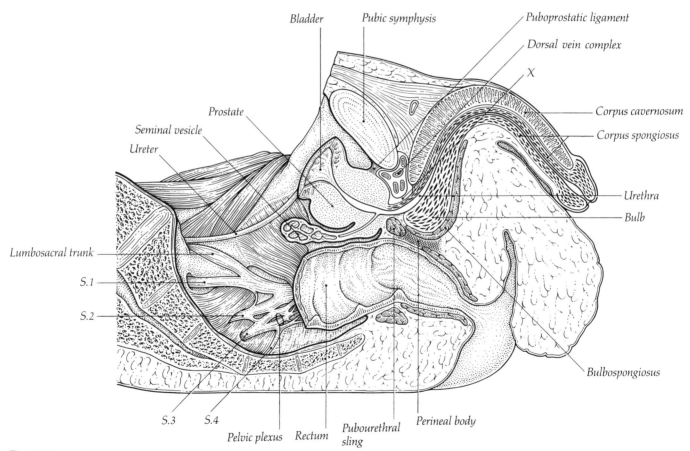

Fig. 3.17
The left half of a hemisected male pelvis (cadaver).

Mobilisation of the prostate and exposure of the subprostatic urethra must, therefore, take these anatomical factors into account. The first step is to incise the endopelvic fascia along its length, all the way back to the lateral pedicle, starting in the natural hiatus anteriorly and keeping lateral (Fig. 3.18), close to the side wall of the pelvis, to avoid damaging the prostatic venous complex that lies under the thicker medial part of the endopelvic fascia.

The incision in the endopelvic fascia is then extended anteriorly by incising the puboprostatic ligament (Fig. 3.19). This must be incised at its origin from the back of the pubis, keeping as close to bone as possible, to avoid damaging the underlying dorsal vein complex and prostatic venous plexus. Before starting this part of the dissection, it is important to ligate and divide the superficial branch of the dorsal vein, in the midline, between the puboprostatic ligaments, and to clear as much as possible of the fatty tissue from the surface of the ligaments and from the undersurface of the pubis, so that the view is not obscured.

Having divided the endopelvic fascia and the pubourethral ligament on each side, the next step is to ligate and divide the dorsal vein complex at the point at which the deep dorsal vein divides into its superficial and lateral branches. This manoeuvre and its importance was first emphasised by Patrick Walsh from the Johns Hopkins Hospital in Baltimore, USA in his description of the technique of radical retropubic prostatectomy. The dorsal vein complex lies in a chunk of connective tissue, between the puboprostatic ligaments above and the membranous urethra below, which is about 1.5×1.5 cm in cross section and is not very well defined. A large calibre

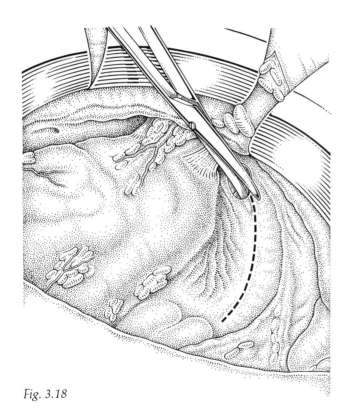

Fig. 3.18

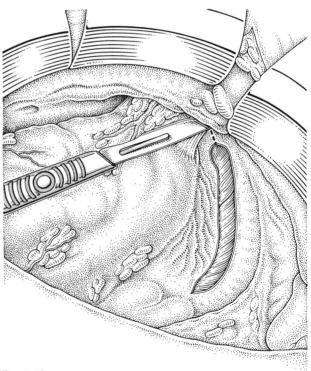

Fig. 3.19

catheter in the urethra helps to define the dorsal vein complex by allowing palpation of the urethra and thereby the groove between the dorsal vein complex and the urethra. Posterior displacement of the prostate using a swab-on-a-stick and good lighting are other essential steps to allow passage and tying of the all-important ligature in the right place in order to avoid troublesome bleeding (Fig. 3.20). Walsh has emphasised (correctly) that there is not sufficient length of the deep dorsal vein to allow either cross clamping and then division and ligation, or the placement of two ligatures and division of the complex between. Only a single ligature can be passed and tied and the dorsal vein complex is then divided proximally. Any back bleeding from the proximal cut ends of the divided vessels on the anterior surface of the prostate is (easily) controlled by diathermy or by suture-ligation.

When the dorsal vein has been divided, the underlying membranous urethra is exposed with the neurovascular bundle on each side. In theory a sling can then be passed around the urethra, isolating it from the neurovascular bundles, so that the urethra can be transected safely. In practice this manoeuvre is usually difficult because of the posterior attachment of the membranous urethra to the rectourethralis and, more distally, to the upper limit of the perineal body. It is easier to incise the anterior wall of the urethra at the apex of the prostate, exposing the catheter within (Fig. 3.21), and then to pull through a length of catheter and divide it, keeping the balloon of the catheter inflated; the catheter can then be used for upward traction of the apex of the prostate, thereby allowing transection of the posterior wall of the urethra (Fig. 3.22). This manoeuvre was also described by Walsh. Having divided the urethra, a

thin but tough layer of fascia with a variable muscle content is exposed posteriorly. This is the rectourethralis and this is divided with scissors to enter the space behind the prostate created from above earlier in the dissection.

The only structures still holding the bladder and prostate in place at this stage are the neurovascular structures. These are the inferior vesical vessels and the pelvic plexus at the base of the bladder on either side proximally, that are continuous distally as the neurovascular bundles to the urethra and the corpora cavernosa. By their attachments they tether the posterolateral aspects of the base of the bladder and prostate before emerging at the apex of the prostate on either side of the now transected urethra.

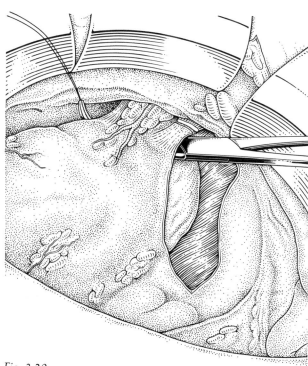

Fig. 3.20

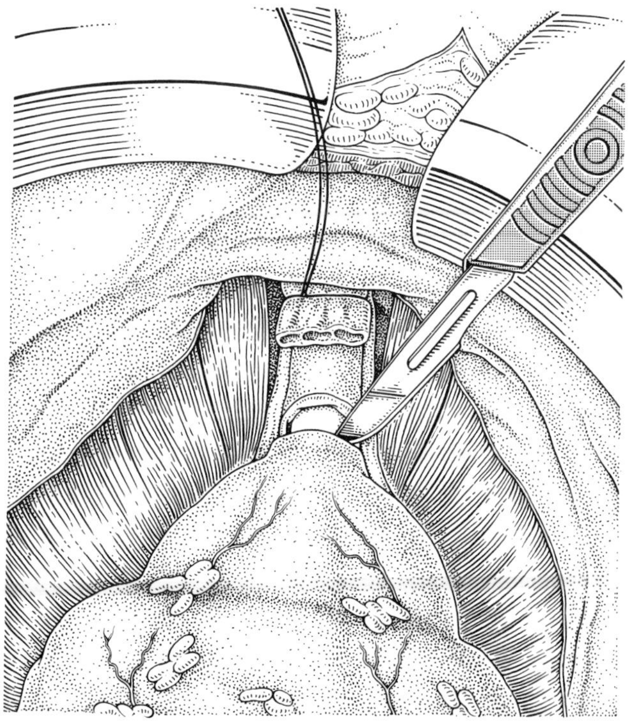

Fig. 3.21

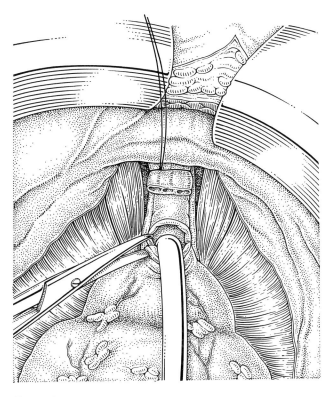

Fig. 3.22

To isolate the neurovascular bundle from the prostate on each side, the vascular branches that run from the bundle to supply the prostate must be carefully ligated and divided. These vessels run within the fascial sheath over the anterior and lateral aspects of the prostate and are defined by passing a Lahey forceps between the prostate and the fascial sheath, working from below upwards. The vessels are then ligated and divided (Fig. 3.23), one at a time, keeping as far anteriorly on the surface of the prostate as possible, until the prostate has been mobilised up to the level of the bladder neck and the inferior vesical pedicle on each side. The two inferior vesical pedicles are now the only remaining attachments of the bladder and these are then ligated and divided close to the bladder (Fig. 3.24), taking care to keep the trauma to the neurovascular bundles and any traction on the pelvic parasympathetic nerves more proximally to a minumum.

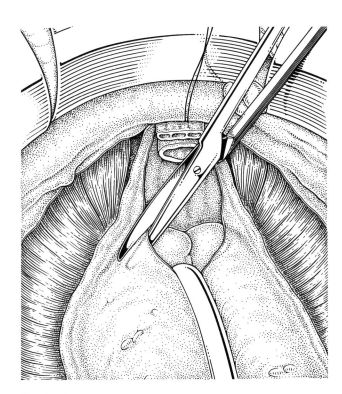

Fig. 3.23

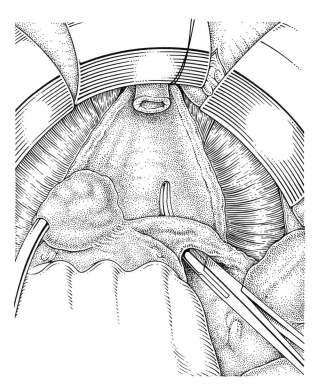

Fig. 3.24

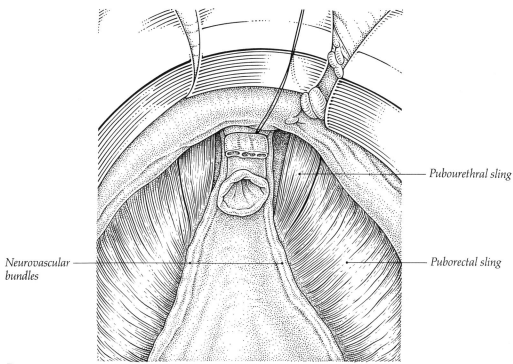

Fig. 3.25

At the end of the procedure the transected membranous urethra will be clearly visible in the anterior midline, with the two neurovascular bundles on each side, all three lying in the pubourethral sling of the levator ani (Fig. 3.25). The neurovascular bundles will be seen to be continuous with the lateral pedicles, and the rectum between them should have an intact anterior fascial sheath. Lateral and posterior to the pubourethral sling, the puborectal sling will also be visible.

In the female, division of the endopelvic fascia and pubourethral ligaments and ligation of the superficial branch of the dorsal vein of the clitoris, performed in the same way as in the male, to avoid damage to the vaginal venous plexus, will expose the urethra lying on the anterior vaginal wall and held down onto it by a triangular fascial layer, which has its base inferiorly and its apex at the bladder neck (Fig. 3.26). To get around the urethra, this fascial layer (which appears to correspond to the

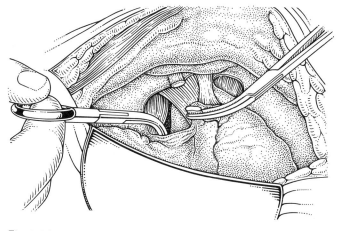

Fig. 3.26
The left pubourethral ligament has been divided with a clip on the proximal end.

chunky dorsal vein complex of the male) must be incised longitudinally, keeping as far lateral as possible to avoid damaging the underlying neurovascular bundles, although preservation of the nerves in the kind of surgery that necessitates this exposure will not often be an important factor. Even without incising this fascial layer, it is possible to pass a Lahey-type forceps around the urethra just below the bladder neck (Fig. 3.27), where a plane of cleavage exists between it and the anterior vaginal wall, for example to create a plane for placement of an artificial sphincter cuff. This is the same plane as that described earlier in this chapter, created by transperitoneal midline dissection between the posterior margin of the bladder and the anterior aspect of the cervix. When dense scarring from previous surgery makes it difficult to develop this plane between the bladder neck and the vagina from one side of the retropubic space directly through to the other, it is often helpful to develop the plane transperitoneally in the posterior midline first and then to break through, under the ureter, to each side of the retropubic space in turn. Similarly, if the posterior wall of the bladder and bladder neck is separated from the anterior vaginal wall between the lateral pedicles from above, and the distal urethra is dissected from the lower part of the anterior vaginal wall through an introital incision, the full length of the urethra and the bladder base can be separated from the anterior vaginal wall without dividing any vessels. This may be helpful to allow the surgeon to pull a section of omentum or a labial fat pad through between the bladder/urethra and vagina as part of a difficult vesico-vaginal fistula repair.

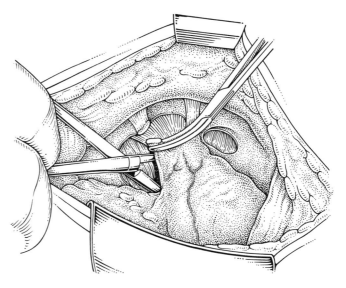

Fig. 3.27

The sphincter-active urethra

The sphincter-active urethra consists of a smooth muscle component and a striated muscle component within the wall of the urethra which, together with the periurethral part of levator ani, the pubourethral sling, produce a zone of sphincteric activity just below the prostate in males and in the distal half of the urethra in females. It is commonly stated that the intrinsic striated muscle component lies maximally in the mid-urethra in females, but John Hindmarsh demonstrated its more distal situation while he was working at the Institute of Urology in London although he has not yet published this work. This area used to be called the external sphincter, the bladder neck being the internal sphincter. Nowadays it is called 'the distal sphincter mechanism' or 'urethral sphincter mechanism' (the bladder neck — described in Chapter

4 — being the proximal sphincter mechanism, although more commonly just called the bladder neck). Of the three components of the distal sphincter mechanism, the striated muscle component within the urethral wall is the most important. This is commonly called the intrinsic rhabdosphincter, and it is this structure that the surgeon usually seeks to attack or avoid when operating on or around the sphincter-active urethra.

One of the most imprecise techniques in urodynamic surgery is endoscopic sphincterotomy because it is difficult to know the extent of the incision to be made to divide the full length of the intrinsic rhabdosphincter and because it is also difficult to know how deep to make the incision. This is because there are few anatomical landmarks visible endoscopically.

Figures 3.28 and 3.29 show the position of the intrinsic rhabdosphincter in the male and female respectively. In the male, the rhabdosphincter has a greater longitudinal extent and although it is predominantly below the verumontanum and in the region of the membranous urethra that is visibly constricted endoscopically by its action, it extends both upwards and downwards to a variable degree. Thus, the only way to be sure of dividing it completely is to incise it in the anterior midline from just below the bladder neck down to the point where the corpora cavernosa indent the bulbar urethra, usually visible in the bulbar urethra by the 'gothic arch' they produce. To divide the full thickness of the rhabdosphincter requires a depth of incision of about 5 mm, but less at the lower limit of the incision. Unscientific though it is, the best guide to the point when the correct depth is reached is bleeding to such an extent that the procedure has to be abandoned in order to control it. Fortunately the bleeding usually stops when a catheter is inserted.

In the female urethra the intrinsic rhabdosphincter lies predominantly in the distal half of the urethral wall (Fig. 3.29) with a variable degree of upward extension. This is therefore the site for a sphincterotomy, bearing in mind the horseshoe configuration of the rhabdosphincter with its posterior deficiency (Fig. 3.30). It is important to bear this configuration in mind for two other reasons. Firstly because a standard Y-V plasty or similar procedure on the bladder neck will only affect the intrinsic rhabdosphincter when it extends the full length of the urethra (a simple anteromedian sphincterotomy is easier for both the surgeon and the patient), and secondly because the urethra can be incised and resutured without necessarily damaging the intrinsic rhabdosphincter if the incision is precisely in the posterior midline (although this is still risky).

The intrinsic rhabdosphincter is the most important component of the distal sphincter mechanism but it is not the only component. Little is known about the other two components in health or

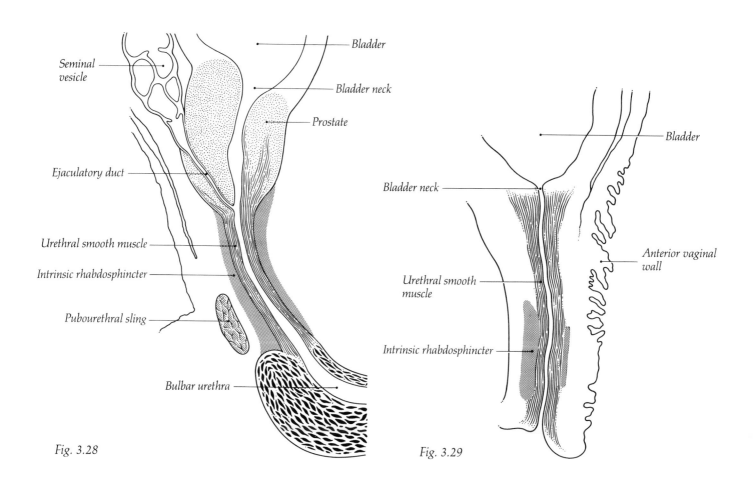

Fig. 3.28

Fig. 3.29

disease — the urethral smooth muscle within the urethral wall itself (like the intrinsic rhabdosphincter with which it is intimately related) and the periurethral part of the pelvic floor musculature. The latter appears rather insignificant in females but is a substantial sling in males. This sling, the pubourethral sling, has already been alluded to above during the description of cystectomy and is described in more detail below with reference to the pelvic floor musculature.

The urethral smooth muscle is intriguing because nobody is sure what it does but everybody believes it is important. It is difficult to study in isolation but evidence from patients with certain types of spinal cord injury suggests that it is under alpha adrenergic control and may be important in certain neuropathic bladder states.

The perineum

The perineal approach to the female urethra has already been covered in previous paragraphs. It therefore remains to describe the anatomy of the male perineum as, for example, in the mobilisation of the bulbar urethra prior to a bulbo-prostatic anastomotic urethroplasty.

Having made a midline perineal skin incision the first anatomical encounter is with the perineal deep fascia which is the posterior extension of the scrotal dartos layer. When this layer is incised fatty tissue bulges through the incision and, with anterior traction on the scrotum, can be seen to be in two halves with a thin midline septum as in the scrotum. If these two halves are separated the bulbospongiosus and underlying bulbar urethra come into view (Fig. 3.31). If the perineal incision is based on palpation of an indwelling urethral catheter, the posterior extent of the bulb of the corpus spongiosum will be surprisingly far back.

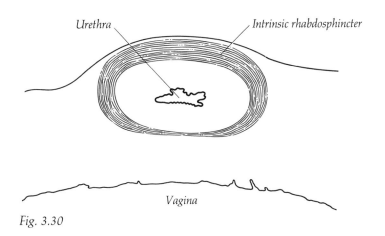

Fig. 3.30

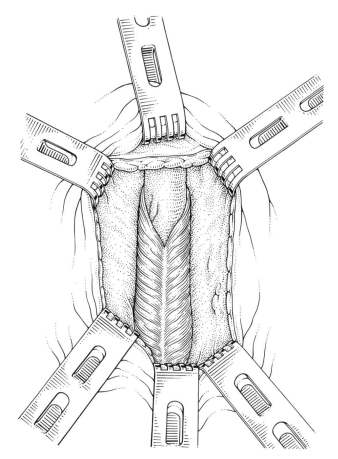

Fig. 3.31

For surgical purposes the bulbar urethra can be described as being that part of the urethra surrounded by the bulbospongiosus. Distal to the bulbospongiosus, the urethra within the corpus spongiosum is ensheathed together with the corpora cavernosa and is tethered to the corpora over half of its dorsal circumference. Within the bulbospongiosus, this fibrous tethering is restricted to that part between 11 o'clock and 1 o'clock, as it would be if the urethra is viewed endoscopically (Fig. 3.32). This tethering of the bulbar urethra is in the form of a fairly thin but tough septum on the deep aspect of the bulbar urethra, when viewed through a midline perineal incision, which is visible when the bulbospongiosus is divided in the midline and reflected off the bulbar urethra on each side and the corpus spongiosum is retracted to one side. This septum runs to the midline between the corpora cavernosa, from distally where the corpora fuse to proximally where they are separated beneath the inferior pubic arch. To approach this posterior midline septum, one must dissect around the lateral aspects of the urethra carefully (Fig. 3.33), to secure with diathermy the fine vessels that run at approximately 1 cm intervals between the corpora cavernosa and the corpus spongiosum. Division of the septum itself is usually bloodless.

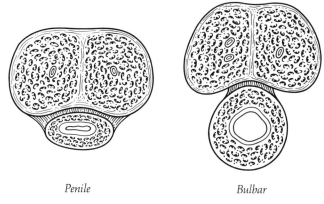

Penile Bulbar

Fig. 3.32

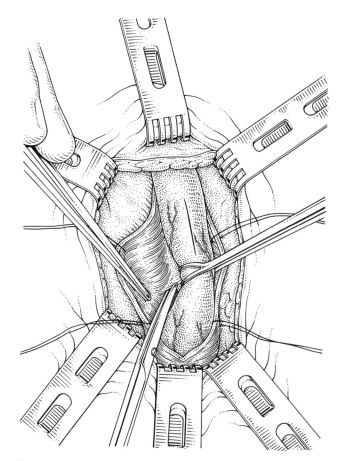

Fig. 3.33

The urethra itself is eccentrically located within the corpus spongiosum that surrounds it. The dorsal aspect of the corpus is thin, whilst the ventral aspect is much thicker, particularly posteriorly where the bulk of the bulb lies (Fig. 3.34). Careful dissection of the posterolateral aspects of the bulb will reveal a fairly superficial arterial branch of the perineal branch of the pudendal artery on each side. These vessels will need to be dealt with during mobilisation of the bulb to avoid troublesome bleeding, but should be left intact if the bulb is to be preserved, as in more distal bulbar urethroplasty procedures or for placement of an artificial sphincter cuff. They are not the main arterial supply to the bulb, which enters much higher up just as the pudendal vessels leave Alcock's canal. These main bulbar arteries are short stout vessels that run directly into the bulb just below the level of the pubourethral sling at the upper end of the bulbar urethra, just below the bulbo-membranous junction, and in front of the perineal body. They are more or less the last attachments to be divided during a cystourethrectomy, lying as they do in the depths of both the suprapubic and the perineal wounds. These should always be looked for as tough bands at 3 and 9 o'clock as viewed perineally, and ligated before division. If not they can bleed furiously.

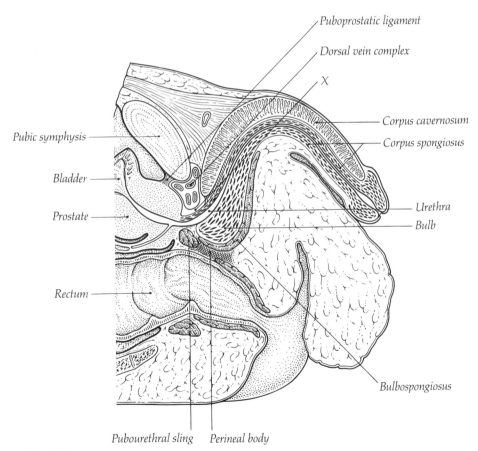

Fig. 3.34

Mobilisation of the bulbospongiosus muscles back to their posterior attachment to the perineal body and division of the midline septum throughout its extent will give sufficient exposure for distal bulbar urethroplasty or for placement of an artificial sphincter cuff in this region (Fig. 3.35). Posterior mobilisation of the bulb of the corpus spongiosum, dividing its attachment to the perineal body all the way up to the prostato-membranous junction (Figs 3.34, 3.36) will be necessary, however, for a proximal bulbar urethroplasty or a bulbo-prostatic anastomosis.

The precise anatomy of the junction between the bulbar urethra when approached from below, and the membranous urethra, when approached from above, is not entirely clear,

particularly as in many instances the appearances are obscured by post-traumatic fibrosis when this combined approach is made (for a urethroplasty). The traditional view is that there is a perineal membrane or urogenital diaphragm or both at this point, but this view has been challenged recently by Chilton and Turner Warwick. Certainly there is no membrane or diaphragm to be found around the membranous urethra when approached from above, as for example during a cystoprostatectomy or radical prostatectomy, that corresponds to the traditionally-described urogenital diaphragm. The question of a perineal membrane is rather less clear, partly because there are a lot of structures in rather a small area with a considerable degree of overlap and partly because

dissection, to a certain extent, creates its own anatomy. Reflection of the bulbospongiosus off the ventral aspect of the corpus spongiosum leaves the perineal body intact posteriorly, behind the bulb of the corpus spongiosum, as a tough band in the coronal plane with a vertical extent equal to the height of the posterior surface of the bulb (Fig. 3.34). The perineal body itself acts as a band of anchorage not only for the bulbospongiosus muscles and the bulb of the corpus spongiosum in front, but also for the perianal musculature behind and for the pubourethral sling, the puboperineal and the transverse perineal muscles above, deeper in where the perineum and pelvis meet. These are tough 'membranous' attachments on the posterior aspect of the membranous urethra, but they do not actually form a

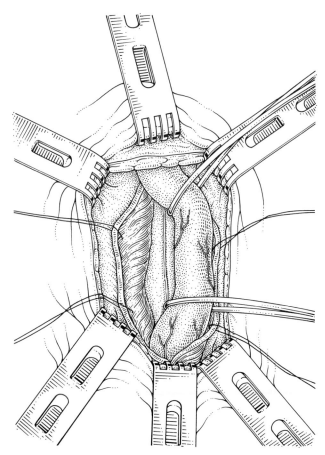

Fig. 3.35

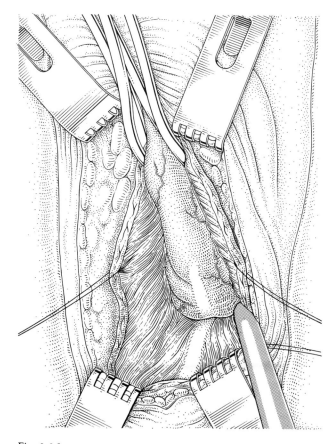

Fig. 3.36

'membrane' or 'diaphragm' around it, only a tough vertically orientated band on its posterior aspect. Anteriorly, having fully incised the midline septum that tethers the bulbar urethra as described above, there is a direct communication at the origin of the bulbar urethra and anterior to it with the plane between the membranous urethra and the dorsal vein complex (Figs 3.34, 3.37), that can be opened up retropubically as described earlier in the chapter. Turner Warwick has called this area of communication between the retropubic and transperineal dissections on the anterior aspect of the subprostatic urethra the 'pre-urethral sub-pubic space' (X in Fig. 3.34). Needless to say, though, this is a potential space rather than a real space and sometimes there is a 'membranous' barrier to be incised to gain access to it, as in Figure 3.37. However, whether this is a perineal membrane or the proximal limit of the midline septum of the bulbar urethra or part of the origin of the bulbocavernous muscles I am not sure. Laterally there are the bulbar arteries forming two substantial bands but again, whether these are individual structures or part of a perineal membrane I am not sure.

On balance I am against the idea of a perineal membrane because in my experience it is inconstant and when apparently present it is of uneven consistency. It is not, however, something I feel strongly about whereas I am quite sure that there is no urogenital diaphragm.

The pelvic floor musculature
The layout of the pelvic floor musculature has, like much else related to the structure and function of the lower urinary tract, been the subject of review in recent years. The concept of a simple muscular diaphragm as described in the standard anatomical textbooks does not stand up in practice. There is indeed a part of the pelvic floor musculature that corresponds to the

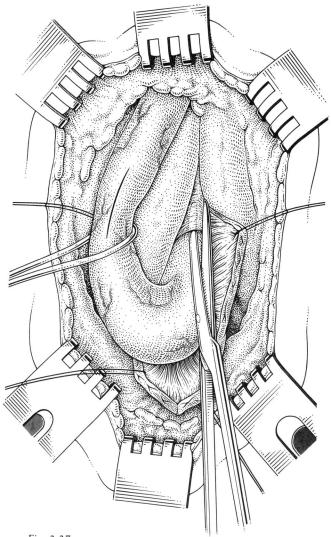

Fig. 3.37

traditional descriptions of pubococcygeus, iliococcygeus, and coccygeus. Together they form a gutter, mainly posterior to the rectum, slung between the pelvic side wall anterolaterally and the lower part of the sacrum and the coccyx posteromedially.

In addition to this 'gutter' layer there is a second component of the pelvic floor musculature, not generally recognised until recently, that corresponds to the anterior part of the traditionally-described pubococcygeus. This component is disposed principally as two slings. These are the

pubourethral sling (or pubourethralis) anteriorly and the puborectal sling (or puborectalis), which is much larger, posteriorly (Fig. 3.25). The pubourethral sling has been mentioned above as visible around the membranous urethra after cystoprostatectomy and is that part of the pelvic floor musculature which contributes to the distal sphincter mechanism. The puborectal sling is likewise an important component of the anal sphincter mechanism, indeed correspondingly more important a component than the pubourethral sling is to the urethral sphincter mechanism.

The pubourethral sling and the anterior part of puborectalis are exposed by division of the endopelvic fascia in the retropubic space. The remainder of puborectalis is posterolateral and posterior to the rectum and can only be exposed by mobilisation of the rectum. If the presacral fascia is incised on either side of the rectum the space between the rectum and the hollow of the sacrum can be entered. This retrorectal space is a large potential space which, when opened widely, allows considerable upward mobilisation of the rectum as, for example, for an anterior resection. The floor of the retrorectal space is the tough fascial layer that binds the anorectal junction to the hollow of the sacrum and which is commonly called Waldeyer's fascia. When this is incised, puborectalis may be found beneath it. Such an exposure may be very helpful during mobilisation and correction of complex gynaecological fistulae involving the rectum.

The other urological relevance of Waldeyer's fascia is that its lateral limits are in close relation to the posterior course of the pelvic parasympathetic nerves as they emerge from the piriformis muscle and before they run into the presacral fascia and thence into the lateral pedicle on each side (described in the next section).

In women the pubourethral sling is absent although there is a slip of muscle that runs deep to the pubourethral ligament between the pubis and urethra just as there is in men in relation to the puboprostatic ligament. Likewise there is in both sexes a muscle slip between the pubis and the perineal body — the puboperineal muscle. This lies deep to the pubourethral sling in males and does not appear to have a significant function in either sex.

The perineal body which is a substantial fibrous body with significant muscular attachments in men — the pubourethral sling, puboperineal muscle, transverse perineal muscles, bulbospongiosus and

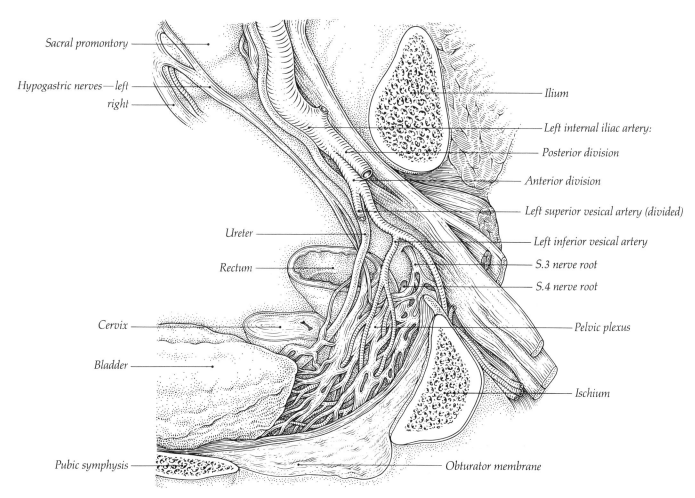

Fig. 3.38
View into the left side of the female pelvis in a cadaver after removing the left side-wall of the pelvis itself.

external anal sphincter — is a rather insignificant fibrofatty structure in women, largely because similarly substantial anterior muscular attachments are lacking.

Pelvic parasympathetic nerves
These have already been referred to with respect to their relationship to the inferior vesical vessels (Fig. 3.38) and their distal course in relation to the posterolateral border of the prostate and the membranous urethra (Figs 3.21, 3.23, 3.25), where they have been described as the neurovascular bundles which ultimately supply the sphincter-active urethra (according to Gosling) and the corpora cavernosa.

Their relationship to the inferior vesical vessels, just below the ureter and just outside the bladder wall, is important in the procedure of transvesical injection of the pelvic plexuses with phenol for the treatment of detrusor instability and hyperreflexia (Ch. 8).

These nerves take origin from the anterior primary rami of S2, S3 and S4, mainly S3 and S4, and run through the piriformis muscle to reach the pelvic surface of the posterolateral side wall of the pelvis (Fig. 3.39), close to the posterolateral aspect of the rectum on each side. From there, the nerves run into the layer of fascia, known as the presacral fascia, that lines the posterolateral side wall of the pelvis, below the common iliac vessels and posterior to the internal iliac vessels (as described earlier). Anteriorly the presacral fascia fuses with the posterior layer of the sheath that surrounds the lateral pedicle (see above), by which route the pelvic parasympathetic nerves come to be within the sheath where they intertwine with the branches of the

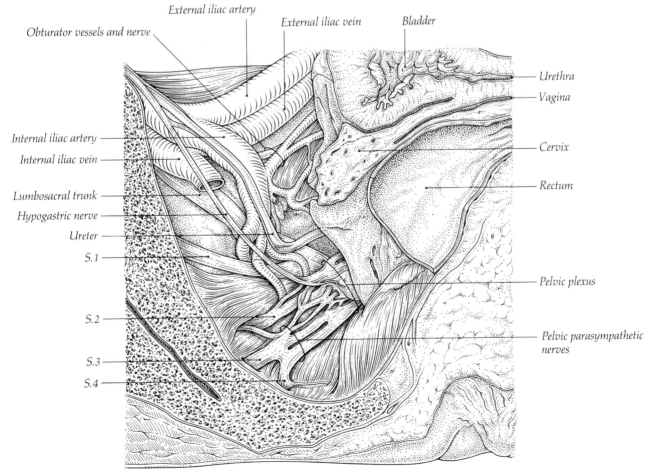

Fig. 3.39
The left half of a hemisected female pelvis with the rectum in its normal position.

inferior vesical vessels. Posteriorly the presacral fascia splits to form a sheath around the rectum. Traction on the rectum, therefore, leads to traction on the pelvic parasympathetic nerves by virtue of their mutual relationship through the presacral fascia (Fig. 3.40) and it is for this reason that a transient or permanent autonomic neuropathy, causing vesicourethral dysfunction, may occur after rectal mobilisation.

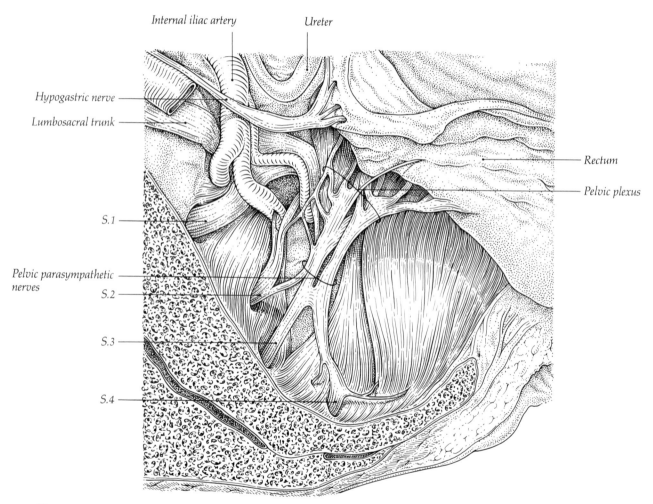

Fig. 3.40
As Fig. 3.39 but with the rectum pulled forward.

REFERENCES

A detailed study of anatomy used to be an important part of surgical training until supplanted by physiology and technology in recent decades. More recently, increasing sophistication of surgical technique has lead to a revival of anatomical 'sophistication' within each surgical subspeciality. Walsh's work is a classic example of this 'sophisticated' approach to anatomy, thereby aiming to refine his surgical technique, in this case radical prostatectomy. The other example is Turner Warwick's anatomical contributions to pelvic and perineal anatomy derived from his experience in urethroplasty. Gosling's work was, and is, from a different point of view — the re-evaluation of traditional academic teaching, using established anatomical methods. One of the important lessons to be learnt from his work is how much can be gained when basic scientists and clinicians work together to try and resolve each others problems.

Uhlenhuth's work is cited although much of it, related to the anatomy of the bladder and the layering of the pelvic floor muscles, is out of date and excessively detailed. His descriptions of the fascial layers and spaces of the pelvis are, however, masterly and unsurpassed. For the surgeon dealing with complex post-radiotherapy pelvic surgery an appreciation of this aspect of anatomy is essential and nobody describes it better than he.

The reference to Chilton relates to the anatomy of the pelvic floor. My own article is concerned with the relationship between the pelvic parasympathetic nerves and the rectum by virtue of their mutual involvement in the presacral fascia.

Chilton C P 1984 The distal urethra sphincter mechanism and the pelvic floor. In: Mundy A R, Stephenson T P, Wein A J (eds) Urodynamics principles, practices and application. Churchill Livingstone, Edinburgh, pp 9–13

Gosling J A, Dixon J S, Humpherson J R 1983 Functional anatomy of the urinary tract: an integrated text and colour atlas. Churchill Livingstone, Edinburgh

Mundy A R 1982 An anatomical explanation for bladder dysfunction following rectal and uterine surgery. British Journal of Urology 54: 501–504

Reiner W A, Walsh P C 1979 An anatomical approach to the surgical management of the dorsal vein and Santorini's plexus during radical retropubic prostatectomy. Journal of Urology 121: 198–200

Turner Warwick R J 1988 Urethral stricture surgery. In: Mundy A R (ed) Current operative surgery: Urology. Bailliere Tindall, Eastbourne, pp 100–218

Uhlenhuth E, Hunter D T, Loechel WE 1953 Problems in the anatomy of the pelvis. Lippincott, Philadelphia

Walsh P C 1986 Radical retropubic prostatectomy. In: Walsh P C, Gittes R F, Perimutter A D, Stamey T A (eds) Campbell's Urology, 5th edn. W B Saunders Co, Philadelphia, pp 2769–2771

URODYNAMIC PROBLEMS

Introduction

The main difference between the treatment of the urodynamic disorders described in this section and the treatment of the reconstructive problems described in the next section is that, with the urodynamic disorders, the results of treatment depend more on an exact urodynamic diagnosis and less on the skill with which the surgical procedure is performed. With a full urodynamic investigation, appropriate to the patient's problem and correctly evaluated, the results of surgical intervention are very satisfactory almost irrespective of technical surgical competence as long as important general principles are adhered to. The procedure required is more or less defined by the urodynamic diagnosis. For reconstructive problems this is not the case — other factors are equally important in getting good results.

Most of the general principles of reconstructive urological surgery are best learnt in the treatment of the urodynamic disorders described in this section because in these disorders individual problems of detrusor overactivity, poor bladder compliance, sphincter weakness and outflow obstruction are more easily definable and seen in a more 'pure' form. By learning the ways to correct these individual problems the surgeon learns how to produce a low-pressure bladder of adequate capacity, a competent bladder outflow and adequate emptying and can then go on to apply these principles to the situations commonly found in reconstructive urology in which multiple urodynamic problems coexist or in which the problems themselves are difficult or impossible to define with any accuracy preoperatively, and can only be anticipated.

The urodynamic disorders discussed in this section are bladder outflow obstruction (excluding strictures), post-prostatectomy incontinence, sphincter weakness incontinence in women (stress incontinence), detrusor instability, sensory bladder disorders, non-neuropathic urodynamic problems in children and finally neuropathic vesicourethral dysfunction. The treatment of bladder outflow obstruction, sphincter weakness incontinence and detrusor instability is the bread and butter of urodynamic surgery. Post-prostatectomy incontinence is fortunately less common but often more complicated because all three of the above problems may coexist. A similar combination of problems is seen in neuropathy, but more commonly and to a more severe degree.

The chapter on sensory bladder disorders is largely concerned with interstitial cystitis. Sensory bladder disorders are poorly understood and some would regard them as only peripheral to urodynamic practice. The treatment of interstitial cystitis does however introduce the technique of substitution cystoplasty and its particular urodynamic problems.

The short chapter on 'Non-neuropathic urodynamic disorders in children' is largely concerned with surgically treatable urodynamic dysfunctions in children. Several of these dysfunctions are similar to the problems seen in adults but less well understood.

Chapter 4

Bladder outflow obstruction

The diagnosis and management of bladder outflow obstruction forms a major part of the workload of all general urologists and is one of the main reasons for the existence of urology as a separate speciality. Given that the reader will be fully conversant with most aspects of the subject, the aim of this chapter is to draw his or her attention to those aspects which pose dilemmas in diagnosis and treatment, and particularly to those problems that are commonly seen following previous treatment of bladder outflow obstruction and how they might be avoided.

BLADDER OUTFLOW OBSTRUCTION IN THE MALE

There are two types of bladder outflow obstruction in male patients that will be discussed here — dyssynergic bladder neck obstruction, that may occur at any age but predominantly in young adults, and prostatic obstruction due to benign prostatic hyperplasia, predominantly occurring in the elderly.

Other causes of outflow obstruction in children, such as posterior urethral valves and so-called anterior urethral valves, are more properly the concern of the paediatric urologist and will not be considered here; neither will outflow obstruction in adults due to carcinoma of the prostate or prostatic abscess. Strictures are discussed in Chapter 11.

Dyssynergic bladder neck obstruction
Anatomically the bladder neck is a mystery. At rest it is closed and acts therefore as a sphincter mechanism; histologically, however, no true sphincter mechanism can be defined although there are changes in morphology at this site which distinguish the area from the rest of the detrusor. The detrusor is composed of interlacing large muscle bundles surrounded by a relatively small amount of connective tissue whereas at the bladder neck the muscle bundles are

smaller, have a more circular orientation and are surrounded by a much larger connective tissue component. Just below the bladder neck, and intimately related to it, there is a second smooth muscle 'collar' surrounding the prostatic urethra above the verumontanum. This second smooth muscle component differs from the bladder neck, which has a cholinergic innervation, by having an alpha adrenergic innervation. Its function is to close off the bladder neck during ejaculation to prevent retrograde ejaculation and it is called the pre-prostatic sphincter.

Normally, when the detrusor contracts the bladder neck opens and when the detrusor is not contracting the bladder neck remains closed. Whether bladder neck opening occurs because it is actually pulled open by the contracting detrusor, or whether it occurs by nerve-mediated relaxation synchronous with nerve-mediated detrusor contraction, is not clear, but indirect evidence suggests that in dyssynergic bladder neck obstruction not only does the bladder neck not open as it normally does, but it may actually contract, as does the detrusor around it. This and other evidence suggests that the bladder neck area has a specific innervation to relax it which is deranged in dyssynergic bladder neck obstruction.

It is also not clear if the obstructing element is the cholinergically-innervated bladder neck smooth muscle proper — common to both sexes — or the adrenergically-innervated pre-prostatic sphincter (PPS) with which the bladder neck mechanism is intimately related in males only. However, as the condition is rare before puberty, when the PPS is comparatively undeveloped, and commonest in the 20–40 age group, after the PPS has developed fully during puberty, and as the condition is extremely rare (maybe non-existent) in female patients, it may be that it is the PPS that is the obstructing factor.

Diagnosis. When bladder neck obstruction presents in children (which is rare), it usually presents as poor bladder emptying, recurrent urinary tract infection, a palpable bladder and secondary upper tract changes in the first year or two of life, although obviously milder cases may present later on in childhood. In adults it more commonly presents with the usual obstructive symptoms of hesitancy and a poor stream.

In children it is usually misdiagnosed as urethral valves until a micturating cystogram shows the absence of valves and indeed that the urethra fills hardly at all because of the 'tight' bladder neck.

In adults the diagnosis is often overlooked because of the very gradual onset and because of the very frequently coexisting detrusor instability. If symptoms of instability are present in a young man it is therefore important to distinguish between idiopathic instability and instability secondary to dyssynergic bladder neck obstruction. A normal free flow rate may help but a video-urodynamic study will usually be necessary, firstly because the implications for fertility of the surgical treatment of a bladder neck obstruction make a substantiated diagnosis important for many patients, secondly because a normal flow rate may be maintained by a detrusor contracting at very high pressures, and thirdly because a restricted bladder capacity due to coexisting detrusor instability makes the interpretation of the flow rate difficult. Finally of course a low flow rate may be due to other causes and particularly anxiety causing failure of opening of the distal sphincter mechanism rather than dyssynergic bladder neck obstruction causing failure of opening of the bladder neck.

The characteristic urodynamic appearance is a bladder neck that fails to open adequately, except perhaps towards the end of voiding, and

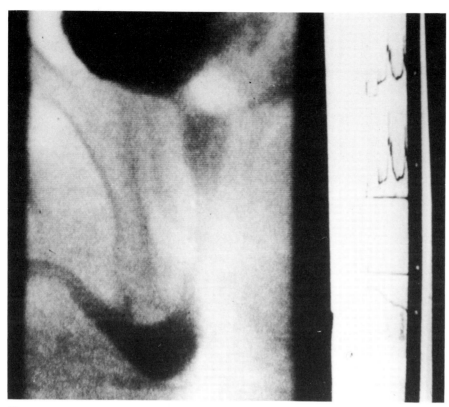

Fig. 4.1

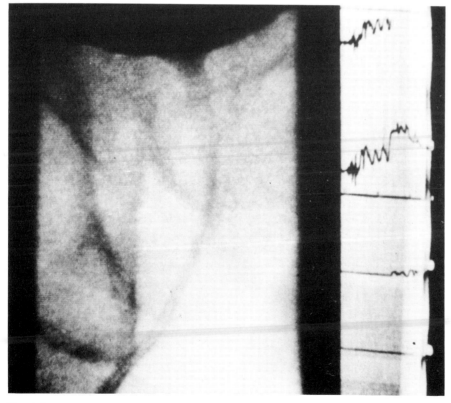

Fig. 4.2

trapping of the urine within the prostatic urethra on interruption of voiding, in the presence of a high voiding pressure and a low flow rate (Fig. 4.1). By contrast, prostatic obstruction produces a more tapered appearance of the prostatic urethra with the same pressure-flow characteristics (Fig. 4.2).

In both adults and children the presence of gross vesico-ureteric reflux or a large diverticulum may make assessment of the bladder neck very difficult because so much of the urine is diverted away from the bladder neck when the detrusor contracts.

Treatment. The treatment of dyssynergic bladder neck obstruction is bladder neck incision. The problem is to decide when it is necessary. When the condition is causing upper tract obstruction or recurrent urinary tract infection and when the peak urinary flow rate is less than 5 ml/s, bladder neck incision is necessary. Unfortunately retrograde ejaculation occurs in at least 10% of patients after this procedure (and substantially more in my own experience). This may be a catastrophe to the patient so the procedure should be avoided where possible until such time as the patient regards this complication as acceptable.

In the very young, a simple bladder neck incision does not always give a satisfactory result and a Y-V plasty of the bladder neck may be necessary.

Bladder neck incision
No special preoperative preparation is required, other than to ensure that the urine is sterile. The endoscopic appearance is of a ring-shaped bladder neck with a prominent posterior lip above a normal prostatic urethra (Fig. 4.3). This is not in itself diagnostic of dyssynergic bladder neck obstruction, only an indication of the site of obstruction — the diagnosis of obstruction must be urodynamically proven.

Using a diathermy point electrode, the bladder neck is incised from the ureteric orifice on one side down to the verumontanum. As the incision is deepened the muscular ring of the bladder neck is disrupted and when this occurs, to reveal extraluminal fat in the depths of the incision, the edges of the bladder neck spring open (Fig. 4.4).

This is a simple procedure, but the critical factor is the complete disruption of the bladder neck ring, which can only be ensured if the incision is carried through to fat. When a bladder neck incision fails to resolve the problem it is almost always because it wasn't deep enough.

A catheter is left in the bladder at the end of the procedure and for 3 or 4 days thereafter, so that extravasation of urine through the incision does not occur when voiding is re-established.

No postoperative follow up is necessary after a postoperative flow study has confirmed the effect of the procedure, except in those with upper tract changes or with secondary urodynamic abnormalities and in children.

Prostatic obstruction

As with dyssynergic bladder neck obstruction, the patient commonly presents with the obstructive symptoms of hesitancy, poor stream and terminal dribbling; the condition is commonly confused with or complicated by detrusor instability; and the diagnosis is made on the basis of a low flow rate. An ultrasound study of the bladder after voiding is a useful additional investigation to assess the ability of the bladder to empty. A large residual urine would suggest that the low flow rate is due to an ineffective detrusor contraction and although this may be secondary to bladder outflow obstruction it suggests that relief of the obstruction may not give a significant improvement in emptying and therefore in symptoms. More elaborate diagnostic

investigation by video-urodynamics is not usually necessary unless the patient presents with overriding symptoms of detrusor instability (in which case the study is more likely to exclude a diagnosis of obstruction rather than to prove it) or if flow rate studies are either equivocal or invalidated by a low voided volume. The treatment is transurethral resection of the prostate.

Transurethral resection of the prostate

The technique of transurethral resection of the prostate (TURP) is well described in several other volumes and will not be described here in detail. There are however a few points worth making in relation to those patients with less than satisfactory results following TURP. Many TURPs are incomplete, even in patients with very satisfactory results, when judged by follow-up endoscopy or by rectal palpation or transrectal ultrasound of the gland. These often reveal a 'V'-shaped wedge of residual tissue which tends to lie (Fig. 4.5):

— at the apex of the prostate, on either side of and below the verumontanum,
— more proximally within the prostatic urethra, usually between 12 o'clock and 3 o'clock when the TURP was done by a right-handed surgeon; between 9 o'clock and 12 o'clock if the surgeon is left-handed,
— at the bladder neck anteriorly.

This is the result of the way in which the procedure is usually performed. The posterior half of the bladder neck is usually completely resected, often as the first stage of the procedure; the right prostatic lobe, at least between 6 o'clock and 10 o'clock, is usually resected before the left (by a right-handed surgeon); tissue at and below the level of the verumontanum is usually left behind to avoid damaging the urethral sphincter mechanism; and little resection is performed anteriorly unless the tissue seems overtly obstructive. As a result of resecting the right lobe first, the left

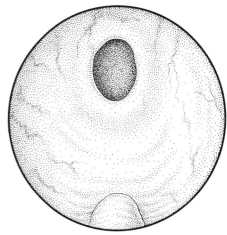

Fig. 4.3

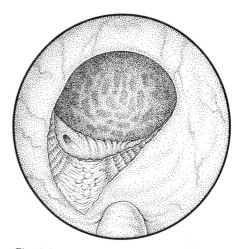

Fig. 4.4

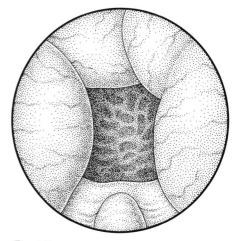

Fig. 4.5

lobe tends to collapse inwards and there is therefore more tissue left anteriorly on the left than on the right. This tissue is sometimes difficult to see at the end of a TURP if the resectoscope is rotated anticlockwise from 6 o'clock to 12 o'clock, but is usually obvious if the 'scope is rotated clockwise.

The key to complete resection is therefore to review the entire prostatic cavity by rotating the resectoscope in both directions before regarding the procedure as complete, and to check the completeness of the resection by rectal palpation.

The problem of residual apical tissue is less straightforward because of the relationship of the tissue with the distal sphincter mechanism. Obviously resecting too little of the apical tissue is not nearly so serious as resecting deeply into the intrinsic rhabdosphincter, and it is therefore better to be safe than sorry. On the other hand, I have never encountered an instance when careful resection of readily palpable apical tissue has led to sphincter damage. Indeed, when the sphincter is damaged by a resectoscope, except when used by a novice, it is usually at 11 o'clock or 1 o'clock where the verumontanum is not visible for orientation, whereas apical tissue is predominantly concentrated laterally on each side where the relationship to the verumontanum is easily checked.

The final point concerns the coexistence of dyssynergic bladder neck obstruction with benign prostatic hyperplasia. Recognising that the key to eliminating the former is the complete disruption of the bladder neck ring through its full thickness and that failure to do this leads to recurrence of the problem or, alternatively, a bladder neck stricture, it is obviously important to recognise when the two problems coexist as a TURP alone may be inadequate. It is therefore important to inspect the bladder neck carefully before a TURP to look for the suggestive bladder neck ring and, if it is present, to perform a bladder neck incision before beginning the resection of the prostate.

It is these points that will need to be attended to in the patient with persistent obstructive symptoms after a TURP, assuming that ultrasound and video-urodynamic studies confirm that the symptoms are due to persistent obstruction and not to detrusor failure. This point is worth stressing — it is pointless to keep doing repeat resections when the cause is detrusor failure or some other non-obstructive problem. In any patient with persistent obstruction the prostate should be completely resected (and any bladder neck obstruction incised through to fat) even if the patient has sphincter weakness incontinence due to a damaged distal sphincter mechanism. Some patients with mild post-prostatectomy incontinence due to sphincter damage (or without endoscopically visible sphincter damage) are improved by resection of residual apical prostatic tissue, presumably because this tissue causes deformity in the area of the intrinsic rhabdosphincter which prevents it from functioning properly.

BLADDER OUTFLOW OBSTRUCTION IN THE FEMALE

Again this may be of two types: bladder neck obstruction or distal urethral obstruction, although the evidence that either of them is truly an obstruction is somewhat tenuous.

Bladder neck obstruction
I have never seen this in a female patient with a contractile bladder and reported instances with good documentation are rare. One commonly sees women with an acontractile bladder and therefore a bladder neck that does not open to allow voiding; such women are best treated by clean intermittent self catheterisation (CISC). If she cannot do this, or if there are problems with CISC, usually due to persistent urinary tract infection despite adequate treatment with antibiotics, a cautious bladder neck incision may be tried. The problems are that even with an adequate bladder neck incision the woman may be unable to relax her distal sphincter mechanism (DSM) appropriately, and the voiding difficulty will therefore persist, or that, on the other hand, the DSM may be intrinsically incompetent (or rendered incompetent by an overenthusiastic incision) leading to incontinence. For these reasons a bladder neck incision should only be performed as a last resort in the two specific instances given above and should never be performed simply because the patient does not like the idea of self catheterisation.

Bladder neck incision
As in men this is a simple procedure, but in women should never be performed posteriorly because of the risk of incising too deeply and causing a vesico-vaginal fistula. It should always be performed in the anterior midline and this has the additional advantage that it is theoretically possible to repair such an incision, through a retropubic approach, if incontinence results.

The procedure is best performed under direct vision using a nasal speculum and a diathermy point to see and incise the bladder neck until it is disrupted at 12 o'clock precisely (Fig. 4.6).

Distal urethral obstruction
As with bladder neck obstruction there is little evidence to suggest that the apparent radiological failure of the distal urethra to open appropriately or adequately during voiding is actually an obstruction. Voiding pressure in such instances is usually normal or low, suggesting that the problem is more a generalised failure of the whole detrusor-urethral unit rather than a localised distal sphincter abnormality. As such the appearances closely resemble the urodynamic picture of a peripheral

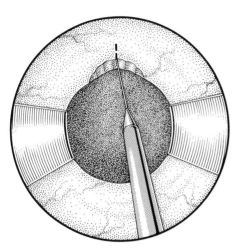

Fig. 4.6

autonomic neuropathy. (One wonders whether this is more than coincidence.) The same comments apply to so-called distal urethral stenosis in young girls although in children the cause of failure to open the urethra to a normal degree is more likely to be due to a failure to relax the distal sphincter normally, whether voluntarily or subconsciously.

Nonetheless high pressure—low flow obstruction is occasionally seen and this responds well to urethral dilatation or 'recalibration'. The normal/low pressure—low flow voiding dysfunction, whatever its cause, certainly is a distinct clinical entity which, like obstruction, responds to urethral recalibration albeit less predictably. Presumably in those that respond the failure of urethral opening is more significant than the failure to generate an adequate detrusor contraction, whereas in those that do not respond the failure to achieve an adequate detrusor contraction is more important.

Urethral recalibration

This is most commonly achieved by urethral dilatation with metal sounds to an empirical level, such as 30 F or 14 Hegar, but this is rather imprecise. I prefer to use an Otis urethrotome without the blade and to wind this up, moving the instrument in and out along the urethral axis, until it is gripped by the urethra. The urethrotome is then expanded to a level 10 F higher than the point at which it is gripped.

The effectiveness of the procedure, as with all the obstruction-relieving procedures described here, is checked by repeating the flow rate study postoperatively. If there has not been a satisfactory response the recalibration is repeated to a degree 10 F higher than on the previous occasion.

Problems of treating bladder outflow obstruction in women

The penalty for overtreating bladder outflow obstruction in women is incontinence. This is unlikely with graded urethral 'recalibration' for distal urethral dysfunction but it is a very real problem with so-called bladder neck obstruction. It is for this reason that clean intermittent self catheterisation is to be preferred for all significant problems of bladder emptying in women, when treatment is necessary. The first question therefore is — 'Is treatment really necessary?'. If the problems of treatment are discussed with the patient she may elect to continue to manage without treatment rather than use CISC or run the risk of incontinence associated with bladder neck incision. If the patient demands treatment but refuses to countenance CISC her motivation must be regarded as suspect. If treatment is necessary because of frequently recurrent symptomatic urinary tract infection but CISC is not possible because of urethral pathology then a Mitrofanoff procedure, as described in Chapter 10, is the best solution.

The theoretical option of urethral sphincteric ablation combined with implantation of an artificial sphincter should only be reserved for those very few patients who are chronically unwell with CISC because of recurrent urinary tract infection despite antibiotic prophylaxis. The reason is that if artificial sphincter implantation is complicated by infection or erosion requiring removal, the patient will be left irretrievably incontinent and she will therefore be substantially worse off than she was to start with. This is too big a risk to take unless there really is no other option.

Chapter 5

Post-prostatectomy incontinence

Post-prostatectomy incontinence is a catastrophe. When it occurs it is usually attributed to surgical misadventure but this is rarely the only factor. Urodynamic assessment of patients with post-prostatectomy incontinence (PPI) has shown that the commonest single abnormality is detrusor instability and that the commonest finding is a combination of detrusor instability and sphincter weakness (Table 5.1). Follow up of patients with PPI has shown that a substantial percentage show improvement or even complete resolution of their incontinence during the first year after prostatectomy.

Table 5.1 The urodynamic abnormalities found on investigating 100 consecutive patients with post-prostatectomy incontinence

Detrusor instability		57
Alone	17	
With sphincter damage	27	
With obstruction	7	
With sphincter damage and obstruction	6	
Sphincter damage		17
Alone	11	
With obstruction	6	
Hypersensitive bladder		14
Alone	8	
With obstruction	6	
Acontractile bladder		6
No abnormality found		6

There are several inferences to be drawn from these observations. Firstly, patients with marked urge symptoms before prostatectomy should be warned that their instability symptoms may persist after the prostatectomy and may worsen temporarily. Secondly, patients with established PPI of a mild degree in the early postoperative period can be reassured that there is a good chance that they will improve spontaneously over the next 3–6 months. Thirdly, further endoscopic surgery should be avoided until the likelihood of spontaneous improvement has passed, unless there is a strong indication. Fourthly, the treatment modality most likely to improve the patient's symptoms, until re-investigation gives a definite diagnosis, is a course of

anti-cholinergic medication for detrusor instability. Finally, both video-urodynamic investigation and endoscopy will be necessary to make a definite diagnosis of the cause of PPI.

ASSESSMENT

The first step is to assess the severity of the symptoms which may vary from relatively normal voiding with stress incontinence between times, to total daytime incontinence with no normal voiding episodes at the other extreme. In those with total incontinence, symptoms suggestive of detrusor instability can only be determined from the pre-prostatectomy symptomatology.

A flow study is the next step, to look for features suggestive of persistent obstruction. This is best obtained after lying down for several hours or first thing in the morning when the bladder has had its best chance of filling to a useful capacity.

Next comes a video-urodynamic study looking for detrusor instability, poor bladder compliance, a reduced capacity, sphincter weakness and outflow obstruction, bearing in mind that sphincter weakness during this study may be a lot less than the patient's symptoms might suggest, because the patient may be able to hold urine during the short period of the study by using pelvic floor activity to augment his reduced sphincter activity.

Finally a cystourethroscopy should be performed to look for a stricture, a damaged sphincter and residual prostatic obstruction and to measure the bladder capacity under anaesthetic for comparison with the capacity under normal circumstances. An associated stricture, either of the sphincter itself or elsewhere in the urethra, is quite common. Sphincter damage is always suspected but not always seen, even when there is proven sphincter

weakness. Presumably the sphincter mechanism can be functionally impaired, possibly as a result of spread of the diathermy current during the prostatectomy, even when it is structurally intact.

MANAGEMENT

Patients with total incontinence, urodynamically confirmed and with obvious major sphincter damage endoscopically are unlikely to improve spontaneously and will require specific treatment for their sphincter weakness. Those with detrusor instability or outflow obstruction should have these treated appropriately; any residual symptoms attributable to sphincter weakness then require specific treatment in their own right. Patients with sphincter strictures should be treated by dilatation (which may improve their symptoms dramatically) until the stricture is stable or by urethroplasty if that fails (Ch. 11). Any residual incontinence is then treated in its own right.

Specific treatment for sphincter weakness incontinence is either to contain the incontinence by use of protective pads, a Conveen pouch or a sheath drainage device, depending on the degree of incontinence, or to cure the incontinence by implantation of an artificial sphincter. Implantation of an artificial sphincter is reserved for those patients with a degree of sphincter weakness incontinence sufficient to interfere with their normal activity who are fit enough to undergo the operation and who have had any obstruction or instability treated or controlled by the appropriate means. The presence of detrusor instability is not a bar to implantation of an artificial sphincter but patients should be warned that the device only controls the sphincter weakness and that symptoms related to the instability will persist and will need to be treated in their own right. They should also be warned that despite careful preoperative urodynamic evaluation detrusor instability may only become apparent after the artificial sphincter has been implanted, presumably because the bladder can then fill to a more normal capacity or 'has something to work against'.

Several artificial sphincters have been marketed, of which the best-known examples are the Kauffman, Rosen and Brantley Scott devices. The Kauffman and Rosen devices both produce uncontrolled occlusive pressures and therefore have lower success rates and higher complication rates than the Brantley Scott device. The alternative procedure of Teflon injection in the region of the membranous urethra to produce an artificial prostate has rarely been successful in my experience and then only temporarily and will not therefore be considered further.

Thus implantation of the Brantley Scott device is the only procedure that will be described here, recognising that at the time of writing other artificial sphincters are being developed, which may eventually replace this device in routine use.

THE BRANTLEY SCOTT ARTIFICIAL URINARY SPHINCTER

The Brantley Scott artificial urinary sphincter (AUS) has developed through various stages. The models currently available are the AS 791 (Fig. 5.1), AS 792 (Fig. 5.2) and AS 800 (Fig. 5.3). Before the AS 800 became available, the AS 791 was intended for cuff placement around the bulbar urethra (Fig. 5.4) and the AS 792 for cuff placement around the bladder neck (Fig. 5.5). The AS 792 was therefore applicable to both sexes and the AS 791 only to males. The AS 791 was essentially for patients with PPI for whom fibrosis around the prostate and bladder neck as a result of their prostatectomy made cuff placement around the bulbar urethra desirable.

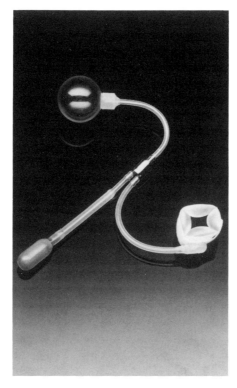

Fig. 5.1

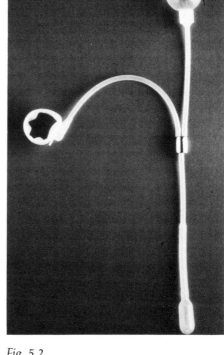

Fig. 5.2

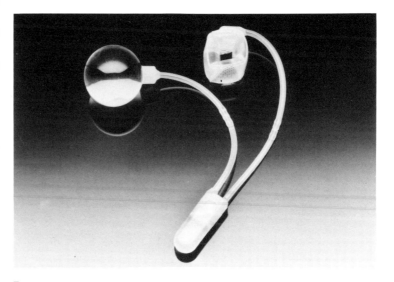

Fig. 5.3

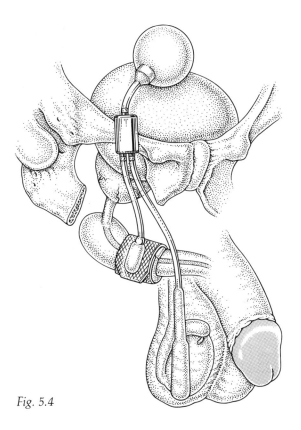

Fig. 5.4

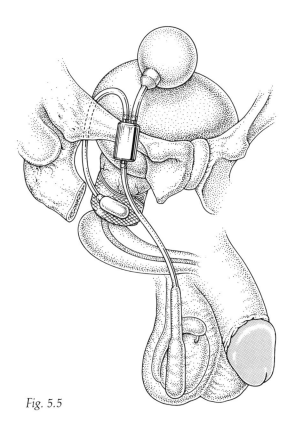

Fig. 5.5

Apart from differences in connecting the various components to the control assembly the AS 791 and AS 792 were identical.

The AS 791 and 792 each consist of four parts — the cuff, the pressure-regulating balloon, the deflation pump and the control assembly. The cuff comes in various sizes from 4.5 – 11 cm, increasing in size by 0.5 cm increments in the lower half of the range and by 1 cm intervals in the upper half, so that it can be fitted accurately around the selected site — either the bladder neck or bulbar urethra. The pressure-regulating balloons are precalibrated during manufacture so that when they are filled with isotonic fluid to a volume of between 16 and 24 ml (approximately), they exert a pressure within a defined range of 51–60 cmH$_2$O, 61–70 cmH$_2$O or 71–80 cmH$_2$O. Balloons with a range of 41–50 or

81–90 cmH$_2$O are available on special request but are not used routinely. The balloon is implanted intra-abdominally and usually extraperitoneally. The pump is placed subcutaneously in the scrotum or labium majus, making it easily accessible to the patient. The tubing from all three components run into the inguinal canal where they are connected to the control assembly (Figs 5.4, 5.5).

The disadvantage of the AS 791/792 is that it can only be deactivated by disconnecting the tubing at some point and it therefore requires a second operation to activate it if it is thought advisable to leave a few weeks between implantation and activation. This is usually the case as the risk of erosion of the cuff through the urethra is much greater if the device is pressurised at a time when the tissues within the cuff are suffering from the effects of operative trauma.

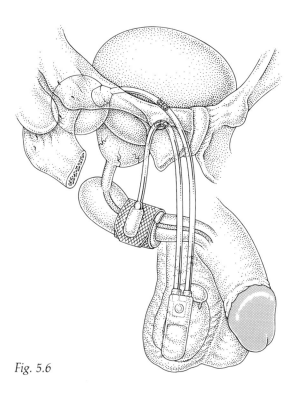

Fig. 5.6

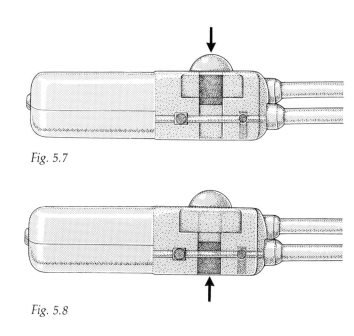

Fig. 5.7

Fig. 5.8

The AS 800 was introduced to get around this problem (Fig. 5.6). The cuff and the pressure-regulating balloon are the same and it works according to the same principles but the control assembly and the deflation pump are incorporated together into a single component (the control pump) which also has a button on it (Fig. 5.7) which, when pressed, deactivates the device (Fig. 5.8) by pushing a plug into the circuit to stop fluid flow. The AS 800 is subsequently activated by 'blowing out' the deactivation valve below the button by giving the pump a firm squeeze. Deactivation and activation can therefore be easily done, whenever necessary, without the need for operative intervention.

The disadvantage of the AS 800 is that the control pump is substantially larger than the deflation pump of the AS 791/792 and too large for young children, especially young girls. The AS 792 therefore has a place in the very young (and is still available at the time of writing, but may not be for much

longer), but for patients in whom the size of the AS 800 control pump is not a problem it is the preferred model because of the deactivation option and it is therefore the most widely used type and has completely replaced the AS 791 in routine use.

The concept is that the AUS is a hydraulic device which produces an occlusive force through the cuff to control continence with a pressure determined by the pressure-regulating balloon. This occlusive force is constantly maintained by the direction of fluid flow from balloon to cuff (Fig. 5.9), except when the deflation pump is squeezed when the fluid is transferred through the pump from cuff to balloon, thereby emptying the cuff and removing the occlusive force so that voiding can take place (Fig. 5.10). Each squeeze of the pump empties 0.5 ml from the cuff and a snugly fitting cuff holds 1–2 ml, so 2–4 squeezes are normally necessary to empty the cuff for voiding.

After it has been emptied, the cuff refills

spontaneously from the pressure-regulating balloon, as this is the normal direction of fluid flow, but this flow is slowed by virtue of the valve arrangement within the control assembly so that it takes a few minutes to occur, thereby giving sufficient time for complete bladder emptying before restoration of the occlusive force.

IMPLANTATION OF A BRANTLEY SCOTT ARTIFICIAL URINARY SPHINCTER

Preparation
The patient is admitted two days preoperatively and undergoes the limited preoperative bowel preparation described in Chapter 2. It is particularly important to ensure that the urine is sterile. Whenever possible an indwelling catheter should be removed several days beforehand.

Blood loss rarely occurs to a significant degree and blood transfusion will not therefore be necessary.

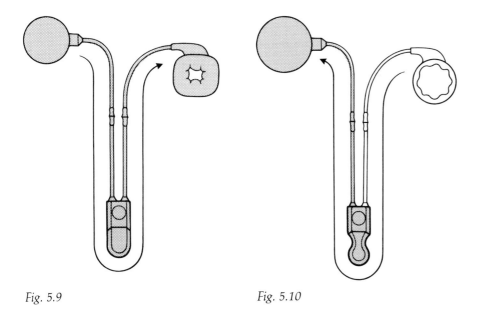

Fig. 5.9   Fig. 5.10

Position

The patient is placed in the low lithotomy position and prepared and draped to allow access to the perineum and the scrotum and to the inguinal and suprapubic regions. The highest standards of sterility must be maintained throughout the procedure to reduce the risk of contamination to an absolute minimum.

Technique

A midline perineal incision is made and deepened down to the bulbospongiosus muscle, which is divided in the midline and reflected laterally on each side to expose the bulbar urethra within (Fig. 5.11). The bulbar urethra is then mobilised over a length of about 3 cm by dividing the deep midline fibrous septum that tethers it to the corpora cavernosa (Figs 5.12, 5.13).

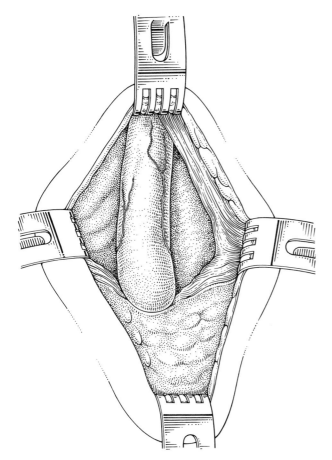

Fig. 5.11

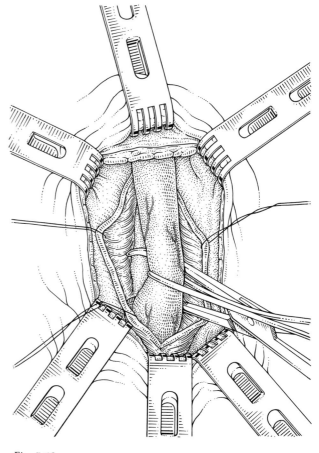

Fig. 5.12

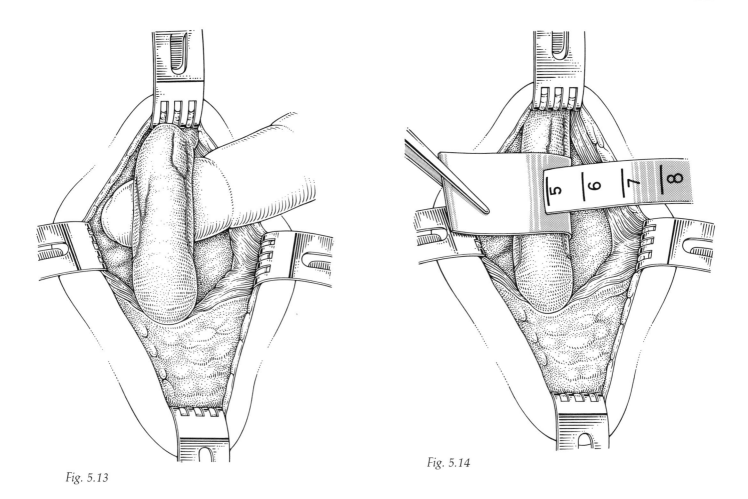

Fig. 5.13

Fig. 5.14

The measuring tape supplied by the manufacturers, which has a width equal to that of an AUS cuff, is then passed around the urethra so that its circumference can be measured (Fig. 5.14). It is usually 4.5 or 5 cm.

A cuff of the correct size (Fig. 5.15) is then filled with fluid to remove the air from the system as far as possible (Fig. 5.16). This fluid should be isotonic so that there will be no net fluid shift through the cuff wall (which is a semipermeable membrane) after implantation and it is advisable to use a radiological contrast solution so that the device can be visualised radiologically during postoperative follow up. A variety of contrast solutions are suitable (Table 5.2). When all the air has been

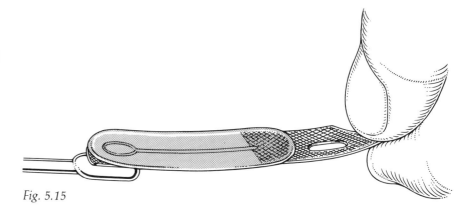

Fig. 5.15

eliminated with the contrast solution, the cuff is deflated. It is then clipped off with a pair of artery forceps which are shod with silicone rubber tubing so that the cuff tubing will not be damaged by the forceps.

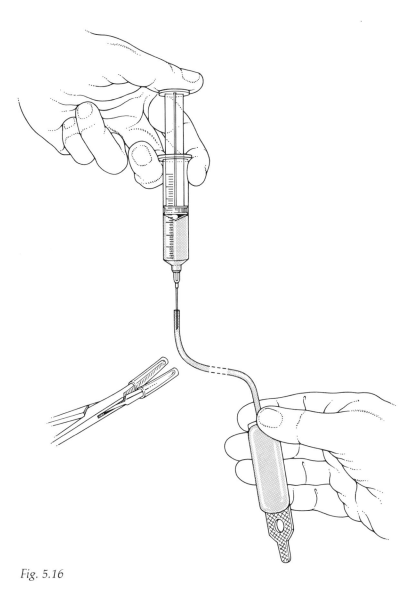

Fig. 5.16

Table 5.2 Suitable isotonic solutions for filling an AUS to allow postoperative radiological monitoring

1. Hypaque 25% (Winthrop Laboratories, New York, NY, USA)
   (50 cc radiopaque dye mixed with 60 cc sterile water).
2. Conray 280 (Mallinckrodt, UK)
   (20 cc radiopaque dye mixed with 60 cc sterile water).
3. Cysto-Conray II (Mallinckrodt Inc, St Louis, MO, USA)
   (60 cc radiopaque dye mixed with 15 cc sterile water).
4. Isopaque-Cysto (Nyegaard & Co, Oslo, Norway)
   (60 cc radiopaque dye mixed with 27 cc sterile water).
5. Iopamiro 300 (Bracco, Italy)
   (47 cc radiopaque dye mixed with 53 cc sterile water).
6. Hexabrix (BYK-Gulden, Germany)
   (53 cc radiopaque dye mixed with 47 cc sterile water).
7. Urografin 30% (Schering AG, Berlin, Germany)
   (49 cc radiopaque dye mixed with 47 cc sterile water).
8. Solutrast 300 (BYK-Gulden, Germany)
   (53 cc radiopaque dye mixed with 47 cc sterile water).
9. Conray FL (BYK-Gulden, Germany)
   (58 cc radiopaque dye mixed with 42 cc sterile water).
10. Telebrix 12 (Laboratoire Guerbet, France)
    (53 cc radiopaque dye mixed with 47 cc sterile water).

N.B. only water for injection should be used. If a patient has a history of a reaction to radiological contrast then isotonic saline should be used on its own but postoperative X-ray monitoring will obviously not then be possible.

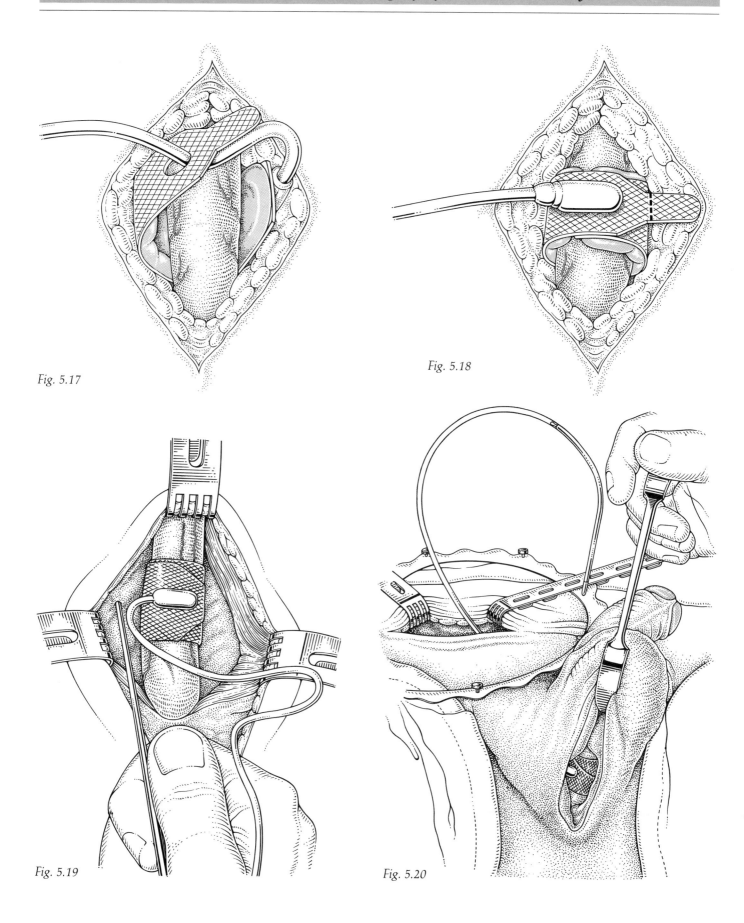

Fig. 5.17

Fig. 5.18

Fig. 5.19

Fig. 5.20

The cuff is then placed around the urethra (Fig. 5.17) and secured in place by threading the tubing through the eye of the cuff so that the eye locks into the groove around the neck of the cuff (Fig. 5.18).

Before and after placing the cuff, I spray it liberally with an iodine spray as a further step to prevent contamination.

Having placed the cuff, a short skin crease incision is made over the internal inguinal ring through which the rest of the components will be placed and all the connections made. The incision is deepened down to the external oblique aponeurosis which is incised to open the inguinal canal.

Using a blunt, purpose-made director needle (a blunted Redivac needle can also be used) the cuff tubing is passed up from the perineum into the inguinal canal (Figs 5.19, 5.20) and reclamped. The midline perineal incision is then sprayed with iodine and closed in layers to reduce the risk of contamination from the perianal region during the rest of the procedure.

The next step is to place the pressure-regulating balloon extraperitoneally and intra-abdominally through the internal ring of the inguinal canal. To do this the internal ring is opened lateral to the point of emergence of the spermatic cord and an extaperitoneal space is created by blunt dissection to a size sufficient to accommodate the balloon. Either a 51–60 or a 61–70 cmH$_2$O pressure balloon may be used; I usually use a 51–60 cmH$_2$O balloon except in younger fitter patients, when a 61–70 cmH$_2$O balloon is chosen. The balloon is then emptied of air by filling it with radiological contrast solution, as with the cuff. The balloon is then sprayed with iodine and passed through the internal ring into the extraperitoneal space created for it. It is then filled to 22 ml with contrast solution and

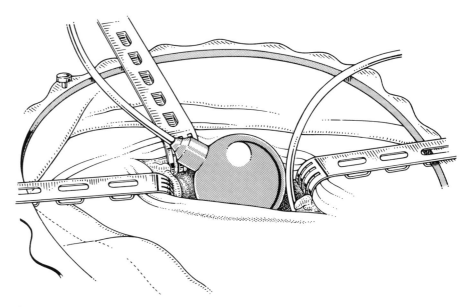

Fig. 5.21
Close up of the right inguinal incision.

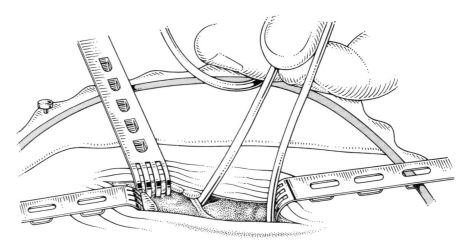

Fig. 5.22

clamped with a pair of silicone-shod artery forceps (Figs 5.21, 5.22). By placing the balloon empty and then filling it, rather than placing it already filled, the hole in the back of the inguinal canal can be kept as small as possible to reduce the risk of subsequent hernia development.

A subcutaneous tunnel is then made from the inguinal canal to the scrotum by blunt dissection, keeping the dissection within the scrotum superficial, between the skin and the dartos layer. A subcutaneous 'dartos pouch' is thereby made in the scrotum for placement of the control pump. The control pump is emptied of air and filled with contrast solution as with the cuff and the balloon. The two lengths of tubing, one to join to the cuff, the other to the balloon, are then clamped with silicone-shod artery forceps and the control pump is sprayed with iodine and pushed into the dartos pouch (Fig. 5.23). To prevent the control pump from riding up out of its pouch during the subsequent manipulations the two tubes from the pump are held in place, through the scrotal skin, with a pair of Babcock forceps (Fig. 5.24). To distinguish between the cuff and the balloon tubes from the control pump, once the pump is in place, the balloon tubing prior to 1989 had a bevelled end (b for bevelled and balloon). More recently the tubing to the balloon from the control pump and also from the ballon itself has been produced with a tight spiral of black thread in its wall (note — b for black and balloon) to make identification easier. The tubing from the control pump to the cuff and of the cuff itself has a clear spiral in it (c for clear and cuff — clever isn't it!). The tubing has also been made kink-proof.

All that remains is to connect the tubes within the inguinal canal (Fig. 5.25) after trimming them to the correct length so that there are no redundant loops that might subsequently kink. Having cut the tubing to the right length, the open ends are flushed with contrast solution so that they are completely filled with fluid. The balloon connections are made using a straight connector, onto each end of which the two appropriate tubes are pushed and secured in place with a 3/0 Prolene tie. Because the two tubes that form the cuff connection both run up into the inguinal canal in the same direction, a straight connector is unsuitable as this would predispose to kinking. A right-angled connector is used, with contrast flushing as before, to exclude any air, and Prolene ties to make the connections secure (Fig. 5.26).

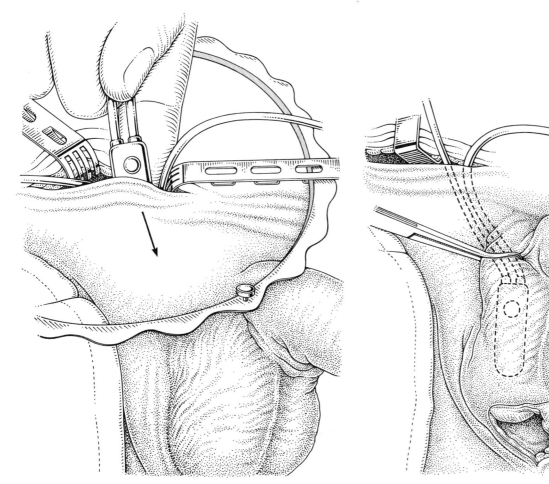

Fig. 5.23

Fig. 5.24

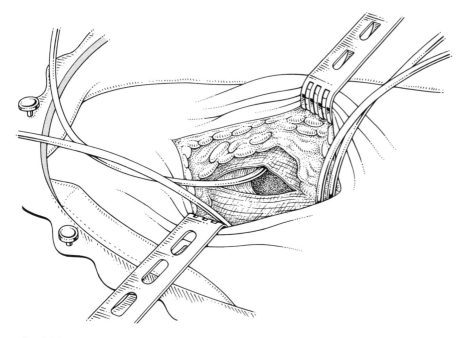

Fig. 5.25

When tying the newer kink-proof tubing on to a connector a stronger tie will be necessary (2/0 Prolene) and extra care must be taken to ensure that a satisfactory connection has been made. kink-proof type, a 'quick-connect' system does not connect naturally to the connectors as well as did the more supple older-style tubing. There is therefore a greater tendency to leak at the connections if the ties are not made tightly enough.

To facilitate connecting the various tubes, particularly of the newer kink-proof type a 'quick-connect' system has recently been introduced by which the connections are made and secured by a purpose-built pair of pliers (Fig. 5.27). This has superseded the previous technique of tie-connection except for revision procedures when the tubing may no longer be sufficiently strong to withstand the rigours of the 'quick-connect' system.

The wound is sprayed with iodine and closed in layers.

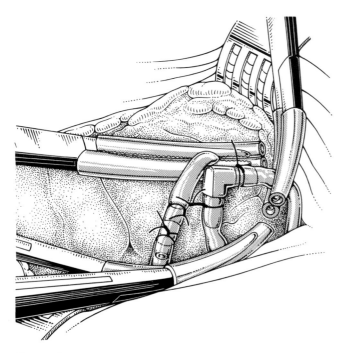

Fig. 5.26

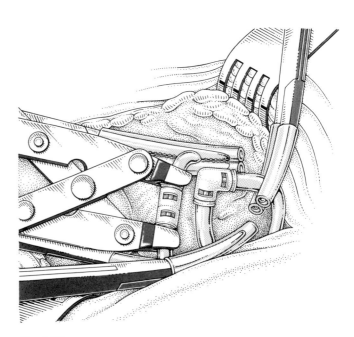

Fig. 5.27

The pump is squeezed to check that the device is working and to note how many squeezes it takes to empty the cuff. With each squeeze the pump empties and refills promptly until the cuff is empty of fluid when the cuff stays flat, refilling only very slowly over the next few minutes. When, having been flat, the pump has just about refilled, the deactivation button on the control block is depressed to deactivate the device.

During the course of the implantation there are four important points to bear constantly in mind. Firstly the various components should only be handled with atraumatic instruments, and the balloon and the inner, thin, inflatable wall of the cuff should never be touched with instruments at all or they may be damaged. Secondly, the tubing should only be occluded with clips that have had the jaws shod with silicone rubber tubing or something similar, again to avoid damage. Likewise only one 'click' of the clip should be used to secure it. Thirdly, when the ends of the tubing are being prepared for connection, blood (and other body fluids) and lint (from swabs) should be kept away because if even tiny amounts get into the device they may interfere with the function of the valves and prevent the device as a whole from functioning. Finally absolute attention should be paid to complete sterility throughout the performance of the procedure.

Postoperative management
The patient should stay in bed for the first 24 hours to reduce the postoperative swelling and discomfort.

The parenteral antibiotic regime that started with the premedication (see Ch. 2) is continued for 3–5 days by which time the patient should be ready to go home, assuming that his temperature is normal and his wounds are healing well. Infection of the device is obviously the main worry and so a normal temperature and satisfactory wound healing are reassuring features.

Occasionally patients develop retention during the first 24 hours postoperatively in which case a fine catheter is passed

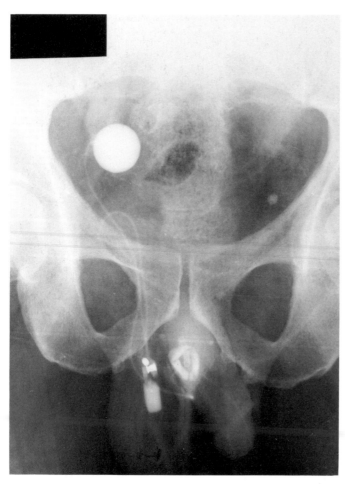

Fig. 5.28

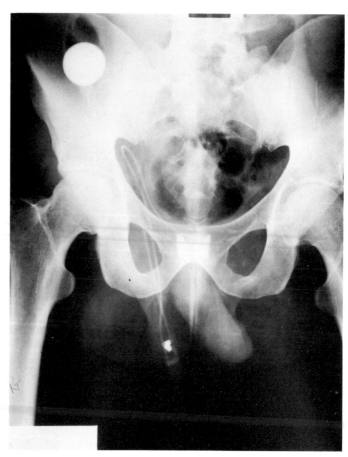

Fig. 5.29

and kept in overnight. It does not occur sufficiently frequently to warrant routine catheterisation.

The timing of activation is debatable. Obviously sufficient time should be allowed for the control pump to be manipulated comfortably. A few weeks additional time thereafter allows the urethra to recover from the trauma of the operation thereby allowing its blood flow to return to its usual level before compression by the cuff is allowed to begin. I feel that this is a more important consideration than getting the patient continent in the shortest possible time and therefore tend to activate my patients 4 weeks after the date of implantation.

Activation is achieved by a firm squeeze of the pump to dislodge the deactivating valve. The patient is then taught how to use the device and kept in hospital for a few hours so that he can use it on at least two occasions to be sure that he is confident with it and that any queries he may have can be answered before he returns home.

Some seemingly very intelligent patients prove to be singularly inept when using an AUS pump for the first time. Very often you just have to get down on your knees in the toilet and do it with them. The four main points to emphasise are: firstly to squeeze the pump as many times as it takes until it no longer refills to ensure that the cuff has been emptied completely; secondly to avoid deactivating the device by pressing the deactivation button on the control pump accidentally; thirdly that if the device doesn't seem to work during these early days then it is probably their inexpertise rather than a malfunctioning of the device (and so is more easily correctable); and finally that if there are any problems at any stage they should telephone or return to see you rather than go somewhere where no-one knows what an AUS is, simply because it happens to be closer to home.

A follow-up plain X-ray to show the device in its entirety is obtained at this time as a baseline for the future, should any problems develop subsequently (Fig. 5.28). For comparison Figure 5.29 shows an AS 800 with a retropubic cuff, Figure 5.30 shows an AS 791 and Figure 5.31 an AS 792.

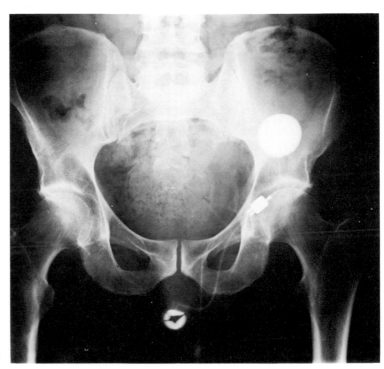

Fig. 5.30

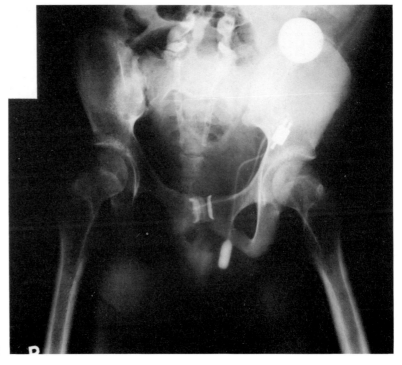

Fig. 5.31

Follow up

The patient is reviewed 3 months after implantation and a video-urodynamic study is arranged to check that the device is working and that the patient is using it properly, to ensure that detrusor behaviour has not changed, and to ensure that bladder emptying is satisfactory.

Complications

The results of treatment of PPI with the AS 800 artificial sphincter are very good, indeed the best results of AUS implantation are in this group of patients. Nonetheless problems do occur from time to time although mainly because of failure to understand the workings and proper use of the device.

It is important that the patient understands that he must squeeze the pump however many times it takes until it does not refill, thereby emptying the cuff completely. Many patients think that they only have to squeeze it once. This is important for two reasons: firstly because although urine will start to flow with the first squeeze the cuff will refill quickly thereafter and this may not allow enough time for bladder emptying; and secondly, in the longer term, because with the passage of time there is often a degree of atrophy of the urethra within the cuff thereby allowing the cuff to hold a larger volume, thereby requiring more squeezes of the pump to empty it. The commonest cause of incomplete bladder emptying, and therefore of frequency and other related symptoms, is failure to squeeze the pump a sufficient number of times to empty the cuff completely, thereby giving insufficient time for complete bladder emptying to occur.

After the first postoperative visit patients are reviewed 6 monthly or if a problem develops. If a problem develops, the plain X-ray and video-urodynamic study are repeated, unless clinical examination reveals an obvious cause. The problems that may develop, other than symptoms related to incomplete emptying as described above, are:

— infection of the device,
— erosion, either internal or external,
— stress incontinence,
— device malfunction,
— symptoms related to abnormal bladder behaviour.

If clinical examination suggests that the device is working normally then it almost certainly is and there will be some other explanation for the patient's problems. Examination may show features of local infection, or that the device has been deactivated accidentally, or that the pump can only be squeezed once and then refills only very slowly in which case there has been a leak of fluid from the system which can be confirmed radiologically. Stress incontinence and abnormal bladder behaviour are apparent from the history and are investigated by video-urodynamics.

When considering the AUS in general terms, rather than in post-prostatectomy incontinence alone, infection and erosion are the most common and much the most serious complications. As the one inevitably leads to the other it is often difficult to know which came first and so in practice they are commonly considered together. Here, for the sake of discussion, they will be considered individually.

Infection of the device. This occurs in about 2% of patients with PPI and rarely occurs except as a result of contamination during implantation. It is therefore usually an early complication, usually manifest by a grumbling fever, by redness, thickening and tenderness of the tissues around the cuff and pump and around the incisions, and by poor function of the device. Although the features may improve with antibiotic treatment, the infection is rarely eradicated completely and it is therefore usually necessary to remove the device and reimplant another one 3–6 months later. If the clinical signs do improve with antibiotic treatment and the problem does not recur, then almost certainly the device itself was not infected.

Occasionally one sees infection as a consequence of untreated urinary tract infection (UTI) complicated by epididymo-orchitis. I have never seen an infection of an AUS in uncomplicated UTI although there is an obvious theoretical risk.

Erosion. This may be due to surgical trauma or to ischaemia of the eroded tissues or to infection of the device and may present as either internal erosion of the cuff through the urethra or external erosion of the control pump or the interconnecting tubing through the skin. Whatever the cause or presentation the entire device rapidly becomes infected if it was not infected already, so the whole thing will almost always have to be removed. Occasionally one is tempted to remove just the eroded component or, if it is the pump or a section of tubing, to reclose the skin over it. This often appears successful for months or even a year or two but inevitably the problem of infection/erosion recurs, the time lag resulting from the low pathogenicity of some contaminating bacteria. Usually when a cutaneous erosion site heals over it is because there has been a second erosion internally so that the infection can decompress itself by discharging into the urinary tract. In these circumstances the apparent benefits of keeping the AUS in for longer are more than offset by the much greater degree of fibrosis and size of erosion that ultimately develop, with obvious implications for implantation of a second device. In any case the function of an eroded device is not usually very satisfactory.

If the urethra was not damaged during implantation of the cuff and infection is not present (which are the commonest reasons for erosion), then urethral erosion is usually a consequence of poor blood flow in the corpus spongiosum secondary to peripheral vascular disease, which is rare. If a second device is subsequently implanted in such a situation, a balloon with a lower pressure range should be used but the patient should realise that erosion may still occur despite the use of such a low pressure.

Stress incontinence. Essentially, the choice of pressure-regulating balloon for patients with PPI is determined by the balance between sufficient pressure to give complete continence on the one hand, and sufficient pressure to cause urethral erosion on the other. The surgeon who routinely uses a 51–60 cmH$_2$O balloon in such patients will have a low incidence of erosion, but a significant incidence of stress incontinence, whereas the surgeon who uses a 61–70 cmH$_2$O balloon will have lower incidence of stress incontinence at the expense of a higher erosion rate. I favour the former statistic and routinely use a 51–60 cmH$_2$O balloon, except in the younger (under 70 years), fitter and more active patient, when a 61–70 cmH$_2$O balloon would be used. This means that 10–15% of patients, with troublesome stress incontinence, will need to have their pressure balloon changed for one with a higher pressure range. This seems to be an acceptable practice in view of the zero erosion rate for bulbar urethral cuffs in my series of patients with PPI since primary deactivation was introduced.

It should be noted that a degree of stress incontinence is likely in all patients. Indeed it is intrinsic in the design of the device that stress incontinence is not compensated for as the valve system of the control pump is specifically designed to slow down filling of the cuff from the balloon to allow adequate time for voiding after the pump has been squeezed whereas rapid transmission would be necessary to compensate in time for surges in intra-abdominal pressure. Thus patients should be warned that a minor degree of stress incontinence is likely and that this does not mean that the device is not working properly. The symptom that patients most commonly complain of is a bit of leakage on standing up from an armchair or getting out of a car.

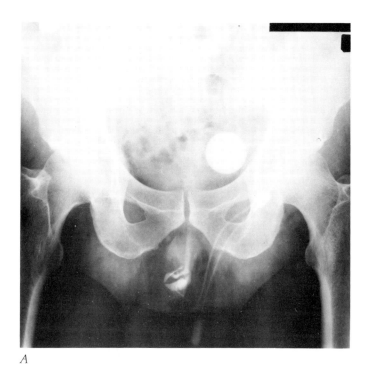

A

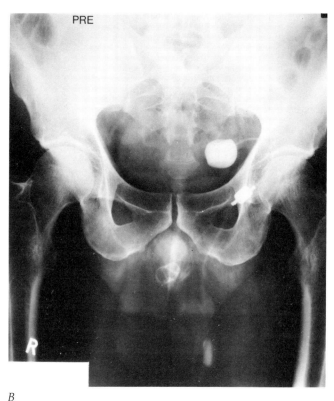

B

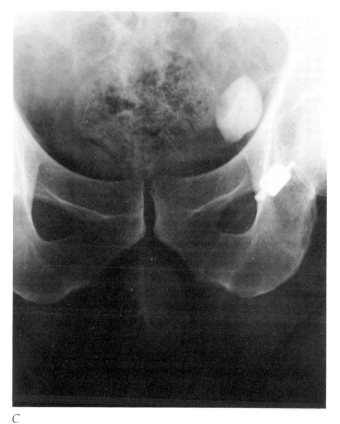

C

Fig. 5.32

Device malfunction. This is rare with currently available components, less than 2% in my experience. The only problem to occur with any regularity, before the method of cuff manufacture was changed to reduce its incidence, was leakage from the seam of the cuff between the inflatable part and its backing, causing a loss of fluid from the system and consequent depressurisation (Fig. 5.32). This is treated by replacing the cuff or, if the device is more than one or two years old, by replacing the whole AUS. These days cuff leaks are less common but they do occur from time to time and are the commonest cause of long-term failure. The usual mechanism, I think, is that creases develop in the cuff (see below) with long-term use and this leads ultimately to perforation.

Leaks may also develop from a connection if this has not been made tightly enough; this particularly occurs when tie connections have been made with modern kink-proof tubing. In this situation, unlike that described in the last paragraph, the leak is a one-way process under the pressure of the system, so the fluid leak is slow, the fluid remains uncontaminated and it never leaks out completely — only until the system is depressurised. Symptoms of loss of function of the device tend to develop within a few weeks or months of implantation and progress only slowly. By contrast, a leak due to a perforation tends to occur much later, progresses rapidly, leads to an almost complete loss of fluid from the system and to contamination of any remaining fluid in the system by yellow-coloured tissue fluid.

The other problems that arise are related to poor technique leading either to instrumental damage of a component during implantation or to kinking of the tubing.

Instrumental damage will inevitably happen from time to time if any of the components of an AUS are handled with instruments. This particularly applies to the balloon and the inner aspect of the cuff. The importance of not over-enthusiastically clamping the tubing and of avoiding contamination of the fluid inside the tubing (whilst making connections) with blood or serum or particles of lint from swabs should also be emphasised.

Kinking of the tubing should no longer occur since the introduction of kink-resistant tubing although it should never occur anyway. Kinks only occur as a result of technical errors — either because lengths of tubing are not kept as short as they should be (Fig. 5.33) or because the position of the control pump is not checked adequately peroperatively so that it is allowed to rotate through 180°. Rotation of the control pump can occur postoperatively (Fig. 5.34) if the patient fiddles with the device before fibrosis and healing have fixed it in position so he should be warned against this. More commonly

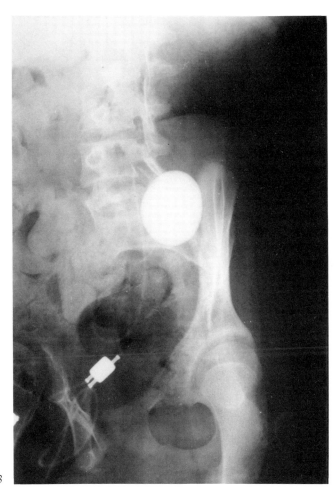

Fig. 5.33

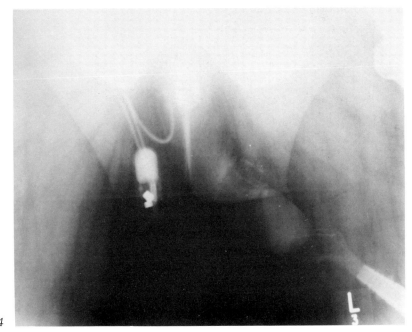

Fig. 5.34

'manipulation' causes the device to ride up the scrotum into the groin, particularly if the tubing was cut too short and the control pump was left a bit too high in the first place.

These points serve to emphasise the importance of attention to detail in the performance of the procedure.

Symptoms relating to abnormal bladder behaviour. For reasons given at the beginning of this chapter and specifically because of the high incidence of associated detrusor instability, this is a relatively common problem in PPI. The patient should be made aware of any urodynamic abnormality as a potential cause of persistent symptoms after implantation of an AUS and should be warned of the possibility even if no abnormality is evident on the preoperative urodynamic study, particularly if he had urge symptoms before his prostatectomy. The reason for this is that detrusor instability seen on the postoperative video-urodynamic study is sometimes not apparent on the pre-implantation study, presumably because it is masked by the sphincteric incompetence.

It is always important to emphasise to the patient that an AUS is only a treatment for sphincter weakness incontinence and nothing more, and that in 60% or more of patients with post-prostatectomy incontinence, sphincter weakness is only a part of their overall urodynamic problem.

PROBLEMS INHERENT IN THE DESIGN OF THE BRANTLEY SCOTT ARTIFICIAL SPHINCTER

The most obvious problem with this device is its cost which, in the UK, is currently £3000 for a complete system (including VAT). This will presumably come down as soon as there is a market competitor.

The problem of persistent stress incontinence (inherent in the design of the device rather than as a result of too low a pressure in the system) has already been mentioned. This is particularly marked in active patients and in patients with obesity or walking difficulties (usually due to osteoarthritis) who therefore have higher than normal intra-abdominal pressures on walking because of the extra effort involved.

A third problem is the relative inability to control the pressure within the system. One never knows whether the pressure in a balloon with a range of 51–60 cmH$_2$O is at the upper, mid or lower part of the range. If, in order to gain better control of incontinence, a 51–60 cmH$_2$O balloon is changed for a 61–70 cmH$_2$O balloon the actual pressure difference after may be as much as 19 cmH$_2$O, which may be sufficient to cause erosion in a compromised urethra, or as little as 1 cmH$_2$O, in which case no benefit is likely to be gained. This problem could be overcome by knowing exactly what pressure each balloon generates at a specific volume or, alternatively, having a pressure-regulating system with a subcutaneous access point in the system with a self-sealing membrane which could be needled for accurate pressure monitoring and adjustment.

Fourthly, it might be possible to reduce the incidence of infection still further if the silicone from which the device is constructed was impregnated with an antibiotic during manufacture.

Finally circumferential pressure, even controlled pressure, is damaging to the enclosed area of the bladder outflow and this situation is made worse because the occlusive force of the cuff is not evenly distributed around its circumference. When inflated the inside of the cuff is not a regular ring but takes up the configuration of three or four cushions. Presumably this configuration gives high pressures at the convexity of the cushions and low pressures between the cushions with a greater propensity for erosion as a result. This configuration also leads to the formation of creases in the cuff wall between the convexities of the cushions that lead in time to perforation. This may be more of a theoretical problem than an actual problem because in real life the cuff is never fully inflated but only partially filled because most of the space within the cuff is taken up by the urethra or bladder neck. Nonetheless it should be relatively easy to manufacture cuffs on a curved template rather than flat as is done at present.

All these difficulties are correctable.

It is perhaps worth noting that even an uninflated cuff exerts some effect, no matter how loosely it is secured. Whether this is due to the cuff itself or to surgical scarring in the area or a combination of factors is not clear, but with high cuff placements, particularly in women, the patient may become continent or develop voiding difficulty or even retention with just the cuff in place, and urethral pressure profiles show a distinct 'pressure zone' in relation to the cuff in all patients. Furthermore pressure profiles show that measured intraurethral pressures (or, with perfusion-type pressure profiles, resistance to flow) bear little relation to the theoretical pressure exerted by the pressure-regulating balloon.

If a cuff is explored (in the absence of infection) a sheath is found around it, and therefore around the urethra, which is lined by a layer of mesothelium — like peritoneum to look at. As the cuff is inflated most of the time the sheath presumably forms in relation to the compressed rather than the uncompressed urethra and is therefore constrictive. Presumably this is how the observed 'pressure zone' develops. This might also explain the observation that changing the pressure-regulating balloon does not make the expected difference, because the sheath must, up to a point, be restrictive to the pressure exerted inwards by the cuff.

REFERENCES

Urological fads seem to go in 2-yearly cycles — currently it is the
Mitrofanoff principle, for the last two years it was detubularisation of
cystoplasties, before that it was the Kock pouch and before that the
artificial sphincter — everyone was doing it! Since the excitement died
down there have been comparatively few publications. The references
given below are to the original publication by Scott, Bradley and Timm
and to three publications from my own unit on selection and results.

Mundy A R 1991 Artificial sphincters. British Journal of Urology 67: in
    press
Mundy A R, Stephenson T P 1984 Selection of patients for implantation
    of the Brantley Scott artificial urinary sphincter. British Journal of
    Urology 56: 717–720
Nurse D E, Mundy A R 1988 One hundred artificial sphincters. British
    Journal of Urology 61: 318–325
Scott F B, Bradley W E, Timm G W 1973 Treatment of urinary
incontinence by an implantable prosthetic sphincter. Urology 1: 252–259

Chapter 6

Sphincter weakness incontinence in women

Table 6.1 Types of sphincter weakness incontinence

1. *Simple* — due to:
   a. loss of urethral support, and
   b. sphincteric incompetence due to partial denervation, in a variable combination usually as a result of childbirth.

2. *Complicated* — by:
   a. urethral disruption as a result of:
      (i) over-enthusiastic urethrotomy
      (ii) excision of a urethral diverticulum
      (iii) inadvertent damage during an anterior repair
      (iv) erosion by a sling;
   b. a 'drainpipe' urethra following multiple previous failed anti-SWI procedures, especially a combination of anterior repairs and retropublic bladder neck suspension procedures;
   c. radiotherapy;
   d. congenital abnormalities:
      (i) epispadias
      (ii) congenitally short urethra
      (iii) idiopathic SWI in childhood
      (iv) bilateral single ectopic ureters (into the urethra)
      (v) following excision of an ectopic ureterocoele.

Sphincter weakness incontinence (SWI) is very common in women, so much so that most women expect to get it to some degree after childbirth. Despite its frequency, its aetiology is poorly understood (Table 6.1) but appears, most commonly, to be related to a loss of support for the urethra and bladder neck combined with incompetence, due to partial denervation, of the distal (urethral) sphincter mechanism, both due to the trauma of childbirth. Whether the associated incompetence of the bladder neck has some similar cause or alternatively is due to a congenital defect is also not known but bladder neck incompetence is a fairly common radiological observation in girls. The commonest manifestation of sphincter weakness is stress incontinence, usually on coughing, laughing or straining or — in severe instances — on running, walking or standing up from a sitting position. Anal sphincteric incompetence is a commonly associated problem but is less commonly symptomatic.

Occasionally one sees SWI following excessive urethral dilatation or over-enthusiastic use of the Otis urethrotome, or in association with a urethral diverticulum or following its surgical excision. Other causes or associations in adults include radical pelvic surgery and radical pelvic radiotherapy.

SWI is sometimes seen in girls and nulliparous women, occasionally due to a congenital abnormality such as epispadias (see Ch. 14) or a congenitally short urethra; sometimes secondary to surgery, as for example following excision of an ectopic ureterocoele involving the bladder neck; or more commonly for no obvious reason. SWI in girls is discussed in Chapter 9.

ASSESSMENT

SWI is so common in women after childbirth that it is easy to overlook other causes of incontinence and proceed to treatment without adequate assessment, sometimes with unfortunate consequences. In theory, in women without any symptoms other than stress incontinence, with demonstrable incontinence on coughing during physical examination, with a normal peak urinary flow rate and flow pattern and complete bladder emptying on an ultrasound study (to exclude an associated voiding dysfunction), and with no history of previous pelvic surgery, no further assessment of bladder and urethral function is necessary. But whenever stress incontinence follows previous surgery, or is associated with other symptoms such as frequency and urgency (as it often is) or voiding difficulty, or occurs in nulliparous women, or is otherwise complicated, then further urodynamic investigation is usually necessary even when overt stress incontinence warrants surgical intervention irrespective of any associated urodynamic abnormality.

In practice, the two important urodynamic considerations, other than to confirm the diagnosis of SWI, are to identify or exclude detrusor instability and voiding dysfunction as they affect adversely the results of surgery. In my experience there is a good negative correlation in premenopausal women between the symptom of urgency and the urodynamic demonstration of detrusor instability — no urgency, no instability — but the positive correlation between the two is poor. In postmenopausal women the correlation, positive and negative, is not nearly so good. Equally, voiding dysfunction is rarely a clinically significant problem associated with SWI in premenopausal women but is commonly so in postmenopausal women. Thus in premenopausal women the theoretical approach to investigation of a patient described above works well in practice but in postmenopausal women a video-urodynamic study is advisable routinely to look for these two associated urodynamic abnormalities. In this way patients with dual urodynamic pathology can be advised not to expect too much from their surgical procedure, particularly when frequency and urgency are the result of coexisting detrusor instability as this, in my experience, can be expected to persist after satisfactory correction of the stress incontinence itself.

In addition to confirming the diagnosis, physical examination (supplemented by urodynamic evaluation when indicated) allows one to determine the degree of urethral mobility and thus, by inference, the degree to which urethral support has been lost. Bearing in mind that this is one of the two main aetiological factors in stress incontinence and that loss of support is easier to correct than sphincter weakness, this has important therapeutic and prognostic implications.

In patients who have had previous surgery to the lower urinary tract, cystourethroscopy is sometimes useful as it may show the presence of more than just simple sphincter weakness, such as the urethral disruption that sometimes follows an excessive urethrotomy, or excision of a urethral diverticulum, or the urethral erosion that sometimes follows sling procedures. Endoscopy is also useful in women with apparently simple SWI who have no apparent loss of urethral support and who therefore presumably have predominantly sphincter weakness. In many such women the urethra will appear normal endoscopically but in some the urethra will appear patulous with little or no visible occlusion anywhere along the length of the urethra but without any surrounding fibrosis (to palpation) that is actually holding the urethra open. This group of patients with a mildly patulous urethra should be identified as a specific group because they may be more suitable for a reduction urethroplasty than for a standard bladder neck suspension.

The other particular problem to look for is the short, rigid, scarred and totally incompetent urethra following multiple previous unsuccessful anti-stress incontinence procedures, particularly combinations of anterior repairs and retropubic anti-incontinence procedures. This type of appearance, commonly known as a 'drainpipe urethra', is also seen following the combination of a Wertheim's hysterectomy and radiotherapy for carcinoma of the cervix. Neither of these two problems responds well to conventional anti-SWI surgery. Even in the absence of a drainpipe urethra, stress incontinence is a common sequel of a hysterectomy and radiotherapy for carcinoma of the cervix and tends to be resistant to standard anti-SWI surgery.

Finally, the presence of any anterior or posterior vaginal wall prolapse should be noted. Stress incontinence and prolapse commonly coexist and persistent prolapse after an otherwise successful anti-incontinence procedure is a regular cause of dissatisfaction, particularly posterior prolapse which is more easily overlooked.

Having differentiated the symptoms of stress incontinence from any other symptoms that the patient might have, and decided that it is of a degree that warrants surgical intervention, and having excluded or identified any associated urodynamic abnormality and discussed its implications with the patient, the next step is to decide which of the many available surgical procedures is most appropriate for that individual.

THE PRINCIPLES OF SURGICAL TREATMENT

The generally accepted aim of surgical treatment for simple SWI is to lift up the bladder neck and support it, thereby stretching and supporting the urethra as well. The results of this, it is thought,

are firstly that pressure transmission to the urethra is improved so that it returns to the normal situation in which it is equal to or greater than pressure transmission to the bladder; secondly that stretching the urethra makes sphincteric activity more effective; and thirdly that supporting the bladder neck and urethra stabilises them and prevents distortion thereby maintaining sphincter function irrespective of position and physical activity. Unfortunately nobody really knows for sure exactly why anti-SWI procedures work, but they do not work by making the incompetent bladder neck competent (a common misconception); they work by allowing the urethral sphincter to work as best it can. In other words, if the distal (urethral) sphincter mechanism is still capable of maintaining continence then stabilising it will cause it to work with maximum efficiency and the patient will usually be cured. If the distal (urethral) mechanism is no longer capable of maintaining continence then stabilising it may help but is significantly less likely to cure the patient.

Hence the importance of distinguishing between two groups of women with simple SWI — those with a hypermobile urethra in whom loss of support can be assumed to be important and those with no excessive mobility and therefore no loss of support in whom loss of urethral sphincter function is more likely to be the dominant aetiological factor. The former group can be expected to do better than the latter group with a standard anti-SWI procedure.

In essence, surgical treatment aims to provide support and stability for the majority of patients with a hypermobile urethra and this generally works well. When there is no excessive mobility and the problem is mainly sphincter weakness then most effective treatments are obstructive either by 'overdoing' a standard supportive procedure or by narrowing the urethra, or by providing a physical obstruction such as an artificial

Table 6.2 Surgery for sphincter weakness incontinence

1. *Simple*
   a. Loss of urethral support (mobile urethra)
      1st line: No significant prolapse —
      Stamey-type procedure
      Significant prolapse — colposuspension
      2nd line: Recurrence (after initial cure and with recurrent urethral mobility) — colposuspension
      persistence (despite adequate urethral fixation) — AUS
   b. Sphincteric incompetence (no abnormal urethral mobility)
      1st line: No patulousness of the urethra endoscopically — Stamey-type procedure
      Patulous urethra — reduction urethroplasty
      2nd line: Persistence or recurrence — AUS

2. *Complicated*
   a. Urethral disruption:
      Minor (i.e. correctable) e.g. post-diverticulectomy — reduction urethroplasty
      Major e.g. sling erosion, trauma — neourethroplasty (Ch. 14)
   b. 'Drainpipe' urethra — AUS
   c. Radiotherapy — Chapter 8
   d. Congenital:
      Structural abnormalities (Ch. 14)
      Functional abnormalities (Ch. 9)

sphincter. Let us start by considering those patients with urethral hypermobility who require support and stabilisation of the urethra.

There are numerous procedures described to achieve this aim, but with one or two exceptions they are all modifications of three basic approaches — the anterior repair, the retropubic bladder neck suspension and the sling procedure. In general it may be said that the anterior repair is the procedure historically favoured by gynaecologists but that the retropubic suspension procedures are much more effective in curing stress incontinence and that the sling procedures are only used if a previous retropubic suspension operation has failed.

In recent years a new(ish) type of procedure has been developed which could be best described as a transvaginal needle suspension of the bladder neck. It is similar in effect to a sling but without an actual sling around the bladder neck. The foremost exponents of this approach are Stamey, and Raz Peyrera although there are other modifications, most of which attempt to turn the procedure into a sort of transvaginal colposuspension.

It should be said that surgeons tend to argue the merits of their own particular favourite anti-SWI procedure with an ardour that approaches passion in its intensity, which can rarely if ever be substantiated by objective evidence. One feels that in most instances they adopt the procedure they feel happiest with first and then justify it afterwards.

My approach to the first-time treatment of 'simple' SWI depends on whether or not there is evidence of loss of urethral support as an important aetiological factor (Table 6.2). In women who have evidence of inadequate urethral support, which is the majority, my preference (or bias) is for a Stamey-type bladder neck suspension when there is no cystocoele or enterocoele requiring simultaneous correction and particularly when the vagina is of reduced capacity or relatively immobile, and for a colposuspension when a cystocoele or enterocoele requires correction at the same time, assuming that the vagina is of good capacity and has a mobile anterior wall.

If there is no evidence of loss of urethral support but the urethra appears to have residual occlusive ability and is not patulous endoscopically I assume that there is some effective residual sphincteric function and advise a Stamey-type procedure to try to enhance it although this is less likely to work than when urethral support has been lost. If the urethra is patulous and non-occlusive endoscopically, which is rare, I assume that there is no effective residual sphincteric function and advise a reduction urethroplasty in an attempt to recreate a zone of urethral resistance that will act as a substitute 'sphincter'.

For 'simple' SWI that has failed to respond to all of these operations, treatment is again based on whether or not there is evidence of loss of urethral support. If there is then I would advise a colposuspension. If there is not — if the urethra is well supported — I would advise implantation of an artificial sphincter (with the proviso described later on). There seems little point in a further 'supportive' operation when the urethra is already surgically supported.

For SWI complicated structually by previous surgery I would be inclined to choose a reduction urethroplasty when urethral incompetence is due to a correctable structural abnormality as, for example, following an over-enthusiastic urethrotomy or a urethral diverticulectomy; or a neourethroplasty for more severe urethral damage; and implantation of an artificial sphincter when a previous adequate anti-SWI procedure has failed due to total urethral functional incompetence, except when due to previous radiotherapy. The treatment of SWI in patients who have had radiotherapy is discussed in Chapter 8.

The treatment of stress incontinence in girls is described in Chapter 9.

The procedures I use most commonly are my own modification of the Stamey procedure and colposuspension in a ratio of about 4:1. Implantation of an artificial sphincter and reduction urethroplasty are much less commonly indicated. I never use slings because they appear to have no theoretical advantage over a

Stamey-type procedure other than by producing obstruction and because the complication of urethral erosion, albeit rare in the expert's hands, is to my mind unacceptable, as it undoubtedly compromises further treatment (see below).

THE MODIFIED 'STAMEY' BLADDER NECK SUSPENSION PROCEDURE

Preoperative preparation
There are no special preoperative preparations other than to ensure that the urine is sterile. Significant blood loss is rare and crossmatching is not therefore necessary.

Position
The patient is placed in the lithotomy position with the legs well apart and the hips slightly flexed. The labia minora are stitched to the skin of the upper thighs to allow a clear view of the meatus and introitus and the patient is draped to allow easy access to the vulva and to the suprapubic area. The perianal region should be excluded as far as possible from the operative field by stitching one of the drapes to the posterior fourchette.

Technique
A 24 F Foley catheter is passed into the bladder and the balloon is inflated to 20 ml. This is sufficient calibre to stretch the urethral wall around it and make the urethra less liable to damage during subsequent stages of the procedure.

A 2 cm horizontal incision is made 0·5−1 cm below the external meatus (Fig. 6.1) and is deepened to separate the urethra and the bladder neck from the anterior vaginal wall (Fig. 6.2). Initially there is a fairly dense fibrous band tethering the distal urethra to the anterior vaginal wall but this becomes progressively thinner as the bladder neck is approached. On either side of the urethra the tissue is easily separated from the anterior vaginal wall. When the bladder neck has been reached (marked with an X in Fig. 6.2), as judged by digital palpation of the junction between the shaft and the balloon of the Foley catheter, the surgeon feels on either side of the bladder neck to ensure that there is enough space on each side for the subsequent placement of the stitches that will hitch up the bladder neck.

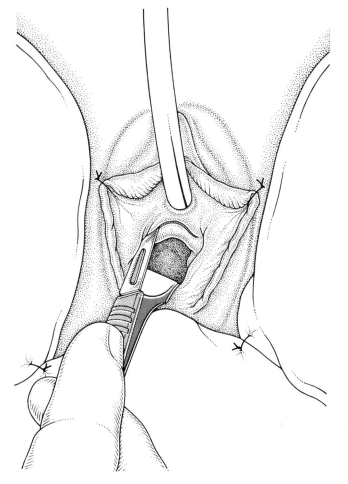

Fig. 6.1

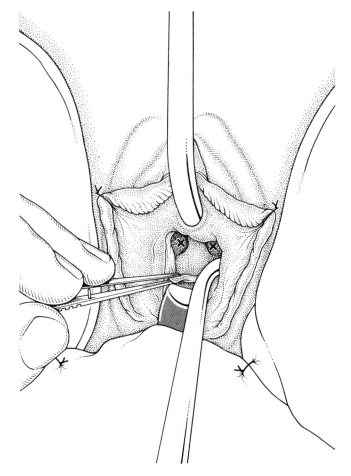

Fig. 6.2

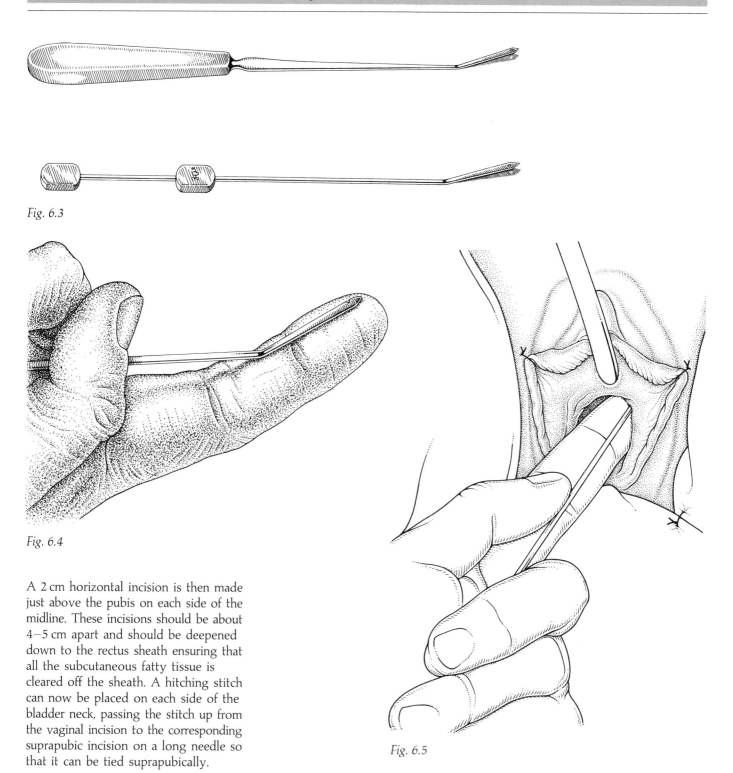

Fig. 6.3

Fig. 6.4

Fig. 6.5

A 2 cm horizontal incision is then made just above the pubis on each side of the midline. These incisions should be about 4–5 cm apart and should be deepened down to the rectus sheath ensuring that all the subcutaneous fatty tissue is cleared off the sheath. A hitching stitch can now be placed on each side of the bladder neck, passing the stitch up from the vaginal incision to the corresponding suprapubic incision on a long needle so that it can be tied suprapubically.

The needle used for this has been specially made with sufficient length to be used in any size of patient and with the end angled upwards to make manipulation easier (Fig. 6.3). The needle is held in the palm of the hand with the shaft along the index finger so that the tip of the needle is at the tip of the finger (Fig. 6.4). Using the finger as a guide (rather like using a Franzen needle for a prostatic biopsy), the tip of the needle is placed at the bladder neck, as close as possible without damaging the wall of either the bladder or the urethra (Fig. 6.5). Traction on the catheter will clearly define the bladder neck as the angle between the shaft and the balloon of the catheter. Keeping the tip of the needle at this point the finger is removed from the incision and the handle of the needle is angled downwards so that the tip can be pushed through the tissues at the side of the bladder neck onto the back of the pubis and then up and over the pubis to emerge at the medial end of the ipsilateral suprapubic incision (Fig. 6.6).

A length of stout nylon is threaded through the eye of the needle and the needle is then withdrawn through the vaginal incision. The nylon is removed from the needle and a 1–1.5 cm length

of 6 mm Dacron tubing, cut from an arterial graft, is slipped over the nylon which is then threaded back onto the needle (Fig. 6.7). The purpose of the Dacron sleeve is to prevent the nylon loop from cutting through the tissue alongside the bladder neck, like a wire through cheese, when the ends of the nylon are subsequently tied. It doesn't really matter what the sleeve is made of—a similar length of silicone tubing would do just as well. I happen to use Dacron because there are a lot of odd bits in my hospital left over by the vascular surgeons.

The needle is then passed back up in the same way from the vaginal to the suprapubic incision but about 2 cm lateral to where it was first passed, to emerge from the lateral end of the suprapubic incision on that side. The nylon is then unthreaded from the eye of the needle which is withdrawn from the vaginal incision leaving the two ends of the nylon emerging from the suprapubic incision and the loop of the nylon at the vaginal incision with a Dacron sleeve over it (Fig. 6.8).

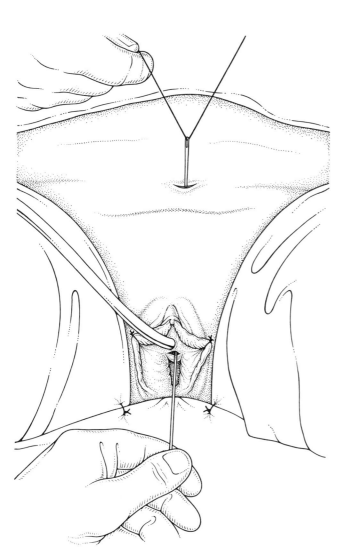

Fig. 6.6

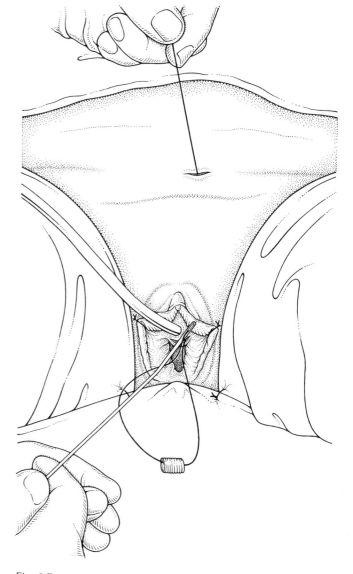

Fig. 6.7

The procedure is then repeated on the other side (Fig. 6.9) so that there is a 'sleeved loop' of nylon accurately placed on either side of the bladder neck with the ends of each emerging from the two suprapubic incisions.

A cystoscope is then passed to ensure that the bladder and urethra have not been perforated by the passage of the needle and also to check that a gentle upward pull of each nylon sling-stitch will cause elevation precisely at the bladder neck.

Before tying the nylon on each side, the vaginal incision is closed with two or three absorbable sutures. If this is delayed until after the nylon sling-stitches have been tied, the elevation that this causes and the consequent retraction of the incision into the vagina makes closure of the incision much more difficult.

The nylon threads are then tied on each side so that the knots lie snugly against the rectus sheath in the depths of the suprapubic incisions. As with the vaginal end, the nylon at the suprapubic end is sleeved with a short length of Dacron tubing to prevent a 'cheese-wire' effect that might cause troublesome postoperative pain. The problem is to know how tightly to tie the knots; in general this is much looser than one might expect. As discussed earlier, the aim of the operation is to support and stabilise the urethra, not to obstruct it. It is easy to show how little tension is necessary by filling the bladder and then producing emptying by suprapubic pressure. Gentle upward traction of the

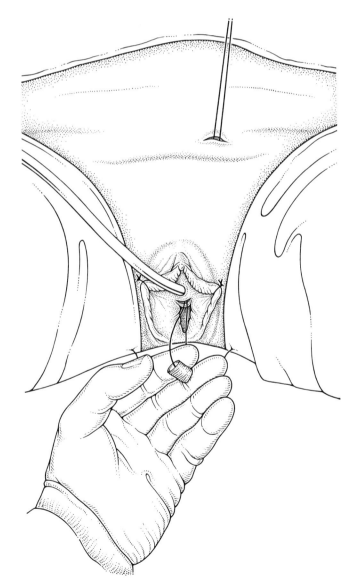

Fig. 6.8

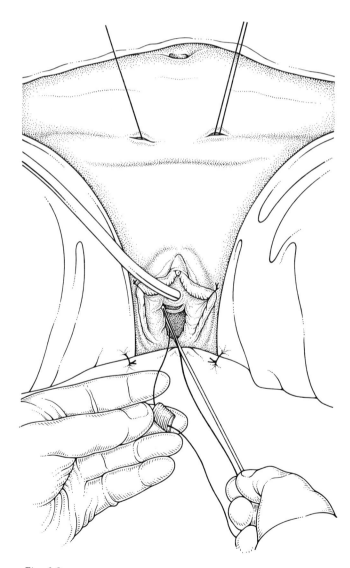

Fig. 6.9

nylon threads together to a degree just sufficient to stop the flow will show the right amount of tension with which the knots should be tied. There is no point in tying them much tighter — either obstruction will result or the stitches will simply cut through the intervening tissue. The suprapubic stab wounds are then closed with one or two interrupted absorbable mattress sutures on each side.

Percutaneous suprapubic catheterisation with a catheter of about 12 F gauge completes the procedure (Fig. 6.10).

If the patient has had one or more previous anterior repairs there is often a lot of scarring between the urethra and the antrior vaginal wall. In such circumstances it is a good idea to interpose a labial fat pad between the two before closing the wounds to prevent this recurring.

Mobilisation of a labial fat pad (Martius procedure). Within the labium majus there is a pad of fat that lies within a thin but definite sheath and receives a blood supply that enters its posterolateral margin from the perineal branch of the pudendal vessels. The vascular supply runs in at the level of the posterior fourchette and the fat pad runs up to the level of the external inguinal ring so it is about 10–12 cm long. The labial fat pad can therefore be used to cover a defect within this sort of radius from the posterior fourchette.

To find it, an incision is made along the length of the labium majus (Fig. 6.11 — N.B. in Figs 6.11 to 6.14 the patient has had a urethral reconstruction as well) through skin and superficial subcutaneous tissue alone, ensuring that the incision extends right up to the external ring to get the maximum possible length of fat pad. The incision is deepened carefully until the plane is

reached between the typically lobulated subcutaneous fat and the flimsy sheath enclosing the fat pad (Fig. 6.12). When the full length of the superficial aspect of the pad has been exposed it is then mobilised by dividing the thin fibrous band that tethers the deep aspect of the sheath to the body and inferior ramus of the pubis. To avoid damage to the fat pad it is best to mobilise it at its upper end first, where it is thinner, and then to work downwards. When it has been mobilised along its length (Fig. 6.13), avoiding the posterolateral aspect where the blood supply enters, it is tunnelled through to the vaginal incision between the inferior pubic arch and the vagina to its desired location (Fig. 6.14) between the urethra and the vagina. The very nature of the fat pad makes it easily damaged so care must be taken during the tunnelling procedure. If one fat pad alone is a little flimsy or if its presence is crucial (for example, if the patient may subsequently require an artificial sphincter in which case the pad acts both to create a plane between the urethra and vagina and to support and help vascularise the urethra) then both fat pads should be mobilised.

Postoperative management

The suprapubic catheter is left on free drainage for about 5 days when it is clamped to allow spontaneous voiding. In most patients this will occur, albeit with varying degrees of residual urine. The voided volume and the residual urine volume are recorded on each occasion until the voided volume is satisfactory and the residual volume is less than about 50 ml, at which time the suprapubic catheter is removed.

If a patient cannot void at all after 2 or 3 attempts at clamping the catheter I send her home with her catheter on either free drainage or 'clamp and release' (I don't think it matters) and bring her back a week later for a further attempt and again a week later if that is also unsuccessful. All patients should be voiding satisfactorily by 3 weeks.

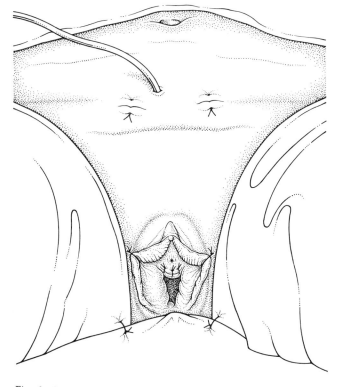

Fig. 6.10

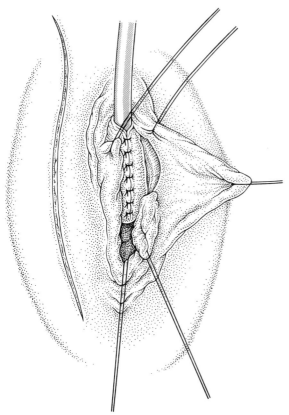

Fig. 6.11

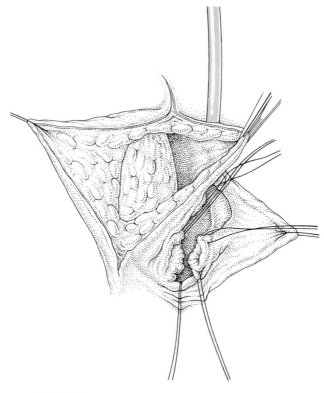

Fig. 6.12

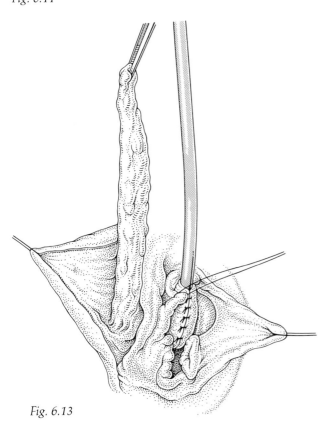

Fig. 6.13

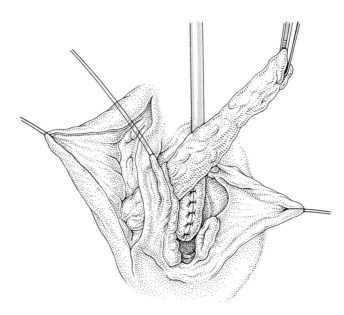

Fig. 6.14

The procedure is such a minor one that some patients are well enough to go home on the first or second postoperative day with their catheters still in. Otherwise they are managed in essentially the same way.

Patients are reviewed at 3 months for evaluation of the result of their operation and this is best assessed by repeating the definitive preoperative investigation, whether this was coughing during physical examination or a video-urodynamic study. In patients with persistent symptoms the VUD study is best deferred for a further 3 months to allow adequate time for a spontaneous improvement later.

There seems little point in following up a patient with a satisfactory result any further beyond reassuring her that she can always come back should problems develop.

Complications
The four main postoperative problems after this procedure are:

— persistent or recurrent stress incontinence,
— persistent frequency and urgency,
— infection of the Dacron buffers in the suprapubic wounds,
— voiding dysfunction due to relative outflow obstruction.

Stress incontinence. Persistent stress incontinence, despite evidence that the urethra has been well supported, is usually associated with a severe degree of sphincteric incompetence as sometimes occurs in uncomplicated SWI but is more commonly seen in 'congenital' sphincter weakness or in the 'drainpipe' urethra (or in neuropathy — but this complication should have been excluded by preoperative examination). In such circumstances implantation of an artificial sphincter may be the only reliable way of eliminating the problem. Implantation of a prosthesis is obviously undesirable

if it can be avoided because of its various inherent problems but equally the complication rate of prosthetic surgery is increased in proportion to the number of previous surgical attempts. It is best therefore to consider it early rather than later if the urethra is relatively immobile and severe sphincteric incompetence is thus the dominant abnormality. In practice I feel that colposuspension is still the 'gold standard' of operations and I tend to advise a colposuspension if a Stamey-type procedure fails to cure simple stress incontinence and reserve the AUS for failures of colposuspension and for the more complicated types of SWI as described below.

Recurrent (rather than persistent) stress incontinence seems to occur rather more commonly after this procedure (c. 11%) than after a colposuspension type of procedure (c. 5%), presumably because it relies far more heavily on the suture material than on surgical scarring to maintain the stabilisation of the bladder neck and urethra. If the stress incontinence was successfully treated for a significant period (years) but recurs, the procedure could be repeated and I have done this, but it is usually better to go on to a colposuspension.

Persistent frequency and urgency. Patients should always be warned before their operation that any preoperative frequency and urgency may persist afterwards, as it does in about 50%. If detrusor instability was present on the preoperative urodynamic study this will almost invariably persist in my experience although other surgeons would not agree with me.

More worrying is the occasional occurrence de novo of detrusor instability after the operation which seems to be more common than after a colposuspension. Interestingly it rarely, if ever, develops in patients who did not have frequency and urgency preoperatively, but only in those who

did, even if they were urodynamically stable at that time. This suggests to me that the instability may in fact have always been present but was previously masked on urodynamic testing by the SWI.

Infection of the Dacron sleeves. When this occurs it almost always affects one of the sleeves in the suprapubic wounds, presenting as a painful red wound, progressing to a chronically discharging sinus. It is treated by removing the sleeve, leaving the nylon stitch intact. In this way any improvement in continence as a result of the procedure can be maintained. The nylon never causes problems — it's always the sleeve. Strangely, infection of the sleeves alongside the bladder neck occurs only rarely.

Voiding dysfunction. This usually presents either as recurrent urinary tract infection or, more commonly, as voiding difficulty and frequency, due to incomplete emptying. Voiding dysfunction is common during the first 3–6 months after operation and can be expected to improve in the majority. In those patients in whom it persists it is often improved by urethral recalibration, if the bladder is contractile. This may not help patients with poorly contractile or acontractile bladders who void by straining. In these patients removal of one of the nylon stitches is often helpful and rarely leads to recurrent stress incontinence. An alternative is to use clean intermittent self catheterisation but this is rarely required in patients who had simple SWI.

The usual cause of voiding dysfunction is outflow obstruction due to tying the stitches too tightly. This is common when one has relatively little experience with the procedure and occurs less frequently when one realises how little tension is required in the stitches to produce the desired effect.

COLPOSUSPENSION

Preparation

The patient is admitted to hospital the day before the operation. Blood transfusion is rarely necessary but cross matching is a wise precaution as bleeding from the pelvic veins is sometimes a problem.

Position

The operation is performed with the patient in the low lithotomy position (Fig. 6.15) with the skin prepared and the drapes placed for a Pfannenstiel or similar incision. A urethral Foley catheter is passed to help identify the urethra and bladder neck. A TUR-Steridrape is useful to allow the necessary peroperative vaginal manipulation without direct contact and therefore with a lower risk of contamination of the operative field.

Technique

If there has been no previous retropubic surgery, a Pfannenstiel incision is used. If there has, a Cherney incision, as described in Chapter 3, is preferred. Having made the incision the retropubic space is widely opened to expose the bladder, urethra, pubourethral ligaments and endopelvic fascia of the pelvic floor all the way round both lateral aspects of the bladder (Fig. 6.16). A ring retractor is then placed to hold the incision open.

The aim of the procedure is to place 3 or 4 stitches on either side of the bladder neck and base that will hitch the anterior vaginal wall on either side to wherever it will comfortably reach on the anterolateral side wall of the pelvis. Ideally this should be to the pectineal ligaments, as these are the strongest structures, so sutures through these are unlikely to cut out; but it is important that the sutures are not under tension, otherwise they will cut out anyway. The two other important points are that there should be direct contact between the vaginal wall and whatever it is sutured to in order to give the best

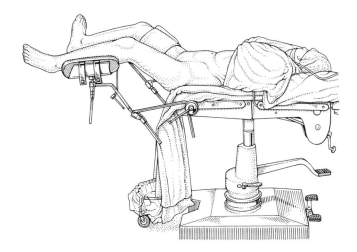

Fig. 6.15

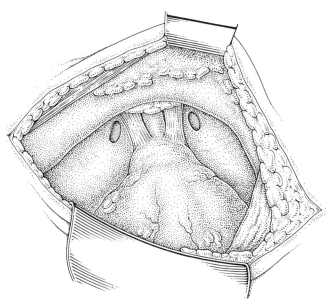

Fig. 6.16

chance of a durable hitch, and that there is no angulation and obstruction of the urethra.

Some surgeons state that for colposuspension to be successful the vaginal wall must reach up to the pectineal ligament on each side and that they can always achieve this without tension. They further claim that it is possible to predict this accurately on preoperative assessment and that

colposuspension is contraindicated if the preoperative assessment suggests that this is not going to be possible. In such cases they would use some alternative procedure. Whereas I would agree that an adequate vaginal capacity and mobility are necessary for a successful outcome following colposuspension, I would strongly disagree that such a degree of elevation is routinely possible, predictable or even desirable.

To assess where to place these sutures the margins of the urethra, bladder neck and bladder base on each side are first defined. This is often made easier by the presence of a Foley catheter to make the urethra and bladder neck more obvious to palpation, but a catheter is not essential. Having defined the margins the bladder base is dissected medially for 0.5 cm or thereabouts by pushing it with a pledget swab against the counter pressure of a finger in the vagina (Fig. 6.17). This has the double effect of defining the bladder margin more clearly and of disrupting the endopelvic fascia so that the anterior vaginal wall can be pushed through. The anterior vaginal wall can then be elevated by a finger in the vagina to see where it reaches comfortably (Fig. 6.18). This shows the surgeon where to place the sutures on the pelvic side wall which may be through the pectineal ligament but may be and often is lower, through the obturator fascia.

The first suture is placed through the vaginal wall just below the level of the bladder neck, the second at the level of the bladder neck and the third and fourth (if possible) along the margin of the bladder base at 1 cm intervals. Each bite of the needle picks up the full thickness of the vaginal wall muscle, but not the mucosa, and to ensure that the bite is at the correct depth the surgeon takes each bite with the index finger of his other hand in the vagina, so that the needle is palpable as it passes through the vaginal wall. The choice of suture material is a matter of individual preference—I use 2/0 PDS but 0 Dexon, nylon or linen are popular alternatives and probably just as good. Each suture is clipped until all the sutures on both sides have been placed. If placing a suture causes bleeding from the vaginal wall that does not stop with gentle upward traction on the suture then the suture is tied to control the bleeding.

When all the sutures on both sides have been placed, the clips holding them are used to pull the anterior vaginal wall on each side out to the side wall of the pelvis. Each stitch in turn is then unclipped and a bite is taken of the pelvic side wall tissue against which the anterior vaginal wall abuts, whether it is pectineal ligament (Fig. 6.19) or obturator fascia. The sutures are then tied.

When all the sutures have been tied (Fig. 6.20), the procedure is complete unless the patient has a degree of posterior vaginal wall prolapse in which case the Pouch of Douglas is obliterated by 2 or 3 purse string sutures, picking up the peritoneum around its margins, starting in the depths of the pouch and working upwards at 2 cm intervals.

Finally a 12 F (or thereabouts) suprapubic catheter and a retropubic tube wound drain are placed and the wound is closed in the usual way.

Postoperative management
Postoperative management is usually straightforward as most patients recover quickly after the procedure. Although some start voiding urethrally within 2 or 3 days, despite having the suprapubic catheter on free drainage, there seems no point in seeking to re-establish spontaneous voiding routinely at this time as most patients will stay in hospital for a week or so in any case.

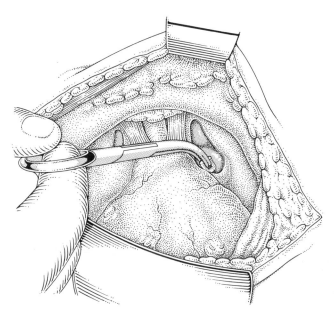

Fig. 6.17

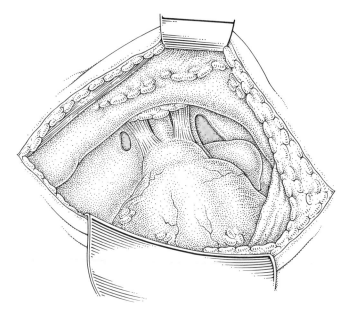

Fig. 6.18

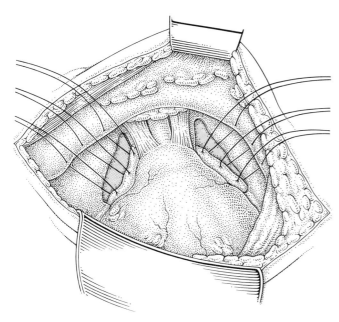

Fig. 6.19

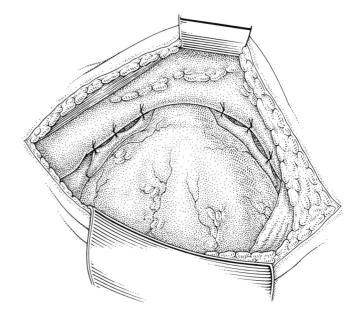

Fig. 6.20

My practice is to clamp the suprapubic catheter on the fifth postoperative day, warning the patient that voiding difficulty sometimes occurs so that she will not be unduly alarmed if it does. The residual urine volume is measured after voiding on 2 or 3 occasions during the 24-hour period of clamping and if the residual urine is less than 50 ml or thereabouts the catheter is removed. With higher residual urine volumes, the suprapubic catheter is retained until voiding efficiency improves.

Dyspareunia is common for the first 2–3 months after colposuspension and patients should be warned of this, but this is unlikely to deter the true enthusiast. They will not come to any harm. Heavy lifting should, however, be avoided and smokers should be warned that coughing may prejudice a satisfactory outcome.

Patients are reviewed at 3 months for evaluation of the result of their operation and this is best assessed by repeating the definitive preoperative investigation, whether this was coughing during physical examination or a video-urodynamic study. In patients with persistent symptoms the VUD study is best deferred for a further 3 months to allow adequate time for a spontaneous improvement later.

There seems little point in following up a patient with a satisfactory result any further beyond reassuring her that she can always come back should problems develop.

Complications
The commonest postoperative problem overall is persistent frequency and urgency, whether or not they were due to instability, and this is the most regular cause of a dissatisfied patient. Hence the importance of ensuring that stress incontinence was the main problem as far as the patient was concerned before operating and of ensuring that she understood that the frequency and urgency might, indeed probably would, persist. Dyspareunia and persistent prolapse as other causes of postoperative dissatisfaction have already been mentioned. Voiding difficulty is usually only temporary; it may persist but rarely to the extent that CISC is required. If troublesome, urethral recalibration usually helps unless the detrusor is no longer capable of effective contraction, in which case CISC is the only option.

Persistent SWI may be due to failed surgery, in which case the urethra will still be mobile (presumably because the stitches cut out in the early postoperative period), or to sphincteric incompetence as the predominant aetiological factor if the urethra has been adequately stabilised. If the stitches have cut out the procedure can be repeated or a Stamey-type procedure can be used as a lesser alternative. If severe sphincteric incompetence is the problem the patient should be considered for implantation of an artificial sphincter.

At 5 years of follow up there is a small but very definite recurrence rate. Patients with recurrence are best treated by a repeat procedure unless there have been multiple previous procedures, in which case they should be considered for implantation of an artificial sphincter.

REDUCTION URETHROPLASTY

I use this for severe urethral sphincteric incompetence due to a structural (anatomical) abnormality of the urethra, although some surgeons use it more routinely for simple SWI. Severe urethral sphincteric incompetence is uncommon in simple SWI; indeed it is uncommon without an associated 'drainpipe' urethra except in women with spinal cord lesions such as spinal cord injury and severe multiple sclerosis in whom the urethra is usually grossly patulous. The other exception is following the over-enthusiastic use of the Otis urethrotome to correct voiding difficulty, using the blade in the posterior midline, in which case disruption of the urethra is seen endoscopically with urothelial healing bridging the gap between the separated urethral margins. The same result sometimes follows excision of a urethral diverticulum. These instances aside there is a group of patients with simple SWI due to urethral sphincteric incompetence in whom there is a minor but definite degree of patulousness of the urethra both radiologically and (particularly) endoscopically. It is for this group that reduction urethroplasty is particularly indicated and the results are acceptably good. This group tends to be older than average with anal sphincter weakness as well, although many patients are embarrassed to volunteer the information unless asked directly.

In patients with a patulous urethra due to neurological disease the patulousness is very much more severe than in the latter group. The results of reduction urethroplasty are not very good, firstly because the neurological disease also affects the bladder, causing problems in its own right, and secondly because the patulousness tends to recur after a year or two even if the result was initially satisfactory. Nonetheless as the alternatives are equally fraught with problems reduction urethroplasty may be a useful way of gaining some improvement.

Whether the urethra is grossly patulous due to neurological disease or of relatively normal calibre, with or without disruption, the principle of reduction urethroplasty is the same and that is to reconstruct the urethra around a small calibre Foley urethral catheter.

Preparation and position

No special preoperative preparation is required. The patient is positioned and draped as for any other type of vaginal surgery, and a large calibre Foley catheter of 24 F or thereabouts is passed into the bladder to define the urethra during the initial stages of the dissection.

Technique

A transverse incision, 2–3 cm long, is made halfway between the external meatus and the introitus and this incision is then deepened to separate the urethra from the anterior vaginal wall up to the level of the bladder neck (as described above for the Stamey-type procedure).

If the urethra is simply patulous then the catheter is removed and replaced with another of 12 F calibre and the urethra is then constricted around the catheter by a series of plicating 3/0 Vicryl sutures along its length (Fig. 6.21).

If the urethra has been disrupted by a previous urethrotomy or diverticulectomy, or is grossly patulous (as in neuropathy) then it will need to be formally reconstructed. A previously disrupted urethra is repaired, having cleanly defined the edges of the urethra, with interrupted 3/0 Vicryl sutures around a 12 F Foley catheter. With a grossly patulous urethra a strip of the posterior urethral wall is excised such that the remaining urethra can be closed in 2 layers around a 12 F Foley catheter (Fig. 6.22). A two-layer inverting closure means that the remaining urethra will need to be slightly less than 2 cm wide, no more, after excision of the strip.

After a reduction urethroplasty the repair should be supported with a labial fat pad (Martius graft). This serves the further purpose of providing a plane of cleavage should the patient have persistent or recurrent stress incontinence requiring implantation of an artificial sphincter.

Postoperative management and complications

Patients having a simple plication with no breaching of the urethral lumen can be managed with just a urethral catheter for about 5–7 days. Those having the more extensive urethral reconstructive procedure are more safely managed with both a urethral and a suprapubic catheter, removing the urethral catheter after about 14 days and then clamping the suprapubic catheter to allow a trial of voiding.

The results of plication of a patulous urethra of a relatively minor degree and of reconstruction of an endoscopically overt urethral defect are acceptably good given the nature of the problem but 20–25% will require further surgery for residual stress incontinence. The results of plication or reconstruction for more severe degrees of patulousness are much less satisfactory as the patulousness tends to recur.

Persistent or recurrent stress incontinence is best treated by implantation of an AUS although a case could be made for a colposuspension if the vagina is of good capacity as it often is in younger patients. If an AUS is implanted great care should be taken to place the cuff around both the urethra and the juxtaposed labial fat pad(s) to keep the cuff away from the reduction urethroplasty suture line and to maintain its vascularity.

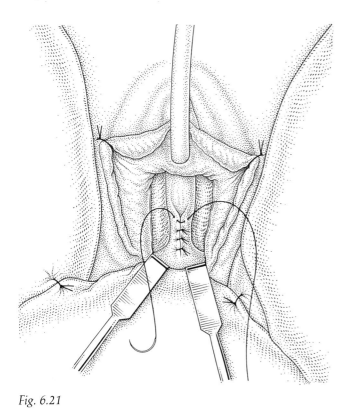

Fig. 6.21

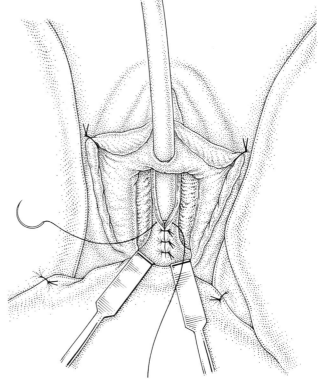

Fig. 6.22

THE ARTIFICIAL SPHINCTER (see also Ch. 5)

The artificial sphincter (AUS) is a treatment for non-neuropathic sphincter weakness incontinence in women when all else has failed — that is generally agreed. The problem is that, theoretically at least, the more surgery there has been around the urethra the more difficult it is to implant an AUS and the more likely there are to be postoperative complications, particularly erosion. A second problem is that it is difficult to know whether, in any individual patient, previous operations have failed to help because the patient was not responsive or because the procedure was performed inadequately. It is difficult therefore to know when to try another standard procedure or to proceed to implantation of an AUS. A more accurate re-statement of the first statement of this paragraph would therefore be that an AUS is a treatment for SWI in women when all else has failed *or is likely to fail.*

The most important first step is to confirm that the patient has stress incontinence rather than just take her word or that of the referring physician, for it. The next step is to show by urodynamic investigation that the bladder is normal and particularly to exclude coexisting detrusor instability. Thirdly an endoscopic assessment with an examination under anaesthetic is performed to look for patulousness or other more severe structural problems and to feel for extensive periurethral fibrosis. Less common but equally important are features of infection around any previously implanted materials such as slings, injected Teflon (horrible stuff — never use it!) or Dacron buffers (used in a Stamey-type procedure) and endoscopic signs of false passages or diverticula or anything else that might make the urethra more than usually prone to peroperative damage or postoperative erosion.

On the basis of these investigations it is possible to select groups of patients for whom AUS is the only feasible type of treatment — for example, those with a 'drainpipe' urethra, those with a totally non-functioning urethra, those with extensive periurethral fibrosis and those with a well hitched-up anterior vaginal wall suggesting that previous surgery was adequately performed. These patients can be offered an AUS.

On the other hand there are those patients with marked urethral and anterior vaginal wall mobility despite previous surgery in whom surgery has obviously been inadequate and those, on the other hand, with features of pelvic sepsis who need to have this eradicated before any further consideration of their stress incontinence; such patients are not suitable for an AUS, at least not in the first instance.

Equally there are two other groups of patients in whom an AUS is actively contraindicated: those who have suffered urethral or bladder neck erosion as a result of a previous sling procedure and those who have had a radical course of radiotherapy to the pelvis. Experience has shown that in these two groups erosion of the AUS cuff is almost inevitable although, when no other option is available, this risk can be reduced by wrapping the urethra with omentum before implanting the cuff (see below). As a general rule, however, an AUS should be avoided if at all possible.

In between are a group of patients in whom a final decision is impossible until the pelvis has been assessed at operation. These patients are offered retropubic surgery which may or may not lead to an AUS. If, at operation, fibrosis is restricted to the anterior bladder wall and bladder neck and the tissues around the urethra are 'virgin territory' (a common finding in such situations, indicating that previous retropubic surgery was inadequate) then a standard colposuspension type of procedure is performed, preceded by a complete division of all adhesions and followed by an omental interposition between the bladder neck and urethra and the pubis. If, on the other hand, fibrosis extends down the front and sides of the urethra, indicating that this area has been fully mobilised and adequately 'hitched' in the past, then an AUS is implanted. If there is any doubt I perform a colposuspension and implant an AUS cuff as well, leaving the cuff tubing plugged off in the inguinal canal for subsequent use if necessary.

Preoperative preparation
The patient is admitted to hospital 4 days before her operation for a full bowel preparation as described in Chapter 2. Given that the main serious complications of the AUS are infection and erosion and that some erosions are due to infection, it is impossible to overstate the importance of doing everything possible to reduce the risk of peroperative contamination. Although

this type of preparation may seem to be overkill it is difficult to know which part or parts of it are important, particularly as the only way the importance of an individual factor can be assessed is by discontinuing it and seeing if a serious complication develops.

Positioning
Positioning is as for a colposuspension. Particular importance is attached to the use of a TUR-Steridrape to allow vaginal manipulation without contamination. A 24 F Foley urethral catheter is passed to help identify the urethra peroperatively.

Incision
Other than in the placement of the cuff the technique of implantation of an AUS is the same as described in Chapter 5. The reader is referred to Chapter 5 for a description of the other more general considerations in AUS implantation.

I prefer a Cherney incision (Ch. 3) because the patient has usually had one or more Pfannenstiel incisions in the past, although reopening a Pfannenstiel incision would suffice in many instances. The retropubic space is widely opened to expose the bladder, bladder neck and the urethra down to the pelvic floor, and the endopelvic fascia and the pubourethral ligaments that constitute the latter (Fig. 6.16). This often requires a tedious, time-consuming division of adhesions and to avoid damaging the bladder or urethra the surgeon should keep as close as possible to the posterior aspect of the pubis but should be careful more laterally to avoid delving too deeply into the obturator fossae.

Discussion with other AUS implanters suggests that most of them implant around the bladder neck: unfortunately this is the area that has been most heavily traumatised by previous surgery, particularly if the patient has also had a hysterectomy causing posterior scarring as well. Dissection often causes bleeding from branches of the inferior vesical

vessels as well as from the para-vaginal veins, and there is a risk of damage to the ureters. My practice is to avoid this area above the pelvic floor and to place the cuff around the urethra after division of the pubourethral ligaments and adjacent endopelvic fascia, thereby exposing relatively normal tissue (at least on the lateral aspects of the urethra) before beginning the rather anxious task of creating a plane between the urethra and the anterior vaginal wall.

To avoid damage to the underlying vaginal veins, it is important to divide the pubourethral ligaments and the endopelvic fascia close to the pelvic side wall. In most patients there is a natural hiatus just behind the ligament on each side at which point incision of these structures can start. The incision on each side needs to be about 5 cm long to allow a clear view of the urethra, instrumental manipulation and digital palpation (Fig. 6.23). In many respects this is the same as in the early stages of a colposuspension when the endothelial fascia is disrupted to push the anterior vaginal wall through. The only difference is that for AUS implantation one is generally being more gentle and precise.

Having made the incision, the urethra can be seen in its upper part close to the bladder neck but the lower half to two thirds is covered by a triangular fascial layer with its apex superiorly which tethers the urethra to the anterior vaginal wall. Sometimes this will need to be divided along the line of the urethral axis to create a sufficient space to work between the urethra and the anterior vaginal wall to create a plane for the cuff. When starting to develop this plane I use blunt dissection, initially at least, and find it helpful to work with a finger in the vagina to feel the thickness (or more usually thinness!) of the vaginal wall as this is the best guide to the correctness or otherwise of the plane of dissection.

In most instances it is fairly easy to open up a plane between the urethra and vagina on each side as far as the midline (Fig. 6.24). In the midline there is normally adhesion between the two, particularly after a previous anterior repair. It sometimes takes a bit of perseverance to work through this by blunt dissection but one should try to resist the urge to use sharp dissection at this stage for fear of damaging either structure. If problems are encountered palpation of the bladder neck by a finger in the bladder often helps. There are two main types of problem encountered at this stage. Firstly there may be a resistance midline band of fibrosis. This can be divided with scissors taking care to lift the urethra off the vagina as far as possible with a Babcock forceps, and taking care to palpate vaginally while doing so to be sure that the vagina has not been tented upwards. Secondly there may be difficulty getting into this plane at all because of extensive previous surgery, particularly when foreign material such as Teflon or Dacron has been implanted. In such instances, when it is particularly difficult to find the right plane from the lateral aspect of the urethra, it may be helpful to open the peritoneum and then to develop from above the plane between the bladder base, bladder neck and upper urethra anteriorly, the vagina posteriorly and the lateral pedicles of the bladder on either side. When this plane has been opened up, down as far as the bladder neck and therefore below the level of the ureters, it will be possible to dissect from the midline laterally under the ureter and out into the retropubic space on each side with relative safety (Fig. 6.25).

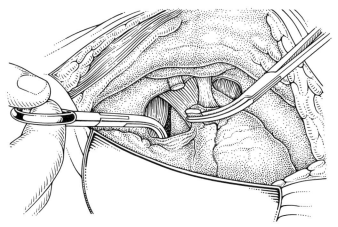

Fig. 6.23
The clip is on the proximal end of the left pubourethral ligament.

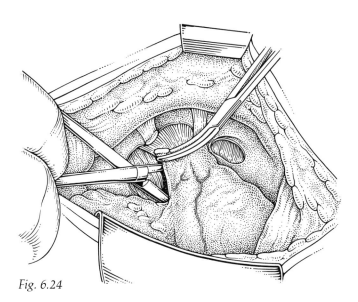

Fig. 6.24

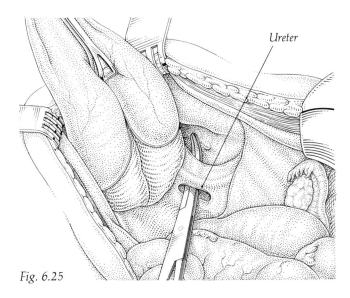

Ureter

Fig. 6.25

Having passed a pair of curved dissecting forceps through from one side to the other (Fig. 6.26) a sling is passed so that further instrumentation is possible with minimal risk of further damage. The vertical extent of the space between the urethra and vagina needs to be at least 2 cm because this is the width of the AUS cuff, so this must be carefully dissected. The manufacturers of the AUS produce a measuring tape (or 'sizer') which not only measures the circumference of the urethra, in order to choose the right size of cuff, but also is of same width as the cuff to ensure that an adequate space has been created (Fig. 6.27).

A cuff is then chosen that will fit snugly but not tightly around the urethra with the 24 F catheter still inside to be sure that there will be enough room for urine to get out during voiding (Fig. 6.28).

The cuff is prepared as described in Chapter 5, so that all the air in it is displaced by isotonic radiopaque contrast solution.

A pressure-regulation balloon with a 51–60 or 61–70 cmH$_2$O pressure range — depending on how difficult cuff implantation was — is similarly prepared and implanted in an extraperitoneal site, either in the right iliac fossa or on the right side of the bladder in the retropubic space.

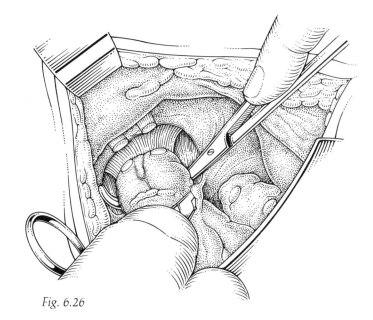

Fig. 6.26

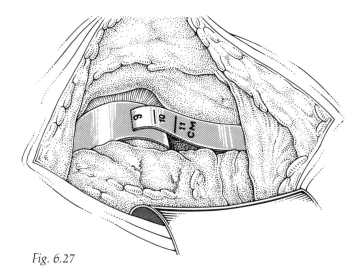

Fig. 6.27

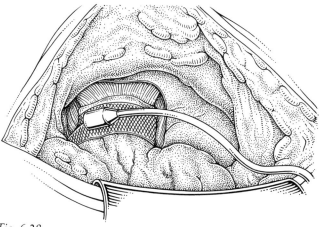

Fig. 6.28

Further dissection into the lower edge of the incision allows the development of a plane down into the right labium majus (if the patient is right-handed). The fascia that encloses the labial fat pad is then opened and an AS 800 control pump is implanted within it (Fig. 6.29). The tubes to join the three components are connected appropriately (Fig. 6.30) and the device is then deactivated.

If there has been any difficulty in mobilising the bladder neck and proximal urethra from the anterior vaginal wall to allow implantation of the cuff then it is a sensible precaution to interpose a tongue of omentum within and around the cuff to reduce the risk of erosion into either viscus.

The omentum is mobilised so far as necessary to allow it to dip down into the pelvis (Ch. 11) and two tongues are created. The first is wrapped around the urethra and held in place with a couple of tacking sutures (Fig. 6.31). The circumference of the omentally-wrapped urethra is then measured and an appropriately sized cuff is implanted.

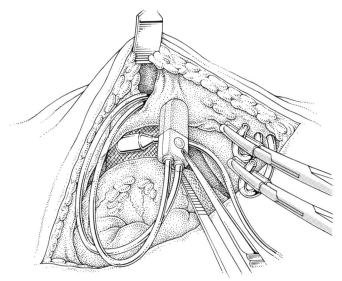

Fig. 6.29

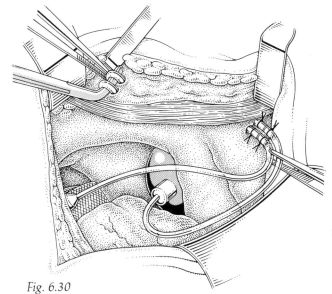

Fig. 6.30

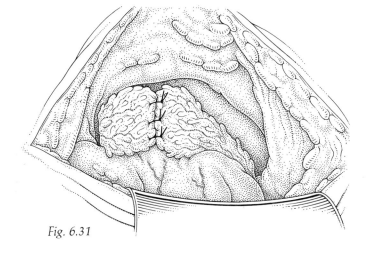

Fig. 6.31

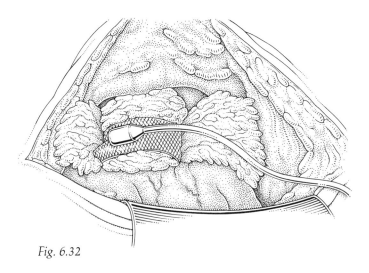

Fig. 6.32

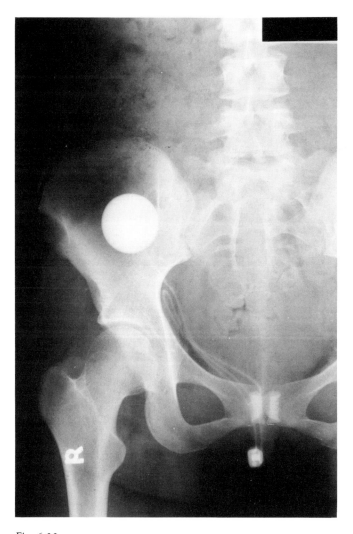

Fig. 6.33

The second tongue of omentum is then wrapped around the cuff, between it and the vaginal wall posteriorly (Fig. 6.32) and separating it (when it has been tacked in place) from the posterior aspect of the pubis anteriorly.

Figure 6.33 shows the typical postoperative radiological appearance.

POSTOPERATIVE MANAGEMENT AND COMPLICATIONS

The subsequent management and complications of the AUS are described in Chapter 5. As with post-prostatectomy incontinence the results of implanting an AUS for SWI in appropriately selected patients are generally very satisfactory and complications are uncommon. The most serious complications, as always, are infection and erosion. Fortunately in this group of patients these are rare occurrences.

The main problem in implanting an AUS in women is in creating a plane of cleavage between the urethra and vagina. The main complication therefore is damage to either of these two structures which may lead to peroperative perforation or postoperative erosion. Hence the importance of taking great care with this stage of the procedure and the desirability of omental wrapping if there has been any difficulty.

If erosion does occur the device will inevitably become infected and, likewise, if infection ocurs erosion will ultimately follow. Infection and erosion are therefore two aspects of the same problem in those instances in which it is impossible to determine which came first.

In male patients who develop infection/erosion the situation is not nearly as serious as in females because a second AUS can always be implanted at a later date with a cuff around the outflow tract at a site remote from the original position. In female patients this is not possible. The seriousness of this is because experience shows that if the urethra has been eroded once then another cuff implanted at the same site will almost certainly erode as well. Urethral erosion in a female is therefore unsalvageable in most cases except by a bladder flap neourethroplasty (Ch. 14). Vaginal erosion is not nearly so serious because this is easily repaired and the urethra may well be intact, in which case another AUS can be implanted at a later date.

Thus if erosion occurs there is a major difference in prognosis between urethral erosion and vaginal erosion, and if infection occurs but erosion has not yet developed it is crucial to intervene urgently before it does — the device must be removed as soon as possible in the hope of preserving the urethra.

If an AUS cuff erodes vaginally it may not be noticed for some time and only discovered when, for example, sexual intercourse is resumed. Although the device will undoubtedly be infected in such a situation, in many instances this is not apparent on examination of the other parts of the device, presumably because infected material can drain out through the erosion. If this is the case, although the device will certainly have to be removed in the end, there is some advantage in leaving it in place for a while. If this policy is followed a significant proportion of the patients who are continent before the device is removed will remain continent afterwards, presumably because a fibrous sheath forms around the urethra at the site of the cuff which acts as an occlusive force. If the whole device is overtly infected with pyogenic bacteria causing swelling, redness and tenderness around the pump or the incision, then obviously this approach will have to be abandoned and the device removed.

If a sphincter has to be removed because of infection or vaginal erosion it is important to fill the channel where the cuff lay so that the plane is kept open for subsequent placement of a new device at a later date, if possible, when everything has settled down.

The obvious way of achieving this is by suprapubic exploration and removal of the AUS with mobilisation of the omentum and wrapping of a tongue of the latter around the urethra in the channel created by removal of the cuff.

A less traumatic way (if the labial fat pads have not been used previously) is to remove the cuff through a short vertical incision in the anterior vaginal wall over the cuff site if infection is the problem and erosion has not yet developed, or through the vaginal erosion if that is the problem, with mobilisation of both labial fat pads to occupy the space vacated. The rest of the AUS can then be removed through a limited groin exposure through the appropriate end of the original incision. This assumes of course that the retropubic space does not require exploration in its own right, to drain a collection of pus, as is occasionally the case.

The artificial sphincter in pregnancy and labour. Most women who have an AUS implanted have had all the children they wish to have or are no longer fertile, but some will still have childbearing potential and will want to know whether the AUS will affect this. Unfortunately there is very little data available.

The two potential problems are pressure from the gravid uterus, during the last trimester and during labour, on the pressure-regulating balloon if this is lying in the retropubic space, and pressure on the cuff during labour causing vaginal or urethral erosion. I have no experience of the first of these problems because I always implant the

pressure-regulating balloon in the iliac fossa (usually the right). As to the second potential problem — cuff erosion following vaginal delivery — this has not occurred in the thirteen patients of mine with an AUS who have delivered vaginally. Caesarean section is an obvious alternative to eliminate or reduce the risk of cuff problems as long as care is taken during the abdominal wall incision to avoid damage to the AUS tubing where it lies subcutaneously over the medial half of the inguinal canal on the side where it was implanted. To reduce the risk of damage to the tubing to a minimum it would be best to use a lower midline incision and to use a diathermy point rather than a scalpel once the skin has been incised.

REFERENCES

In the pre-Stamey era, Stanton took Burch's colposuspension and made it his own. He has written numerous articles on the subject — the one referred to here is a recent review. This procedure has been partly superseded by the Stamey-type procedure and again a recent review of my own is given of my own modification.

Other procedures are rarely required. The May 1985 issue of *Urologic Clinics of North America* covers 'Female Urology' in general and is worth reading in its entirety. More specifically it includes a review by Scott of the AUS in women and, for the sling enthusiasts, an article by McGuire, who is probably the foremost protagonist. The article from Raz's group on his approach to stress incontinence is also worth reading to get another point of view.

Mundy A R 1988 The Stundy procedure. In: Mundy A R (ed) Current operative surgery: Urology. Balliere Tindall, Eastbourne, pp 75−82

Stamey T A 1986 Endoscopic-suspension of the vesical neck. In: Stanton S L, Tanagho E A (eds) Surgery of female incontinence, 2nd edn. Springer Verlag, Berlin, pp 115−132

Stanton S L 1986 Colposuspension. In: Stanton S L, Tanagho E A (eds) Surgery of female incontinence, 2nd edn. Springer Verlag, Berlin, pp 95−103

Chapter 7

Detrusor instability

Patients with frequency and urgency or urge incontinence (the urge syndrome) can be divided by the nature of their symptoms into two groups. In one group the urgency is due to the sensation that the bladder is about to empty involuntarily — that is motor urge. In the other it is due to the sensation of pain or discomfort in what they perceive as a full bladder — this is sensory urge. In the motor urge group most but by no means all patients can be shown urodynamically to have involuntary detrusor contractions to account for their symptoms and in the absence of a definable neurological cause for these involuntary detrusor contractions this condition is called detrusor instability. Detrusor instability may be secondary in males to bladder outflow obstruction, either dyssynergic bladder neck obstruction or prostatic obstruction (rarely a stricture), otherwise it is idiopathic. In women there is no correlation with bladder outflow obstruction and all cases of detrusor instability are idiopathic.

Sensory urgency or urge incontinence may also be either idiopathic or secondary. Causes of secondary sensory urge include urinary tract infection, urethrotrigonitis, a bladder stone, a bladder tumour, interstitial cystitis, irradiation cystitis and any other cause of bladder hypersensitivity which can be defined by radiological, bacteriological, endoscopic or histological means. In the absence of a definable cause sensory urge is idiopathic. Thus, up to a point, idiopathic sensory urge tends to be a dustbin diagnosis — a group into which patients with the urge syndrome are thrown when there is no definable cause for their problem.

This is a rather cynical view of idiopathic sensory urge because on urodynamic evaluation there is a characteristic early first sensation of filling and a reduced bladder capacity, and electronic testing will usually confirm the clinical impression that there

is an associated urethral hypersensitivity to catheterisation. In other words, I have no doubt that idiopathic sensory urgency is a distinct clinical entity, albeit one that at present we know very little about. On the other hand, this view of sensory urge does have the important clinical consequence that there is considerable diagnostic overlap between the group of patients with symptoms of motor urge but no demonstrable detrusor instability, the group with idiopathic sensory urge, and normality, not to mention the overlap of all these groups with such conditions as the urethral syndrome, prostatitis and the bladder problems due to affective disorders — all of which are equally poorly defined conditions. Furthermore there is the practical therapeutic point that, of all the conditions mentioned so far, the only one that can be cured predictably is detrusor instability.

Thus the thrust of clinical evaluation in a patient with the urge syndrome is to identify detrusor instability by urodynamic testing and then to satisfy oneself that the patient's symptoms are due to that urodynamic abnormality and not to any other associated problem of which affective disorders are the most common type.

If detrusor instability is excluded by adequate and, if necessary, repeated urodynamic evaluation, and if demonstrable causes of sensory urge such as urinary infection, bladder stone, bladder tumour or interstitial cystitis (which is discussed in detail in Ch. 8) have been excluded by the appropriate investigations, it is usual practice to treat those with an idiopathic urge syndrome in much the same way as those with defined detrusor instability, at least in the first instance.

The problem with this approach arises when a patient fails to respond to the conservative treatment for detrusor instability with bladder drill and anticholinergic medication with

oxybutynin. Given that in general terms the only available options left are surgical, the one minor (the phenol technique) the other major (augmentation or 'clam' cystoplasty), all patients require re-evaluation to be sure that all of their symptoms are attributable to the bladder. Having satisfied oneself that this is so it seems reasonable, for reasons given below, for all female patients to try the phenol technique (it is contraindicated in males because it may cause impotence) irrespective of whether or not detrusor instability has been urodynamically demonstrated because it is such a minor procedure, but it is my opinion that it would be foolhardy to perform a 'clam' cystoplasty on a patient with no overt urodynamic abnormality, however severe the symptoms.

From the foregoing comments the reader will have gathered that the indications for surgery in patients with urge incontinence are refractory detrusor instability in either sex and refractory idiopathic sensory urgency in women; refractory meaning a failure to respond to bladder drill and oxybutynin or terodilin.

Before oxybutynin became available the surgical procedure of choice was bladder transection but when oxybutynin became available it became clear that patients who failed to respond to oxybutynin did badly after bladder transection and the only ones who did do well were those who responded to oxybutynin but who could not take it because of side-effects or would not take it in the long term. Furthermore the phenol technique (see below) is a much lesser procedure and therefore has completely supplanted bladder transection in women, and clam cystoplasty is more predictable in men. Thus bladder transection is now a thing of the past.

The aetiology of detrusor instability is unknown and so surgical treatment is

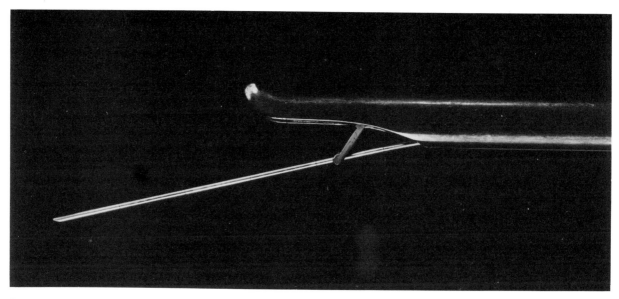

Fig. 7.1

empirical. The two techniques currently used are transvesical injection of the pelvic plexuses with phenol which aims to decentralise the bladder, and 'clam' cystoplasty which aims to make involuntary bladder contractions ineffective. The phenol technique is a minor, almost day case procedure, with minimal morbidity if properly performed and (as yet) no mortality. For these reasons I think it is justifiable to try it in female patients with either motor urge incontinence or idiopathic sensory urge incontinence that has proved to be unresponsive to conservative methods of treatment although results are somewhat variable and never very satisfactory. Unfortunately only women are suitable as there is a risk (albeit mainly anecdotal) of impotence in men. Clam cystoplasty is therefore reserved for men with refractory detrusor instability after failed conservative treatment and for women with detrusor instability after failed conservative treatment and phenol injection. I would not treat sensory urgency by clam cystoplasty although I believe it has been done.

THE PHENOL TECHNIQUE

Anybody who is fit enough to have a cystoscopy is fit enough for this procedure. Suitable patients are those with detrusor instability (or hyperreflexia — see Ch. 10) that has failed to respond to oxybutynin and terodilin. No special preoperative preparation is required.

The technique involves passing a 30 cm long flexible needle up a cystoscope with an Albarran bridge as for ureteric catheterisation (Fig. 7.1). The needle is then pushed through the bladder wall, halfway betwen the bladder neck and the right ureteric orifice, to a depth of 2 or 3 cm (Fig. 7.2).

It should be emphasised that the site of injection is below the ureter, not under the trigone. If the phenol is injected in any quantity underneath the trigone there will not be enough room to contain it and a vesico-vaginal fistula may result. When injected under the ureter the phenol enters the inferior hypogastric sheath (see Ch. 3) where the pelvic plexus is situated and where there is plenty of room for the volume of phenol to be injected.

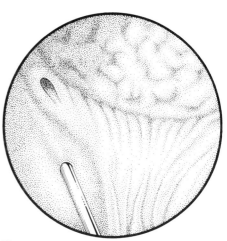

Fig. 7.2

10 ml of 6% aqueous phenol is injected — slowly and under direct vision to be sure that it is extravesical; in other words, nothing should be seen cystoscopically. The bolus of phenol is almost always palpable through the anterior vaginal wall but dissipates rapidly if it has been injected in the correct place. The needle is then removed and the procedure is repeated on the other side.

Care should be taken during the procedure to be sure that the syringe containing the phenol is firmly luer-locked into the needle so that phenol does not get squirted out into the surgeon's eyes. Protective goggles are another sensible precaution. Injecting the bolus of phenol in the right place usually involves downward deflection of the tip of the needle with the Albarran bridge to engage it in the bladder wall and then elevation of the working end of the cystoscope (by standing up) to get the needle through the back of the bladder and into the region of the pelvic plexus.

The patient is usually discharged from hospital the next day with the warning that transient haematuria is common. Transient acute retention for the first 12—24 hours after injection occurs occasionally, requiring a short period of catheterisation.

In patients who have had the phenol injected in the correct place, there have been no other complications. Three patients have passed sloughed pieces of bladder wall, presumably because the phenol has been injected into the bladder wall, rather than deep to it.

The overall subjective response rate of this procedure is only 36% but, when the results are broken down for age, the response rate is 16% in those aged less than 55 years and 68% in those aged 55 years and over (although this is not every surgeon's experience). Objective analysis shows that 64% of those with

a useful subjective response changed from unstable to stable detrusor behaviour. It should be noted that stable behaviour is not necessarily normal behaviour. Indeed in successfully treated patients the urodynamic appearance is that of a peripheral autonomic neuropathy — mildly impaired compliance, low voiding pressure, low flow rate, incompetent bladder neck and residual urine. In other words the phenol technique rarely cures the patient, strictly speaking, although it usually 'cures' the symptoms. It simply converts a socially incapacitating bladder abnormality to a socially acceptable one.

The response rate in patients with idiopathic sensory urge is about 15—20%. It is worth emphasising that the technique should not be used in patients with sensory urgency due to interstitial cystitis or who have had radiotherapy or any other form of inflammatory pancystitis on bladder biopsy. I have seen such patients, treated in this way elsewhere (of course), who have had catastrophic degrees of sloughing of the bladder wall as a result.

'CLAM' CYSTOPLASTY

This is a much bigger procedure than the phenol technique; hence the reason for trying the phenol technique first in younger women even though the response rate in this group is low.

Many patients who come to cystoplasty have more than just simple detrusor instability. A high proportion of young men have post-obstructive instability (associated with dyssynergic bladder neck obstruction) and a high proportion of women have mixed stress incontinence and detrusor instability. In the women a mild to moderate degree of stress incontinence is often an advantage as it reduces the likelihood of postoperative voiding dysfunction (see below). In men with bladder neck obstruction, the obstruction must be

eliminated completely before proceeding to cystoplasty. Indeed, every now and then one sees a patient in whom a *complete* resolution of obstruction leads to resolution of their instability as well, so it is sensible to allow sufficient time (about six months) for this to occur.

Apart from the usual complications of any major operation, there is one particular problem associated with augmentation cystoplasty which must be anticipated and discussed with the patient before the operation. That problem is voiding imbalance. This is almost universal after any type of cystoplasty in men assuming that bladder neck competence is unimpaired; it is less common in women because sphincteric incompetence is a common associated abnormality. Voiding imbalance occurs because augmentation cystoplasty acts to make involuntary detrusor contractions ineffective in causing involuntary voiding and in so doing it makes voluntary contractions similarly ineffective in causing voluntary voiding. For this reason it is advisable to warn male patients that they may require a bladder neck incision at some stage after cystoplasty and if the potential side-effect of retrograde ejaculation is regarded as unacceptable then cystoplasty should be deferred.

As indicated above, women with sphincter weakness incontinence (SWI) are very unlikely to run into problems with voiding difficulty after a cystoplasty, perhaps not surprisingly. Furthermore mild to moderate degrees of SWI tend to disappear or reduce to an insignificant level spontaneously after a cystoplasty, perhaps because the distal sphincter mechanism no longer has to contain the excessive detrusor activity. For these reasons the surgeon should not attempt to correct any SWI at the time of cystoplasty. He should however warn patients with severe SWI that they may require a Stamey-type procedure at a later date should troublesome symptoms persist.

Any residual voiding imbalance after the cystoplasty in either sex can be managed either by sphincter rebalancing or preferably by intermittent self catheterisation (see below). It is important to warn patients about the possibility of postoperative voiding dysfunction before their operation. Otherwise patients who reasonably expect this operation to be their last may be resentful or disappointed about having to have further treatment to correct residual problems.

An occasional cause of voiding dysfunction after a cystoplasty is diverticulisation of the cystoplasty segment. This is due to contraction of the suture line by which the cystoplasty segment is sewn in place. The result is an 'hour glass' deformity with the cystoplasty segment acting like a diverticulum. It is prevented as described below by an almost complete bisection of the bladder before inlaying the cystoplasty segment.

Preoperative preparation
Patients are admitted to hospital 2 or 3 days before their operation. The

preoperative regime consists of a mechanical and antimicrobial bowel preparation as described in Chapter 2.

The urine should be sterile and two units of blood should be cross matched although it is not usually required.

Technique
A variety of different techniques have been described using a variety of different cystoplasty patches. The technique described here uses ileum. In some situations it may seem easier to use the colon, particularly the sigmoid colon, to get a patch down into the pelvis on a vascular pedicle, but colonic anastomoses are more prone to complications than ileal anastomoses and, coupled with the theoretically higher risk of a carcinoma developing in a colonic segment when it is in contact with urine in the long term (see below) and the higher pressures generated by colonic segments, this makes an ileocystoplasty preferable. However, in about 10% of patients it proves impossible to get ileum to reach sufficiently far down into the pelvis and sigmoid colon has to be used. This

usually only occurs in patients with spina bifida and a marked lumbar lordosis who have a prominent sacral promontory and a short mesentery but is occasionally seen in non-neuropathic patients, usually when they are overweight.

Any lower abdominal incision may be used but I prefer a Cherney incision (Ch. 3) (Figs 7.3, 7.4) in thin female patients or a lower midline incision otherwise, as these provide wide and therefore easy access to the pelvis.

The repropubic space is widely opened to expose the pelvic floor all the way around the front and both lateral aspects of the bladder, and a ring retractor is placed to hold the incision open.

The urachus and obliterated umbilical arteries are then ligated and divided together just above the dome of the bladder and the peritoneum is opened. Blunt dissection on either side of the urachus will open up the plane of cleavage on each side between the fascia on the lateral aspect of the bladder wall and the fascia and overlying peritoneum

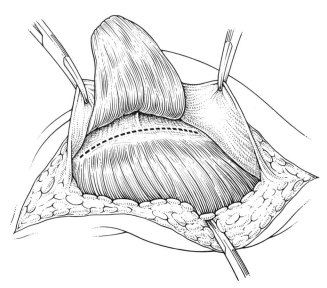

Fig. 7.3

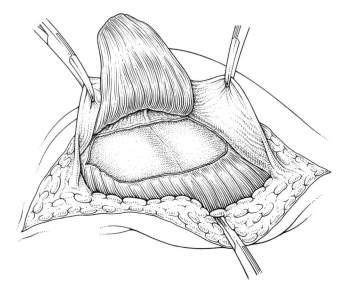

Fig. 7.4

on the dome of the bladder at the point where these two fascial layers join together to form a single sheet which runs to the brim of the pelvis along the line of the iliac vessels (Fig. 7.5). This plane of cleavage is developed down along the lateral margin of the bladder towards the bladder neck. This exposes the maximal circumference of the bladder and allows the large veins that run in the fascia on the lateral bladder wall to be secured without much bleeding. Indeed keeping the blood loss down is the only advantage of opening this plane. That aside, the bladder could be bisected in any plane.

When the maximal circumference of the bladder has been exposed in this way, the bladder wall can be incised around its maximal circumference from a point one to two centimetres in front of the ureteric orifice and about one centimetre lateral to the bladder neck on one side to a similar point on the other side. It is easiest to do this by picking up the bladder in the midline just in front of the urachus with two Babcock forceps and opening it between them. The incision in the bladder can then be extended downwards from the dome to the base, on one side at a time, with a clear view of the ureteric orifices on the inside of the bladder (Fig. 7.6). In this way the bladder is almost completely bisected leaving intact only about 1 cm of the bladder neck on each lateral aspect (Fig. 7.7).

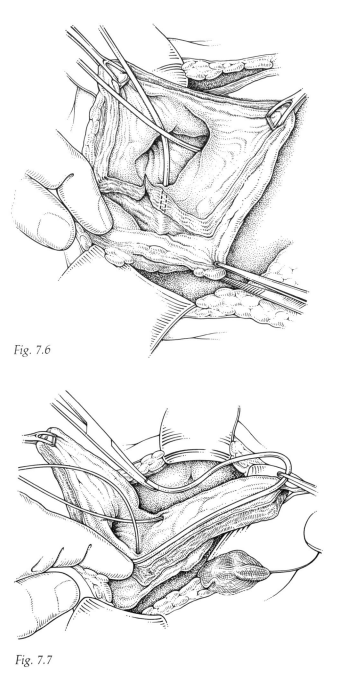

Fig. 7.6

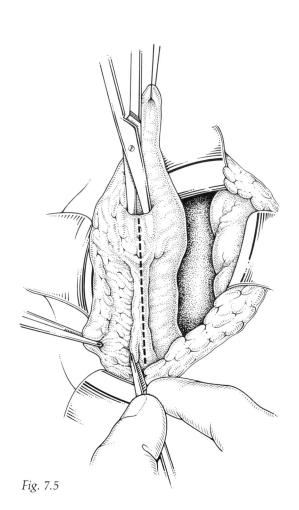

Fig. 7.5

Fig. 7.7

The circumference of the bisected bladder is then measured (Fig. 7.7 — in this case with a length of silicone tubing) and haemostasis is secured, particularly at the two ends of the incision in the bladder wall in the region of the superior vesical pedicles where a few significant vessels may be encountered.

The next stage is to define and isolate a section of ileum on its vascular pedicle. A convenient section of ileum is selected that will drop down easily into the pelvis and reach, without tension, to both apices of the bladder bisection. The ileal segment should preferably be 25 cm or more proximal to the ileocaecal valve to avoid interference with valve function and to leave as much as possible of the terminal ileum intact as this is functionally the most important section. If an ileal segment will not reach, then a sigmoid segment will have to be used but this is very unusual in the absence of neuropathy. The ileal segment must be equal in length to the measured maximal circumference of the bladder (which is usually about 25 cm) and have a well defined vascular arcade supplying it (Fig. 7.8). The segment is isolated and the ileum on either side of it is reconstituted in the usual way, anterior to the isolated segment — I use a single

layer of inverting vertical mattress sutures of 3/0 Vicryl, knotted on the inside — and the mesenteric defect is closed to prevent the development of an internal hernia. The ileal segment is then opened on its antimesenteric aspect to produce a patch (Fig. 7.9).

The ileal patch is now sewn into the bisected bladder. There is a tendency for the margins of the bladder to contract during the course of the procedure leading to an overlap between the ileal edge and the bladder edge during the anastomosis of the patch to the bladder. To prevent this happening, or at least to reduce its extent, each suture line is first halved and then quartered with stay-sutures and each quarter is then sewn up individually (Fig. 7.10). The posterior suture line is dealt with first so

the first stay-stitch is placed to tack the mid-point of the inferior margin of the ileal patch to the mid-point of the posterior bladder wall at the dome (B in Fig. 7.10). The second and third stay-stitch tack the two ends of the ileal patch to the apices of the bladder incision alongside the bladder neck (A in Fig. 7.10) and the fourth and fifth stay-stitches tack the ileum to the bladder half way along either side (C in Fig. 7.10). The ileum is then anastomosed to the bladder with a continuous 3/0 Vicryl stitch picking up the full thickness of the bladder and ileal wall, starting at the apex of the bladder incision in front of the ureter and working up on each side to the dome from inside the bladder, locking to each of the 'quartering' stay-stiches in turn as they are encountered (Fig. 7.11). The

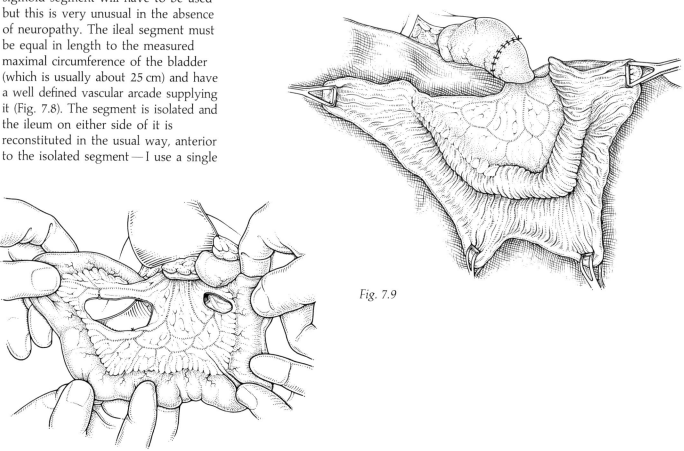

Fig. 7.9

Fig. 7.8

procedure is repeated to sew the other (upper) edge of the ileal patch to the margin of the anterior half of the bladder. Once again the two edges are tacked together with stay-sutures to halve and quarter the line of anastomosis (Fig. 7.12) which is then closed, preferably from inside the bladder to invert the suture line, with a continuous full thickness Vicryl stitch locking to each stay-stitch in turn until the ileocystoplasty is complete.

A wound drain is left in the retropubic space and a 20 F suprapubic catheter (large enough not to be blocked by the ileal mucus in the urine) is left in the bladder. The catheter should be brought out through the anterior bladder wall and not through the suture line between the bladder and the ileum because a hole in the bladder wall, when the catheter is

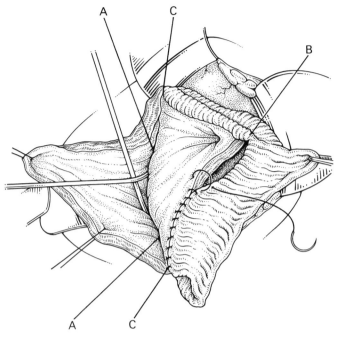

Fig. 7.10

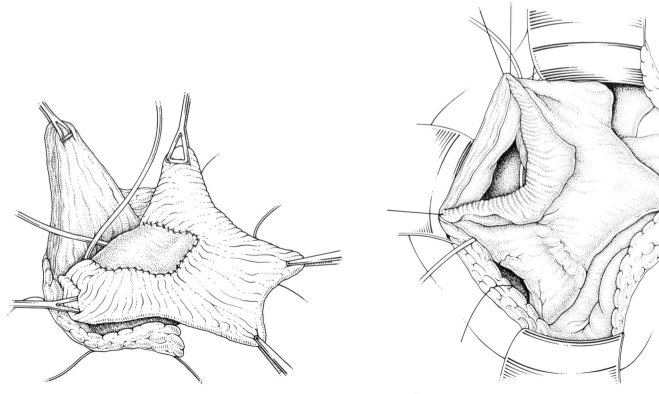

Fig. 7.11

Fig. 7.12

subsequently removed, closes and heals much more quickly than a defect in the suture line.

The wound is then closed (Fig. 7.13).

Postoperative management
The wound drain is removed when it stops draining and the suprapubic catheter is clamped for a trial of voiding on about the eighth postoperative day by which time the patient should be fully mobile. The parenteral antibiotic regime is continued for the first 3–5 days.

When the suprapubic catheter is first clamped and the patient starts to void spontaneously a voided volume chart should be kept noting the time and volume passed and, on two or three occasions, the residual urine volume. Assuming that the patient is voiding satisfactorily, the catheter is removed after 24 hours and the patient is discharged home the next day by which time the suprapubic catheter exit site should be closed. Any excessive urine leakage from this site is dealt with by 24 hours of indwelling urethral catheterisation. Persistent or recurrent urine leakage from the suprapubic site usually means that there is either significant bladder outflow obstruction or alternatively a communicating abscess.

If the patient has difficulty in establishing spontaneous voiding it is usually because the discomfort of the lower abdominal wound prevents the patient straining sufficiently. There are three options — either to keep the indwelling suprapubic catheter on free drainage for a week or two longer before trying again; or to use a 'clamp and release' system to get the augmented bladder used to filling and emptying, and to encourage the patient to void spontaneously as much as possible; or to use clean intermittent self catheterisation (CISC) until spontaneous voiding is satisfactory. As voiding

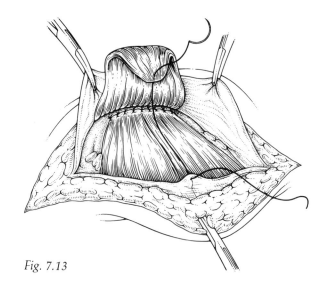

Fig. 7.13

FLOW RATE 0–50 ml/sec

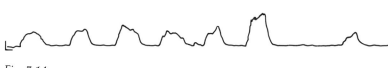

Fig. 7.14

difficulty does not usually persist for very long in non-neuropathic detrusor instability any of these three options would be reasonable but as it occasionally does persist I prefer CISC particularly as it rids the patient of the rather cumbersome indwelling suprapubic catheter at the earliest opportunity.

Complications
When the patient goes home, and on subsequent follow up, he or she will usually be passing reasonable volumes with a relatively normal frequency. If not, the usual cause is a large residual urine volume. This may cause problems in two ways: by restricting the effective capacity of the bladder, thereby causing frequency, or by predisposing the patient to recurrent urinary infection. The residual urine volume is measured either directly by catheterisation or

indirectly by ultrasound and if this suggests a voiding imbalance it is then confirmed by a video-urodynamic study. A low flow rate and an interrupted flow pattern is another sign of voiding imbalance (Fig. 7.14). At about 3 months a follow-up video-urodynamic study should be obtained routinely to serve as a baseline for the future.

At this time patients should have stabilised and learnt how to use their augmented bladders. Some patients will have had all detrusor activity abolished but most retain some detrusor contractile activity (Fig. 7.15A and B shows the preoperative appearance and Fig. 7.16A and B the postoperative VUD appearance of a typical patient). Even if the detrusor does still contract, at least part of voiding will have to be achieved by straining and some residual urine is common.

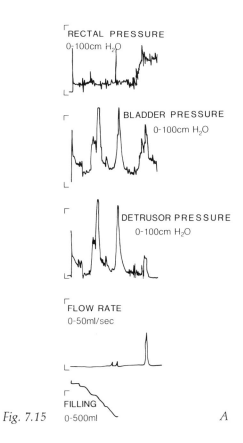

RECTAL PRESSURE
0-100cm H$_2$O

BLADDER PRESSURE
0-100cm H$_2$O

DETRUSOR PRESSURE
0-100cm H$_2$O

FLOW RATE
0-50ml/sec

FILLING
0-500ml

Fig. 7.15   *A*

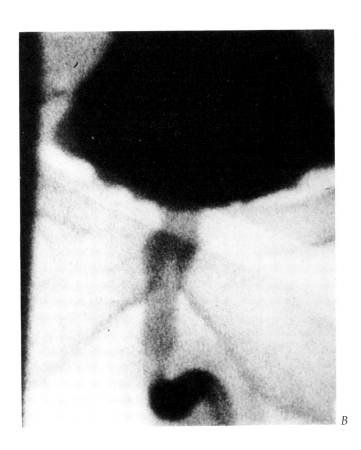

B

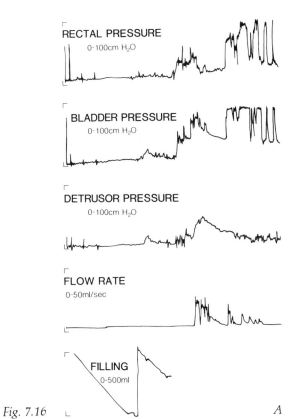

RECTAL PRESSURE
0-100cm H$_2$O

BLADDER PRESSURE
0-100cm H$_2$O

DETRUSOR PRESSURE
0-100cm H$_2$O

FLOW RATE
0-50ml/sec

FILLING
0-500ml

Fig. 7.16   *A*

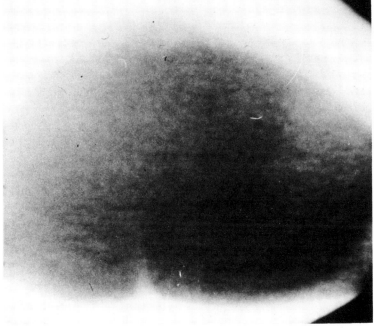

B

In essence the difference between those who empty their augmented bladders well and those who do not is the greater ability to empty by straining in the former group, and further treatment in the latter group is directed towards improving that means of emptying. This is often achieved simply by letting the patient watch his or her own video study to see the residual volume to be eliminated; they thereby learn to void by double micturition. Otherwise there are two options: either to 'relax' whichever of the two sphincter mechanisms is the objectively demonstrated site of the functional obstruction (usually the distal mechanism) or to use intermittent self catheterisation.

The real question, however, is to decide when treatment is necessary, and in the asymptomatic patient with sterile urine it is probably not necessary. Sphincter rebalancing, either by graded Otis sphincterotomy or by bladder neck incision, whichever is objectively deemed appropriate, or clean intermittent self catheterisation is therefore reserved for the occasional patient with persistent postoperative symptoms due to a large residual urine volume or with recurrent urinary tract infections. These days I rarely use 'sphincter rebalancing' procedures and tend to rely much more on CISC, particularly as most patients only need to perform CISC once or twice a day (first thing in the morning or last thing at night or both) with spontaneous voiding during the day time.

It is worth emphasising that voiding difficulty requiring CISC is rare after a cystoplasty in non-neuropathic detrusor instability but this is not the case in neuropathic detrusor hyperreflexia (see Ch. 10) where significant voiding dysfunction is regularly seen after a cystoplasty and CISC is commonly required.

Other than voiding difficulties and associated urinary tract infection, and the problems associated with incorporation of a gut segment into the urinary tract discussed below, complications should be rare. There are of course the complications of any major abdominal procedure — cardiovascular, thromboembolic, respiratory and gastrointestinal — which may disturb the postoperative course of 15% or so of patients but these are generally minor and transient.

The problems that do occur are generally the result of either poor selection or poor technique. The best results come from adequate bisection of the bladder and interposition of an adequate patch of bowel in a well motivated patient with proven detrusor instability. A poor result is usually because one or more of these four criteria has not been satisfied. If this is the case, at least an adequate bisection or a small patch can be corrected by reoperation; a poorly motivated patient with a dubious diagnosis cannot. Although we have all succumbed to the constant entreaties of our emotionally more fragile patients 'to do something' against our better judgement, we have generally wished we hadn't and this instance is no exception. A whingeing patient with bladder symptoms is one thing but a whingeing patient with bladder symptoms who you have made dependent on self catheterisation is an altogether worse proposition. If the patient is inadequately motivated or the diagnosis is suspect then a clam cystoplasty is not indicated (if the patient is not right for the operation, the operation is not right for the patient — Mundy's law of surgery).

PROBLEMS DUE TO INCORPORATION OF INTESTINAL SEGMENTS INTO THE URINARY TRACT

Most of the complications of 'clam' cystoplasty have already been mentioned. There are, however, some other effects that have not yet been discussed all of which relate to the incorporation of an intestinal segment into the urinary tract. These effects occur whatever the type of intestinal segment and however it is incorporated. Thus the following discussion applies equally to ileal or colonic conduits as to ileal or colonic cystoplasties, and to substitution as well as to augmentation cystoplasties.

The problems arise mainly because the gut segment continues to behave like gut after transposition to the urinary tract. Absorption of fluid and electrolytes, and secretory and motor activity continue unabated. In addition to this lifelong continuation of intestinal function within the urinary tract there are infective and histopathological problems that also occur.

Fluid and electrolyte problems
Both ileal and colonic cystoplasty segments absorb water and electrolytes. Secretion also occurs but the net result is usually absorption. Electrolyte absorption seems to be greater in colocystoplasties although this may simply be a reflection of their greater size (I tend to use ileum for augmentation and colon for substitution). Chloride absorption imposes an extra burden on renal function and tends to produce a metabolic acidosis although development of an overt hyperchloraemic acidosis does not appear to be directly related to renal function.

The metabolic abnormality is not usually apparent on routine serum electrolyte analysis of venous blood as only about 16% of patients are hyperchloraemic.

BLOOD GAS ANALYSIS RESULTS

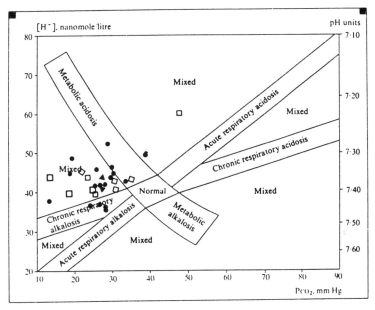

- ● Caecocystoplasty

- ◻ Ileal augmentation

- ▲ Colon augmentation

Fig. 7.17

Stones

In my series of patients with cystoplasties, 6% have developed bladder stones during follow up. The cause of these stones is not clear. In almost all instances they have developed in colocystoplasties but they do occur in ileocystoplasties. The time of onset has varied from 6 months to 8 years after the cystoplasty and as yet no definite pattern has emerged to suggest the underlying pathophysiology.

Stones have been reported after continent diversion in relation to staples used in the construction of the neobladder pouch but it may be that such stones would have developed anyway. Perhaps either mucus or staples could act as a nidus around which stones could develop, either as a result of chronic infection or as a consequence of disturbed calcium homeostasis secondary to chronic acidosis.

Infection and histopathological changes

Other than mucus the main secretory product of both ileum and colon is immunoglobulin (Ig) A. The colon appears more active than the ileum in cystoplasty segments, particularly for IgA secretion. IgA may be important in reducing the incidence of frank urinary tract infection after a cystoplasty but bacteriuria with a mixed growth of organisms is still all too common. It is found in about 50% of augmentation cystoplasties (usually ileocystoplasties) and about 75% of substitution cystoplasties (usually colocystoplasties). This may be of great importance in the long term because associated with this mixed bacterial growth are high levels of urinary nitrosamines which are chemical compounds derived from secondary amines and nitrates in the diet. Nitrosamines are not normally present in the urine because nitrate must first be converted to nitrite and the nitrite must then react with the secondary amines but both these reactions can be catalysed or otherwise

The abnormality is always obvious however on arterial blood gas analysis if the results are plotted on a graph as shown in Figure 7.17. The most common abnormalities are either a frank metabolic acidosis or a metabolic acidosis with respiratory compensation. At its worst this may cause hypocalcaemia and hypokalaemia and become symptomatic with weakness and tingling of the fingers as the most common manifestations. Whether, in the long term, the acidosis may also cause demineralisation and abnormalities of bone metabolism, particularly in growing children and middle-aged women, is not known but it is certainly a possibility because in chronic acidosis bone plays an important part in the buffering process and calcium is mobilised from bone as a result. Early results of studies of bone density in such patients at Guy's Hospital suggest that although calcium may indeed be mobilised from

bone as a result of the acidosis after cystoplasty, an ileal cystoplasty segment can itself absorb calcium from the urine in the bladder and so calcium is not lost and demineralisation does not usually occur, in adults at least. This does not seem to be the case however with children after any type of gut interposition in the urinary tract but particularly with colonic cystoplasty segments — children after colocystoplasty seem to grow less satisfactorily and seem more prone to orthopaedic problems — although it is still too early to be sure about this. Either way, if a patient does develop symptoms or signs related to acidosis or its secondary effects on calcium or potassium metabolism the treatment is with oral bicarbonate. Calcium or potassium supplements are useless unless bicarbonate is given as well and are usually unnecessary if bicarbonate is given in adequate doses.

induced by bacteria. Nitrosamines as a group are widely recognised as carcinogens in an increasing number of situations of which gastric cancer in achlorhydria is probably the best known. Nitrosamines are also believed to be carcinogenic in patients with ureterosigmoidostomies, causing adenocarcinoma at the anastomosis, and are associated with squamous cell carcinoma in the bilharzial bladder. Indeed the levels of urinary nitrosamines found in patients with chronic mixed bacteriuria after cystoplasty are far higher than those found in the urine-faeces mix after ureterosigmoidostomy and in bilharzia. These findings are all the more worrying because follow-up biopsies of patients with cystoplasties show histological features of chronic inflammation and squamous metaplasia in a disturbingly high percentage of patients. The significance of these observations has yet to be established but they suggest that there is a distinct potential for the development of tumours in patients with cystoplasties, particularly colocystoplasties in which there is a low but definite incidence of keratinising squamous metaplasia and of transitional epithelial mucin distribution, both of which are regarded by some authorities as being associated with malignant transformation. Given that nitrosamines are implicated in normal gastrointestinal cancer and that gastric cancer is commoner than cancer of the sigmoid colon which is commoner than cancer of the right side of the colon with ileal cancer a very rare occurrence, it would seem the ileum is the safest choice for a cystoplasty. The right colon would be second best, sigmoid colon should only be used if there is no choice and gastrocystoplasty should be abandoned (it always seemed a ludicrous idea to me anyway unless there is no alternative).

The other implication from these findings is that long-term antibiotic prophylaxis might be advisable in those patients with chronic mixed bacteriuria

in an attempt to sterilise the urine although such efforts are by no means always successful.

Mucus

Mucus production is not usually a problem in the long term once patients (and their family doctors) get used to its presence and do not confuse it with pus. The average daily production from both ileum and colon when used as a cystoplasty segment is about 35–40 g and this usually washes out easily during voiding, although the occasional patient produces large plugs of inspissated mucus which can cause urethral obstruction (Fig. 7.18). Mucus production may be a problem in the early postoperative period after cystoplasty, when spontaneous voiding is being established after the immediate postoperative period of indwelling catheterisation, and in patients on intermittent self catheterisation (CISC). In such circumstances a mucolytic agent is

helpful to dissolve the mucus or break it up into smaller fragments. The most useful agent is 30 ml of 20% acetylcysteine used as a bladder washout either as a one-off or occasional procedure, or regularly in those with recurrent problems on CISC. Orally administered mucolytic agents do not appear to be useful although Ranitidine appears to reduce the production of mucus and this may be more suitable than regular instillations of acetylcysteine in those patients with recurrent mucus obstruction. Acetylcysteine takes about 45 minutes to dissolve mucus in vitro so it is best instilled into the bladder by urethral catheterisation and retained for at least an hour (longer if possible) to allow maximum dissolution.

Unusually high mucus production with retention of mucus in the bladder may lead to recurrent urinary infection in the traditional sense rather than the chronic mixed bacteriuria discussed in the last

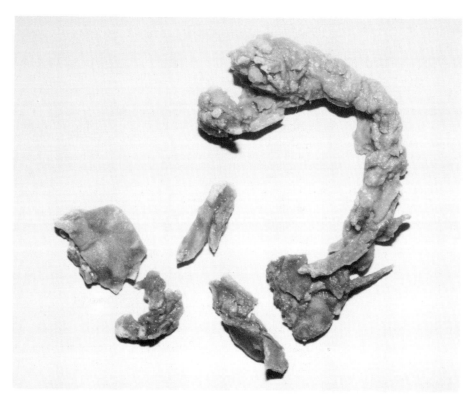

Fig. 7.18

section. This is particularly so in patients on CISC. Eliminating the mucus problem usually helps but when it does not, anti-infective agents will need to be used. Standard antibiotic prophylaxis with drugs such as trimethoprim is not always helpful and when it fails methenamine (Hiprex) — which is not an antibiotic and therefore preferable — or one of the newer quinolone antibiotics, ciprofloxacin, taken one week on and one week off (to prevent the emergence of resistant strains), usually work.

Contractile activity

Problems from gut contractions are rarely a problem in augmentation cystoplasty except in patients with neuropathy. Gut contractile activity is much more of a problem with substitution cystoplasty and will therefore be discussed in the next chapter.

Suffice it to say that in the absence of neuropathy most ileal patches are docile and generate no pressure at all and those that do generate pressures of less than 30 cmH$_2$O. Colonic patches generate pressures of a higher amplitude, in the range of 30–50 cmH$_2$O, and on a more regular basis. In neuropathy these pressures are higher in both instances and occur more frequently.

Nutritional consequences

Resection of the terminal ileum reduces the absorptive area of the ileum and interferes with the enterohepatic circulation of bile salts. The greater the resection and the more distal the resection, the greater the problem, so problems are more likely with substitution cystoplasty but can occur with any type of cystoplasty.

Loss of the absorptive surface may lead to malabsorption of vitamin B$_{12}$ which, after the liver stores have been depleted, may cause problems of macrocytic anaemia or neuropathy after a few years. Once the neuropathy has developed it may be irreversible so B$_{12}$ deficiency

must be looked for and treated before a deficiency becomes manifest.

Loss of greater lengths of ileum, or loss of even quite a short length in otherwise compromised bowel such as after previous gut resections or after radiotherapy, may cause malabsorption of fat or fat soluble vitamins.

Finally malabsorption of bile salts may lead to gallstone formation and hyperoxaluria which in turn may lead to urolithiasis particularly in association with the acidosis-related disturbance of calcium metabolism, recurrent urinary infection, and the presence of mucus as a nidus.

Diarrhoea

Bile salt malabsorption, malabsorption of fat and bacterial colonisation of the terminal ileum as a result of loss of the ileocaecal valve are all established causes of diarrhoea. In patients who were previously constipated there may be no apparent change in bowel function or even an improvement, but diarrhoea can be troublesome. This is particularly so in patients with neuropathic bladder (and bowel) dysfunction who have had their 'stable state' disturbed by their pre-operative bowel preparation and the relative starvation of the perioperative period. In them, post-operative diarrhoea may be catastrophic and take several weeks to settle.

In the longer term, those with established diarrhoea require investigation to determine the exact cause and direct treatment. An empirical trial of cholestyramine to correct bile salt diarrhoea is the most likely to help.

Pregnancy after cystoplasty

It is obviously of some concern to know how to deal with a female patient who becomes pregnant after augmentation cystoplasty, particularly with reference to the vascular pedicle of the cystoplasty segment and its relationship to the gravid uterus.

My experience is that vaginal delivery is not complicated by the presence of a cystoplasty. In two patients who had caesarian sections (for unrelated obstetric reasons) delivery was also uneventful, presumably because the vascular pedicle of the cystoplasty was pushed over to one side by the expanding uterus. My view, based on this, is that a normal vaginal delivery is to be preferred and can be expected to be straightforward. The risk of damage to the vascular pedicle of the cystoplasty makes caesarian section undesirable if it can be avoided, but if it is necessary it should be straightforward if reasonable care is taken in the knowledge of the patient's previous urological surgery.

For obvious reasons particular care should be taken during the pregnancy to watch for urinary tract infection and increased voiding difficulty.

REFERENCES

For an up-to-date review of detrusor instability my review in 1988 is as
good as any (he said modestly).

The phenol technique was originally described by Ewing et al (1982) but
the largest experience was published by Blackford et al (1984) from the
combined units of Guy's and Cardiff Royal Infirmary.

The 'clam' technique was described by Bramble (1982) but again the largest
published experience comes from the Guy's and Cardiff series reported by
Mundy & Stephenson (1985).

The complications of incorporating intestinal segments into the urinary tract
were described by Murray et al (1987) and Nurse & Mundy (1988,
1989). Almost all the work alluded to in the section on the problems of
incorporating intestinal segments into the urinary tract was done by
Diane Nurse at Guy's Hospital. The other unit with a major interest in
the subject is Scott McDougal's in Nashville, Tennessee. The reference
listed here (Koch et al 1991) is the latest in a line of interesting studies.

Blackford H N, Murray K H A, Stephenson T P, Mundy A R 1984 The
results of transvesical infiltration of the pelvic plexus with phenol in 116
patients. British Journal of Urology 56: 647–649

Bramble F J 1982 The treatment of adult enuresis and urge incontinence by
enterocystoplasty. British Journal of Urology 54: 693–696

Ewing R, Bultitude M I, Shuttleworth K E D 1982 Subtrigonal phenol
injection for urge incontinence secondary to detrusor instability in
females. British Journal of Urology 54: 689–692

Koch M O, McDougal W S, Thompson C O 1991 Mechanisms of solute
transport following urinary diversion through intestinal segments: an
experimental study with rats. Journal of Urology 146: 1390–1394

Mundy A R 1988 Detrusor instability. British Journal of Urology 62:
393–397

Mundy A R, Stephenson T P 1985 'Clam' ileocystoplasty for the treatment
of refractory urge incontinence. British Journal of Urology 57: 641–646

Murray K, Nurse D E, Mundy A R 1987 Secreto-motor function of
intestinal segments used in lower urinary tract reconstruction. British
Journal of Urology 60: 532–535

Nurse D E, Mundy A R 1988 Metabolic complications of cystoplasty.
British Journal of Urology 63: 165–170

Nurse D E, Mundy A R 1989 Assessment of the malignant potential of
cystoplasty. British Journal of Urology 64: 489–492

Chapter 8

Sensory bladder disorders

INTRODUCTION

Sensory bladder disorders are a major problem in urological practice, mainly because the majority of patients defy an exact diagnosis and because the treatment for this majority is so unsatisfactory. This chapter neatly sidesteps this issue by concentrating only on those relatively few patients for whom treatment is possible.

In some patients, of course, bladder sensitivity is secondary to bacterial urinary tract infection, bladder stones, bladder tumours or some other relatively well understood condition. If this group is excluded, two groups remain. The first is that group of conditions in which the pathological problem could be described—albeit somewhat simplistically—as pancystitis. The bladder in these patients, and sometimes the urethra as well, is diffusely involved throughout its circumference and throughout its thickness in a chronic inflammatory process due to a number of conditions of which interstitial cystitis and irradiation cystitis are the most widely recognised. It is this group of problems that this chapter seeks to address.

The other group of patients are those with the same symptoms as the latter group — principally frequency, urgency and a painful bladder — but with no endoscopic or histological bladder abnormality. This group is unfortunately the largest group, the group that makes sensory bladder disorders such an unsatisfactory group to treat, and a group who, in my opinion, are not candidates for surgical treatment with currently available treatment methods except perhaps the phenol technique described in Chapter 7. They will not be considered further.

PANCYSTITIS

These patients, usually middle-aged women, present with frequency, urgency and bladder pain. This pattern of symptoms usually leads to endoscopy rather than urodynamic studies as the first line of investigation. On endoscopy there are usually two striking features — firstly, and most importantly, pain on bladder distension causing the patient to gasp or moan despite the general anaesthetic, and secondly the appearance of the bladder wall.

The gross appearances are variable. There may be a diffuse inflammatory change, discrete areas of bullous oedema, discrete so-called Hunner's ulcers that bleed on distension, or evidence of suburothelial bleeding variously described as petechial haemorrhages, ecchymoses or 'glomerulations'. When bleeding such as this does occur it is often more obvious when the bladder is allowed to empty than it is during filling. Sometimes the bladder appears more or less normal and it is important to remember this because a normal endoscopic appearance does not exclude the possibility of pancystitis.

Deep biopsies are mandatory, firstly to give a histological diagnosis and secondly — and most importantly — to exclude a carcinoma in situ or tuberculosis or some other condition with a specific treatment.

The histological appearance may be classified as:

1. Interstitial cystitis,
2. Chronic non-specific cystitis (without the mastocytosis that is thought to be specific for interstitial cystitis),
3. Eosinophilic cystitis,
4. Irradiation cystitis (in a patient who has had previous pelvic radiotherapy, usually for carcinoma of either the bladder or cervix).

The other endoscopic parameter to quantify is bladder capacity which is often reduced, sometimes dramatically to give a so-called 'end-stage bladder', as a result of chronic fibrosis. Occasionally in a burnt-out case the low capacity is the only striking endoscopic feature.

Urodynamic studies are principally to exclude other causes of frequency and urgency although endoscopy is usually sufficient for this purpose. Common findings in interstitial cystitis, other than pain and a reduced capacity are poor compliance and sphincter weakness (for which there is no satisfactory explanation at present).

After a full evaluation along these lines, patients can be allocated to one of five groups:

— those with interstitial cystitis,
— those with chronic non-specific cystitis who in severe and intractable cases are treated in the same way as interstitial cystitis,
— those with eosinophilic cystitis,
— those with irradiation cystitis,
— those with burnt-out bladders in whom pain may be absent and who have poor compliance and a restricted bladder capacity as their only significant objective abnormalities.

There are of course other causes of a poorly compliant bladder such as longstanding bladder outflow obstruction, often with detrusor decompensation, but in the majority of such patients the bladder capacity is normal or even increased. For descriptive purposes the poorly compliant, 'burnt-out' bladder considered here refers to those who also have a significantly reduced capacity whatever the underlying cause.

Eosinophilic cystitis is a rare condition. It usually causes bullous oedema of the bladder base and trigone, commonly obstructs the ureteric orifice(s), sometimes responds to steroid treatment and is not treated surgically as it always (?) burns itself out, leaving bladder capacity intact. It will not therefore be considered further. A similar more generalised chronic cystitis is occasionally seen in systemic lupus erythematosus and may be treated as for interstitial cystitis if all else fails as it usually affects the bladder dome rather than the bladder base.

INTERSTITIAL CYSTITIS

Interstitial cystitis is a poorly understood condition or group of conditions which can cause debilitating symptoms. It usually affects middle-aged or elderly women and is rare in men. Much attention has been focused recently on the aetiology and pathology and for a review of this work the reader is referred to the publication by Holm Bentzen.

There are two main symptoms of interstitial cystitis — pain and frequency. The pain is typically associated with a full bladder and relieved by voiding and, if voiding is deferred, may be associated with haematuria due to overdistension of the bladder wall. The frequency may be due to the pain or due to a restricted bladder capacity as a result of extensive fibrosis of the bladder wall. In the latter instance particularly, the frequency is the frequent and regular passage of consistent small volumes of urine by day and night, rather than the irregularity in both timing and volume typically associated with detrusor instability.

Cystoscopy shows one of two patterns of involvement. The first is of discrete scars — so-called Hunner's ulcers — predominantly in the dome of the bladder, which bleed on distension and cause pain even under a general anaesthetic. The second is a more diffuse 'cystitis' pattern which involves the bladder more generally causing one of the various types of suburothelial

bleeding described above. Whatever the gross or microscopic appearances of the bladder by far the most important diagnostic feature in either group, in my view, is the moaning with pain through the general anaesthetic. The correlation between symptoms and histopathological findings is so poor that this is the best objective sign with which to substantiate the patient's symptoms of a 'painful bladder'. In the absence of this sign I would be very reluctant to consider surgical intervention unless the patient had a small capacity, poorly compliant 'burnt-out' bladder.

Conservative treatment modalities include bladder distension, oral steroids and intravesical instillations, of which dimethyl sulphoxide (DMSO) is the most widely used and most effective.

Bladder distension often helps in milder cases when the bladder capacity under anaesthetic is well preserved. Oral steroids have been advocated for those patients who fail to respond to bladder distension but I cannot remember seeing a patient in whom they helped. DMSO seems to help some of those with the more diffuse type of 'cystitis', particularly when pain and pain-related frequency are the main symptoms, but is not generally very helpful. When frequency is due to a restricted bladder capacity nothing makes much difference.

Severe symptoms are usually associated with a small bladder and this type of bladder is usually poorly compliant. Despite this predictability, urodynamic studies are important not only to look for this but also to look for sphincter weakness which is extremely common but which is usually asymptomatic because it is overshadowed by the pain and frequency of the interstitial cystitis. It may however become a problem after the latter has been eliminated and it is wise to anticipate this.

The phenol technique does not help

interstitial cystitis and may cause an alarming degree of sloughing of the bladder wall; augmentation cystoplasty is contraindicated because it leaves behind the source of the symptoms and because a shrinking bladder continues to shrink until only the augmentation is left and the original symptoms begin to recur. The only surgical treatment for severe interstitial cystitis is subtotal cystectomy and substitution cystoplasty.

The aim of subtotal cystectomy is to remove that part of the bladder which is involved in the disease but to leave enough of the trigone and bladder neck to give adequate bladder sensation and preserve the function of the bladder neck. (It is also important not to leave too much bladder behind to prevent the cystoplasty from subsequently being converted into a diverticulum, as discussed below.) It therefore follows that if the trigone is involved in the interstitial cystitis then even a fairly radical subtotal cystectomy may be insufficient to relieve the patient of her symptoms and that if the urethra is also involved then the only way to be sure of curing the symptoms is by cystourethrectomy which will in turn require total substitution of the lower urinary tract.

Thus, before advising a subtotal cystectomy and substitution cystoplasty for interstitial cystitis it is important to biopsy the trigone to see if it is involved. If it is, the state of the urethra should be checked as well. If these are both involved then subtotal cystectomy is likely to be insufficient. The alternatives then are either more radical surgery — cystourethrectomy and substitution cystourethroplasty — or for the less heroic patient a continent or conduit urinary diversion. All these options should be considered and discussed with the patient. Subtotal cystectomy and substitution cystoplasty is a major operation but in patients whose outflow tract is not involved the results are predictably good with few postoperative complications. Cystourethrectomy is not as such a much more formidable undertaking but the problems in substitution cystourethroplasty of creating an even-calibred urethra and a satisfactory continence mechanism make it much less predictable in outcome and much more prone to postoperative problems. The same two problems apply to continent diversion although the range of alternative solutions is greater because the siting of the external 'meatus' is for the surgeon to choose rather than predetermined as it is in substitution cystoplasty. For those wanting the simplest solution to their problem an ileal conduit urinary diversion would be much more appropriate. Given these alternatives the patient may decide to live with her symptoms.

Substitution cystoplasty for interstitial cystitis is best performed with an unmodified segment of the right colon. In recent years there has been a burst of enthusiasm for 'detubularisation' in bladder substitution but this is fraught with problems in interstitial cystitis as discussed later on in this chapter.

Before finally embarking on subtotal cystectomy and substitution cystoplasty, it is worth trying an empirical course of doxycycline or oxytetracycline for 6 weeks to see if this gives any improvement. Some patients with chronic non-specific cystitis and a more mild, diffuse pattern of bladder involvement do improve sufficiently to avoid surgery.

SUBTOTAL CYSTECTOMY AND SUBSTITUTION CYSTOPLASTY

(For patients with interstitial cystitis without trigonal or urethral involvement — generally Hunner's ulcer.)

Preoperative preparation
The patient is admitted to hospital 4 days preoperatively for a full 'bowel prep' as described in Chapter 2. 4 units of blood should be cross matched.

Position
The patient is placed supine and draped for a lower midline incision from the pubic symphysis to a point approximately halfway between the umbilicus and the xiphisternum. The upper limit of the incision is governed by the need to mobilise the hepatic flexure and gain access to the middle colic vessels for the substitution cystoplasty.

Procedure
The lower midline incision is deepened down to the peritoneum and the retropubic space is opened to expose the anterior and lateral aspects of the bladder and the pelvic floor all the way round from one lateral pedicle to the other.

The peritoneum is then opened in the midline just below the umbilicus to

allow ligation and division of the urachus and the obliterated umbilical arteries together. The peritoneum is then incised on either side, lateral to the obliterated umbilical arteries (Fig. 8.1), down into the pelvis to the lateral pedicles where the obliterated umbilical arteries originate from the superior vesical arteries. A ring retractor is then placed to hold the incision open and the abdominal contents are packed out of the way with wet packs.

The first part of the procedure is the subtotal cystectomy and the initial stage of the dissection is the mobilisation of the bladder and the clear definition of the upper two thirds of the lateral pedicles.

Firstly the peritoneal incisions on each side are extended over the lateral pedicles and then medially to meet with each other along the line of the posterior margin of the bladder. In women this is along the base of the broad ligaments on each side and over the anterior aspect of the cervix/anterior vaginal wall between. In men it follows the course of the vas on each side and the upper margins of the ampullae and seminal vesicles between. The peritoneal incision is then deepened to open up the space between the bladder base in front and the genital structures behind and between the lateral pedicles on either

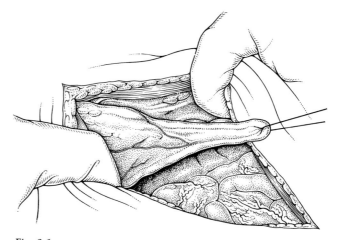

Fig. 8.1

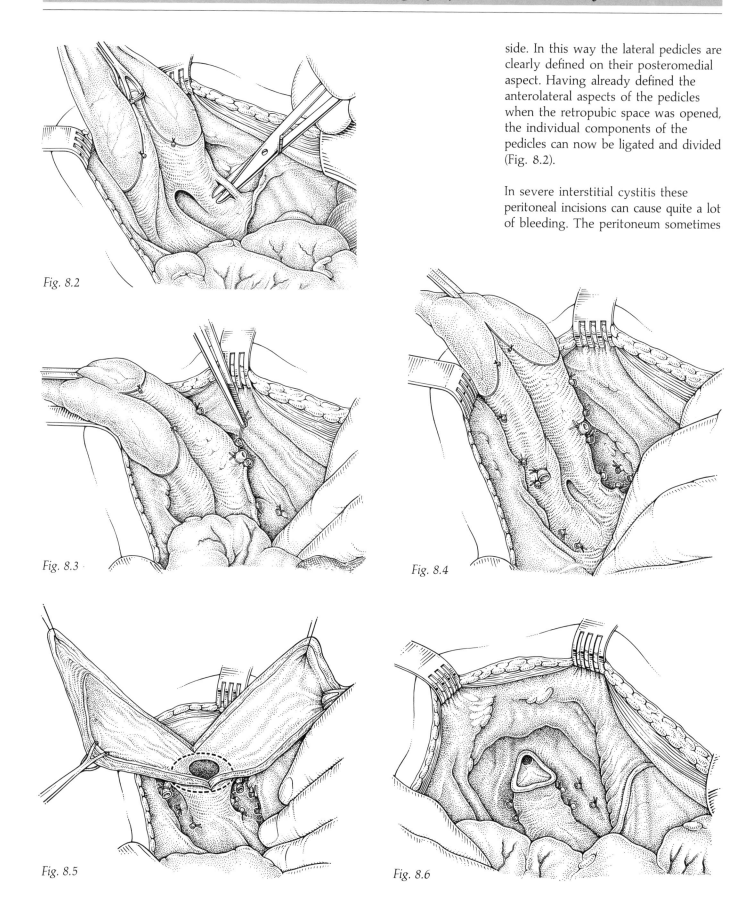

Fig. 8.2

Fig. 8.3

Fig. 8.4

Fig. 8.5

Fig. 8.6

side. In this way the lateral pedicles are clearly defined on their posteromedial aspect. Having already defined the anterolateral aspects of the pedicles when the retropubic space was opened, the individual components of the pedicles can now be ligated and divided (Fig. 8.2).

In severe interstitial cystitis these peritoneal incisions can cause quite a lot of bleeding. The peritoneum sometimes appears the same as the bladder with subperitoneal 'glomerulations' and when this is the case there is often a considerable increase in the vascularity of the connective tissue layer immediately deep to the peritoneum. I sometimes wonder how much this 'interstitial peritonitis' appearance contributes to the pain in severe cases.

It is descriptively convenient to divide the lateral pedicles into four parts — the obliterated umbilical artery, the rest of the superior vesical vessels, the ureter, and the inferior vesical vessels. The first three of these, down to and including the ureter, are ligated and divided in turn. When these have been ligated and divided on both sides (Figs 8.3, 8.4) the bladder above the level of the trigone can be excised. This is most easily achieved by opening the dome of the bladder and then extending down the incision in the sagittal plane so that it is bivalved from the bladder neck anteriorly to the interureteric bar posteriorly (Fig. 8.5). The two ends of this incision can then be extended around the margins of the trigone and bladder neck to excise each half of the bladder in turn (Fig. 8.6).

It is easy to leave too much of the bladder behind particularly if the surgeon intends to leave the ureters in place. If the ureters are left and the margin of the subtotal cystectomy is close to the ureteric orifices then vesico-ureteric reflux is the usual consequence, which may cause postoperative problems in its own right. On the other hand if enough bladder is left to avoid compromising the function of the vesico-ureteric junctions there is a much greater potential for interstitial cystitis in the residual bladder to cause persistent symptoms. More importantly there may be enough residual bladder to cause the cystoplasty to behave as if it were a diverticulum, particularly if there is contracture of the cystoplasty anastomosis. It is surprising to see, at a subsequent cystoscopy, how much of the bladder remains even when you think you have done a really radical excision. It is important therefore to make a distinct effort not to leave any more of the bladder behind than just enough of the trigone to preserve sensation and so the ureters must be disconnected from the trigone and reimplanted into the cystoplasty later in the procedure. The line of excision of each half of the bladder is therefore from the anterior end of the bivalving incision just above the bladder neck,

along the lateral border of the trigone to just below the ureteric orifice, and then along the interureteric bar to the posterior end of the bivalving incision.

Sometimes there is considerable bleeding from the edges of the bladder remnant, in which case the edges are overrun with a running, locking stitch to control it. When haemostasis has been secured the right side of the colon is mobilised for the cystoplasty.

The peritoneum of the right paracolic gutter is incised along the white line lateral to the caecum and ascending colon and this incision is extended around the hepatic flexure above and around the caecum and terminal ileum below. This incision includes the underlying fascia and particularly the so-called phreno-colic ligament at the hepatic flexure. The terminal ileum, caecum, ascending colon, hepatic flexure and transverse colon can then be retracted medially (Fig. 8.7) to expose the ileocolic, right colic, middle colic and interconnecting marginal vessels on the posterior aspect of the colonic 'mesentery' (Fig. 8.8). The duodenum and head of the pancreas, inferior vena cava, ureter and gonadal vessels are thereby clearly exposed.

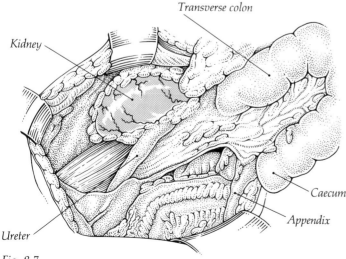

Fig. 8.7
Viewed from the patient's left.

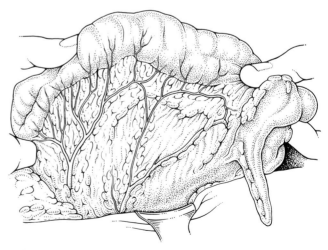

Fig. 8.8
Viewed from the patient's right.

To give a colonic segment of adequate length to act as a substitute bladder of good capacity, and one that will reach easily down to the pelvis for anastomosis to the bladder remnant, bearing in mind that the axis of rotation of the cystoplasty segment is around the ileocolic artery, the colon is divided at the level of the middle colic vessels.

The middle colic artery and accompanying vein usually bifurcate early into distinct right and left branches. The right branch runs down to the right colic and ileocolic as the marginal artery and the left branch runs to anastomose with the inferior mesenteric, also as the marginal artery. The gap between the two branches of the middle colic vessels therefore provides a suitable point to divide the colon, and the right branch of the middle colic artery is a suitable point to divide the vascular pedicle. This is carefully ligated and divided (Figs 8.9, 8.10) and the mesentery is then divided back to the ileocolic vessels, dividing the right colic vessels when necessary.

The vessels of the terminal ileum are then dealt with in a similar way to give a length of ileum of about 5 cm from the ileocaecal valve (Fig. 8.11). The selected points of the ileum and colon are divided to isolate the cystoplasty segment on its vascular pedicle (Fig. 8.12). Intestinal continuity is then restored in the usual way anterior to the cystoplasty segment — I prefer a one-layer closure of inverting interrupted 3/0 Vicryl mattress sutures with the knots on the inside.

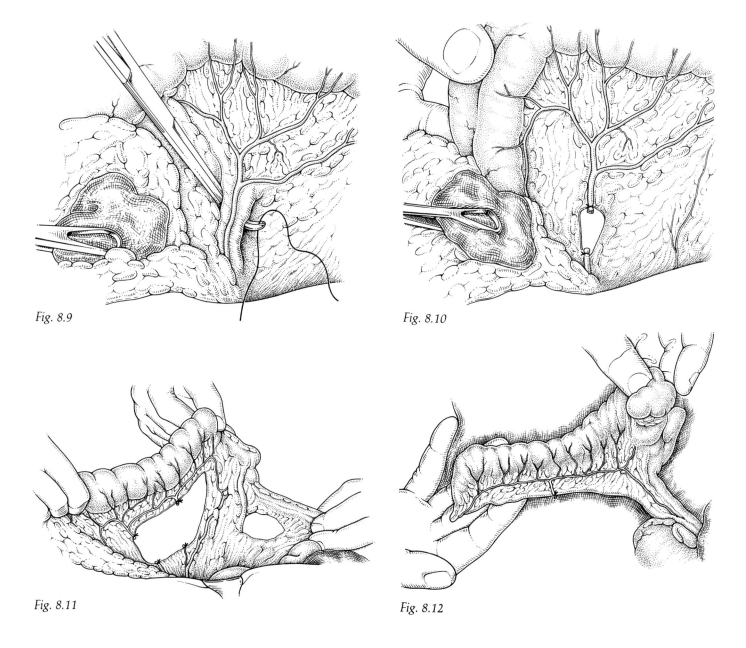

Fig. 8.9

Fig. 8.10

Fig. 8.11

Fig. 8.12

The ileocolonic segment is then washed out with saline to clear away any faecal residue (Fig. 8.13 shows the segment full and gives some idea of its capacity) and rotated through 180° so that the open end of the colon can be anastomosed to the bladder remnant and the ileal tail can be anastomosed to the ureters.

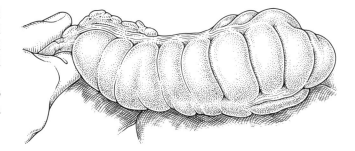

Fig. 8.13

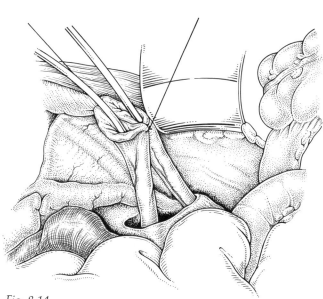

Fig. 8.14

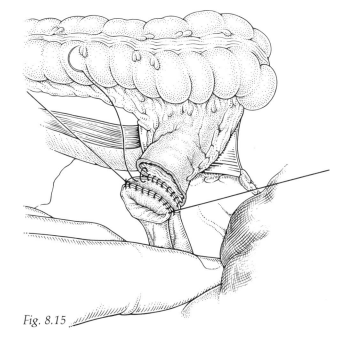

Fig. 8.15

The left ureter is mobilised and brought through to the right side deep to the sigmoid mesocolon and the two ureters are sutured together with interrupted 4/0 Vicryl sutures to give a common ureteric orifice (Fig. 8.14) just above the right common iliac vessels. The common ureteric orifice is then anastomosed to the terminal ileum of the cystoplasty segment (Fig. 8.15). Before completing this anastomosis, splinting tubes (see Ch. 2) are passed up each ureter and then sutured to the common ureteric orifice at some convenient spot to anchor them firmly. The tubes are then passed through the ileocaecal valve and out through the stump of the appendix alongside a cystoplasty catheter (Fig. 8.16) which may need to be trimmed to a length appropriate to the size of the cystoplasty segment.

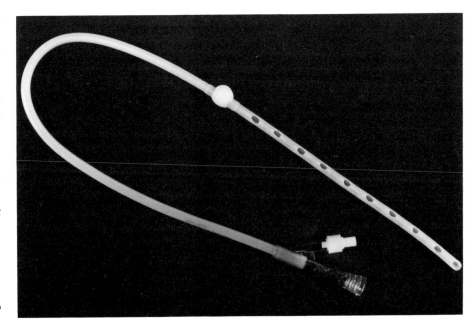

Fig. 8.16

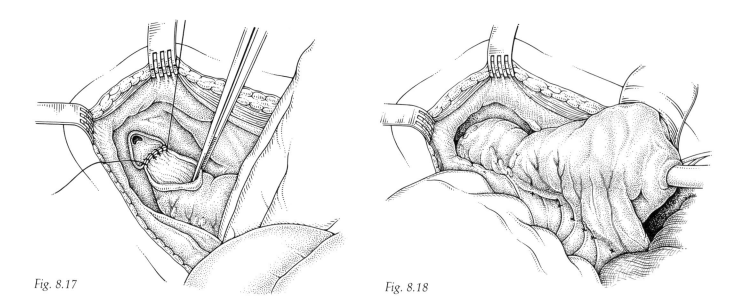

Fig. 8.17

Fig. 8.18

The colonic end of the segment is then anastomosed to the bladder remnant having first made sure that the segment lies comfortably with no undue or excessive twisting of its vascular pedicle. The anastomosis is performed with a running 3/0 Vicryl suture locking at two or three places to prevent constriction of the anastomosis. It is convenient to begin with two lengths of Vicryl in the posterior midline and then to run one around to the right and the other around to the left (assuming the surgeon is on the patient's left side) (Fig. 8.17), knotting them together anteriorly (Fig. 8.18). Each bite should pick up the full thickness of both the bladder and colonic walls to ensure mucosal apposition, inversion of the suture line and haemostasis.

Finally the omentum is brought down to cover the anastomosis and wrap around the cystoplasty segment and all mesenteric defects are closed (Fig. 8.19). A tube drain is left in the retropubic space to drain any oozing or extravasation.

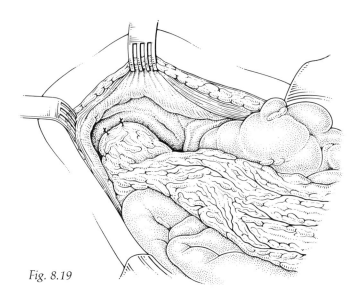

Fig. 8.19

Postoperative care
The drain is removed when it ceases to function. The catheter is clamped on the eighth postoperative day to allow spontaneous voiding. When the patient has been voiding for 24 hours without incident and assuming that measured residual urine volumes are insignificant, the catheter is removed and the patient is discharged home. A follow-up video-urodynamic study is performed 3 months later to ensure that the result is satisfactory.

Complications
The cystoplasty-related problems that might occur are voiding difficulty, frequency, urge incontinence, stress incontinence, bedwetting, urinary mucus and urinary tract infection. The mucus, infective and metabolic problems related to the presence of a bowel segment within the urinary tract have been described already in the last chapter, to which the reader is referred for a more detailed discussion.

Voiding difficulty is unusual unless the patient is male with a competent bladder neck, or a female who has had previous stress incontinence surgery or simply does not realise that she has to strain to void. If 2 or 3 trials of voiding fail, the patient is sent home for a break to return in a fortnight's time for a further trial of voiding. The problem rarely persists. Minor degrees of residual voiding dysfunction may be treated by urethral recalibration as described in Chapter 4.

Frequency is the rule until the patient learns to recognise altered bladder sensation and may persist if there is a significant degree of sphincter weakness or if too large a bladder remnant was left (Fig. 8.20A shows the bladder remnant on VUD with the cystoplasty as a 'diverticulum' in Fig. 8.20B), or if the residual bladder, whatever its size, contains residual interstitial cystitis. It is a disturbingly common problem when the trigonal remnant is involved by the interstitial cystitis — this is unfortunately common in the more generalised type of the disease but fortunately rare in the Hunner's ulcer type of disease. In the patients with residual disease both the frequency and the pain persist. Frequency may also be due to colonic contractions (in which case pain is not an associated symptom) and this is sometimes helped by drugs such as Lomotil, Imodium or Colpermin. Otherwise further surgery is required as described below.

It has to be said that, when frequency was the main indication for the cystoplasty, postoperative frequency is disturbingly common. As a general rule the best results of cystoplasty for interstitial cystitis are in patients with pain as the main symptom or when bladder capacity was grossly restricted by fibrosis.

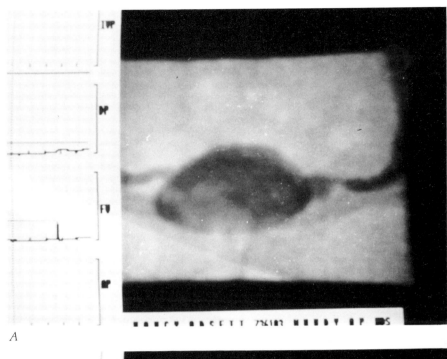

A

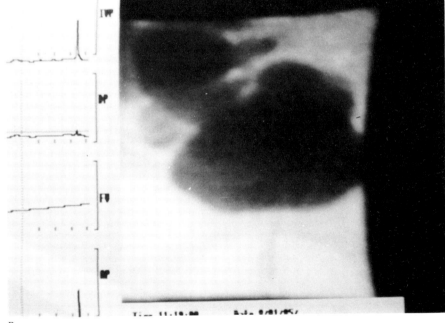

B

Fig. 8.20

Urge incontinence is usually the result of colonic overactivity in association with sphincter weakness. It is rare because a normal (or relatively normal) sphincter should be able to contain the usual degree of colonic activity but, given the preponderance of interstitial cystitis in middle-aged and elderly women and the high incidence of associated sphincter weakness, this ability may be impaired.

There has been a great deal of discussion in the last 2 or 3 years about 'detubularisation' of bowel segments for cystoplasty. The suggestion is that this will eliminate all gut contractile activity and the impression given is that this should be done as a matter of routine.

In the absence of neuropathy or outflow obstruction, isolated but otherwise intact gut segments only generate significant pressures in 50% of right (ileo-)colonic segments and 75% of ileal or sigmoid segments when incorporated into the urinary tract as cystoplasties. The remainder generate no pressure — they are 'docile'. When active segments do generate pressure waves, peak pressures are usually 30–60 cmH$_2$O in the right colon and ileum and 50–100 cmH$_2$O in the sigmoid colon. Detubularisation will usually reduce peak pressures to less than 20 cmH$_2$O in the right colon and ileum and 30–50 cmH$_2$O in the sigmoid colon. In neuropathy, gut segments are much more commonly active and peak pressures may reach 100 cmH$_2$O in the right colon and ileum, and as much as 200 cmH$_2$O in the sigmoid colon although not usually as high as this. Detubularisation in neuropathy generally reduces pressures to the levels seen in 'straight' cystoplasties in the absence of neuropathy but does not entirely eliminate contractile activity in either group.

What detubularisation does achieve is that it gives the maximum potential capacity for any given length of bowel by giving the maximum diameter of the patch thereby produced. If the surgeon's aim is to keep the length of the cystoplasty segment to a minimum — as for example when ileum is being used, to minimise the risks of nutritional disturbance — then detubularisation will give the maximum achievable capacity. When the length of the cystoplasty segment is not critical, as when colon is being used, then the same capacity can be achieved simply by using a longer segment and there is not the need for detubularisation — at least not for reasons of capacity.

My experience with subtotal cystectomy and substitution cystoplasty in patients with non-neuropathic problems is that if the patient has normal bladder sensation (from the preserved trigone) and a normally functioning distal sphincter mechanism, then gut contractile activity in an adequately sized 'straight' cystoplasty is rarely a problem and detubularisation is unnecessary. Of these

two factors a normally functioning distal sphincter mechanism is the more important. Patients with 'straight' substitution cystoplasties following total cystoprostatectomy for bladder cancer have no sensation in the normal sense and have to rely entirely on sphincter function to become continent, as they almost always do (see Ch. 13). Thus although sensation of bladder fullness from a preserved trigone is undoubtedly an advantage, it is not as important as a normally functioning distal sphincter mechanism.

If on the other hand there is deficient sensation from the trigonal remnant or no sensation at all; if the sphincter is not normally innervated or not normally functioning; if the patient has an artificial sphincter; or if the patient has a neuropathy in which case, irrespective of the above factors — most of which are likely to be operative — the bowel is likely to be hypercontractile, then detubularisation is indicated to reduce intravesical pressures to a minimum and get maximum capacity from the neo-bladder. Detubularised substitution cystoplasty will be discussed in the chapter on neuropathic bladder dysfunction (Ch. 10).

The problems with detubularisation are: that there is greater blood loss both peroperatively and postoperatively, increasing the morbidity; that more of the terminal ileum is lost with possible long-term nutritional consequences; and that for the same reason troublesome diarrhoea may be an annoying postoperative problem although all of these can be overcome by variations in technique. More problematic is voiding difficulty which almost always occurs whereas it is rare after a 'straight' cystoplasty. This means that CISC will be necessary much more often. In interstitial cystitis this can be a great problem because the urethra is often hypersensitive, sometimes exquisitely so, making CISC painful or even impossible.

In summary then, detubularisation is a way of getting the largest possible capacity out of a length of bowel, particularly when the available length is restricted. It may coincidentally reduce intravesical pressure in the neobladder but that is arguable. It is reasonable to suggest that in most instances a neobladder should be detubularised as in most instances there is either no bladder sensation (e.g. following total cystectomy) or abnormal sphincter function (e.g. neuropathy, congenital structural anomalies). But in interstitial cystitis the much higher requirement for CISC with a detubularised bladder means that a straight cystoplasty is much to be preferred as hypersensitivity to urethral catheterisation is so common in this condition and problems from neobladder contractibility are so uncommon by comparison.

Patients who do have problems from gut contractions in their cystoplasty who do not respond to Colpermin, Lomotil or Imodium are treated by 'patching' the cytoplasty. The cystoplasty is exposed and opened along its length and an appropriate segment of bowel with a length equal to the length of the incision is isolated on its vascular pedicle, opened to form a patch and sewn into the cystoplasty to form a 'pouch' (Fig. 8.21). The success of this procedure can almost be guaranteed although intravesical pressures are not necessarily reduced to zero.

I have only had to 'patch' a cystoplasty in this way twice (5%) for interstitial cystitis. The vast majority of patients (95%) therefore do not require a detubularised or 'pouch' type cystoplasty and the crucial factor is a normally functioning distal sphincter mechanism.

Stress incontinence. This is not usually a problem in its own right but may be so when associated with colonic activity in the cystoplasty segment as discussed above. Many women seem quite happy to accept a mild degree of stress

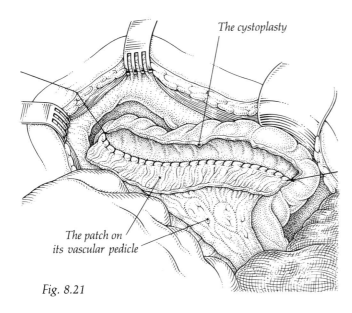

The cystoplasty

The patch on
its vascular pedicle

Fig. 8.21

incontinence after cystoplasty, presumably because they are pleased enough by being rid of the frequency and pain of the interstitial cystitis. This is just as well because sphincter weakness is difficult to treat satisfactorily after a cystoplasty without causing voiding difficulty and its attendant problems.

Bedwetting. This is very common to start with and all patients should be warned to expect it. Presumably it occurs because the zone of bladder sensation is reduced to just the area of the trigone, which should be all that is left of the bladder. Given the relative hypersensitivity preoperatively, this reduction in sensation is all the more profound assuming the trigone itself is not involved. Again the element of sphincter weakness, in conjunction with colonic activity, plays a part. Bedwetting resolves in the majority over about 3 months as the patient re-learns the nature of the bladder sensation.

Some people ascribe bedwetting to reduced urethral pressures at night but this is probably less important than loss of the normal afferent stimulus in the bladder wall that causes a reflex rise in urethral pressure as the bladder fills.

This — combined with loss of awareness of bladder filling, a degree of sphincter weakness and contractile activity in the cystoplasty segment — causes persistent bedwetting in about 10% of patients, particularly in the elderly. When bedwetting does persist then the most important factor to check is bladder capacity. If there is daytime sphincter weakness then an artificial sphincter should be considered but for most patients containment with a condom drainage device in men or appropriate pads and pants will be more suitable.

Urinary mucus. This is rarely a problem — it just takes a bit of getting used to — but patients and their family doctors must be told that it is mucus and not pus. The only times it has been a problem in my experience is firstly when, 7–10 days postoperatively, the suprapubic catheter is clamped and spontaneous voiding starts, because of the accumulation of a week's worth of mucus in a largely recumbent individual, and secondly when intermittent self catheterisation is being used for bladder emptying in children having the operation for neuropathic bladder dysfunction. In both instances bladder irrigation with 30 ml of 20%

acetylcysteine retained in the bladder for about an hour will break up the mucus.

Urinary tract infection. An asymptomatic low growth of mixed organisms is common after a large bowel cystoplasty, occurring in nearly 75% of patients. An overt infection with a single pathogen is not common and suggests an underlying voiding imbalance which should be investigated and treated. The usual cause is a large bladder remnant with 'diverticularisation' of the cytoplasty.

An asymptomatic mixed bacterial growth may not be quite as innocuous as it has hitherto been assumed to be. In Diane Nurse's work, described at the end of the last chapter, it was found that a mixed bacterial growth in colocystoplasties was associated with high urinary nitrosamine levels and the two together were associated with chronic inflammatory changes and epithelial metaplasia in the cystoplasty, the bladder remnant and at the junction between the two. As nitrosamines are known to be the carcinogens responsible for tumours in patients with ureterosigmoidostomies this is a worrying finding which will require further investigation. Suffice it to say that sterilisation of the urine may turn out to be a desirable goal in all patients with cystoplasties, not just those with symptomatic infections and pure bacterial growths on culture.

A summary of the management of a patient with problems following a cystoplasty for interstitial cystitis
From what has been said in the foregoing paragraphs the commonest persistent symptoms are frequency and incontinence and the commonest causes are active disease in the bladder remnant, too large a bladder remnant, sphincter weakness or excessive colonic activity in the cystoplasty.

The first step is urodynamic and endoscopic re-evaluation. If the bladder remnant is too large it will have to be excised down to the bladder neck, assuming that the trigone is free of disease. If biopsies of the trigone and bladder neck area show active disease, irrespective of the size of the bladder remnant, then either the bladder and urethra must be removed with substitution urethroplasty (see below) or the cystoplasty should be converted into a surface diversion depending on the patient's general condition and inclination.

Sphincter weakness incontinence (SWI) may be a problem in its own right or in association with excessive colonic activity in the cystoplasty which is rarely a problem without SWI as well (in my experience). Sphincter weakness can be corrected by a Stamey-type of bladder neck suspension but this may cause voiding difficulty requiring CISC thereafter. It is important therefore to check preoperatively that the patient is willing and able to perform CISC without undue discomfort. It would obviously be a disaster if the patient was subsequently found to need CISC but felt it to be intolerably painful.

Excessive colonic activity on its own is rare — it is usually only a problem when combined with SWI. As discussed above the best way to deal with it seems to be by 'patching' the cystoplasty with a segment of ileum. This will usually correct the problem without the need for a bladder neck suspension which should in any case be avoided because of the likelihood that CISC may be required thereafter. Bladder neck suspension should therefore be reserved for those patients with persistent SWI despite a satisfactory reduction of intravesical pressure by 'patching' the cystoplasty.

CYSTOURETHRECTOMY AND SUBSTITUTION CYSTOURETHROPLASTY

(For female patients with interstitial cystitis involving the trigone and urethra — generally the diffuse non-Hunner's type of the disease.)

This is a larger undertaking than subtotal cystectomy and substitution cystoplasty with a higher risk of complications and an almost certain requirement for CISC to empty thereafter. A surface or continent diversion may therefore be in the patient's best interests, assuming of course that she doesn't decide that she will tolerate her bladder symptoms after all. If a diversion is performed there is no need to remove the bladder. When urine no longer enters the bladder the pain goes away (usually).

The crucial factor in substitution cystourethroplasty is the creation of a continence mechanism. This almost always involves an anastomosis between the neourethra and the neobladder by means of tunnel technique to create a flap valve which — like a Leadbetter — Politano ureteric reimplantation in reverse — will prevent urine entering the neourethra but will allow catheterisation through it to empty the bladder.

The neobladder is best constructed from the ileocolonic segment as described earlier in this chapter with an ileal 'patch' to detubularise the segment to increase its capacity and reduce its contractility. The choice of structure for the neourethra depends on what is available, and this factor and the degree to which the proposed neourethra can be mobilised in turn determine the siting of the 'external meatus'. The simplest situation is the use of the appendix with the proximal end detached and reimplanted into the ileocolonic segment with a tunnel technique and the other end brought out at the site of the natural external meatus. Sometimes the relevant structures are not sufficiently mobile to allow this although of course, the 'external meatus' could always be fashioned on the abdominal wall as a continent diversion.

If the appendix is inadequate or insufficiently mobile or has been removed a suitable alternative neourethra can be constructed from the segment of colon adjacent to that used for the substitution cystoplasty. Another less satisfactory alternative is a labial skin tube neourethroplasty as described in Chapter 12. Both of these guarantee a near normal site for the external meatus because the ileocolonic segment for the cystoplasty can then be rotated through 180° around its vascular pedicle to allow the transverse colonic end to reach down comfortably for the anastomosis of the neourethra. When the appendix is used as the neourethra the anastomosis obviously has to be to the caecal end of the cystoplasty which means that the whole ileocaecal segment has to be more than usually mobile to allow it to drop down low enough into the pelvis for anastomosis of the neo-meatus to the perineum.

The disadvantage of a colonic or labial neourethra when compared with the appendix is that a surgically constructed tube is not as smoothly lined and therefore easily catheterisable as the appendix. In any case a small or atrophic labium may not allow the formation of a skin tube of adequate length for the purpose.

These are the types of consideration that must be taken into account when discussing cystourethroplasty and the patient must be warned that the operative findings may dictate a course other than that which is hoped for.

Position

The low lithotomy position will be necessary to allow anastomosis of the neourethra to form the neomeatus.

Procedure

The preoperative preparation is the same as for subtotal cystectomy and substitution cystoplasty. Having described cystourethrectomy in Chapter 3 and subtotal cystectomy in the last section I will not bore you by describing it again but I should point out that the whole urethra should be removed right out to the external meatus. This is because the neourethra must be anastomosed to the exterior not to a urethral stump, however short. The risk of stenosis of the relatively narrow calibre anastomosis that would result is too high.

With the cystourethrectomy complete the right colon is mobilised as for a substitution cystoplasty. It will then be apparent what the choices are. If the segment has a sufficiently long vascular pedicle to allow the caecum to reach right down to the pelvic floor and if the appendix is reasonably normal in length and calibre then it will be possible to use the appendix as the neourethra.

The appendix is circumcised from the caecum taking a small cuff of caecal wall to make a good wide external meatus when anastomosed to the perineum (Fig. 8.22). The caecal wall and the ileal stump are both closed. Great care is taken to preserve the mesentery of the appendix.

The tip of the appendix is then incised or excised to allow catheterisation with a 12 F or 14 F catheter. One of the caecal taeniae is incised carefully down to the mucosa to create a trench 4 or 5 cm long in which the appendix and its mesentery will lie (Fig. 8.23). The mucosa at the upper end of this incision is then opened. This will become the 'internal meatus'. The tip of the appendix is then sutured to the hole in

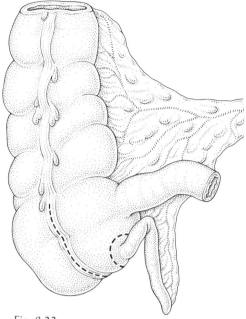

Fig. 8.22
The illustrations for the rest of this Chapter show a non-detubularised right colonic bladder substitute for clarity of presentation. The neo-bladder is actually detubularised along its posterior taenia coli and patched by folding colon down from above or ileum up from below.

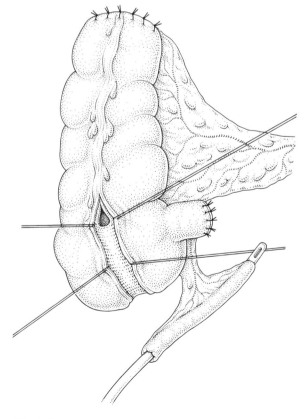

Fig. 8.23

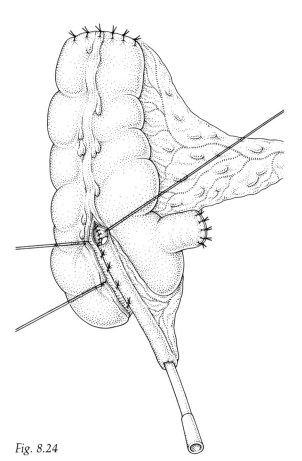

Fig. 8.24

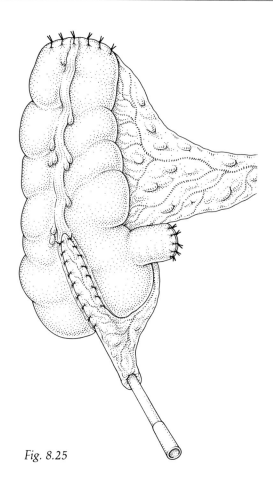

Fig. 8.25

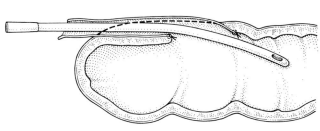

Fig. 8.26

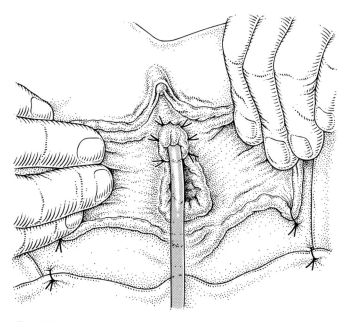

Fig. 8.27

the mucosa with 5 or 6 interrupted 4/0 Vicryl sutures (Fig. 8.24) and the catheter is passed through into the cystoplasty. The appendix is then laid in the gutter created by incising the taenia and held in place by a series of tacking sutures on each side (Fig. 8.25) which also act to make that part of the appendix lying in the trench intramural (Fig. 8.26). In this way is created a continence mechanism resembling the anti-reflux mechanism of Leadbetter—Politano ureteric reimplantation.

The caecal end of the appendix is then trimmed to size and anastomosed transperineally to form a neomeatus (Fig. 8.27). The ureters are then trimmed to length and anastomosed to the cystoplasty segment, again using a tunnel technique, and the cystoplasty is closed with a 22 F suprapubic catheter to ensure adequate urinary drainage.

If the appendix has been removed or is too shrivelled up or otherwise unsuitable, or if the ileocaecal segment is not sufficiently mobile in its natural orientation to reach comfortably to the pelvic floor then this approach will clearly not be possible. If the appendix is satisfactory but mobility is lacking then one solution is to construct the system just described but bring the appendix through to the skin of the abdominal wall as a continent catheterisable stoma, preferably in the umbilicus where it will be concealed.

The other alternative so as to achieve an orthotopic reconstruction is to construct a neourethra from the distal end of the cystoplasty segment. The distal 5 cm or so is carefully separated (Fig. 8.28) from the remainder of the cystoplasty segment, carefully preserving the marginal artery (Fig. 8.29). This 5 cm segment is then trimmed to size so that it can be closed in two layers around a 14 F catheter to form the neourethra, checking before proceeding that it is readily catheterisable — it is much easier

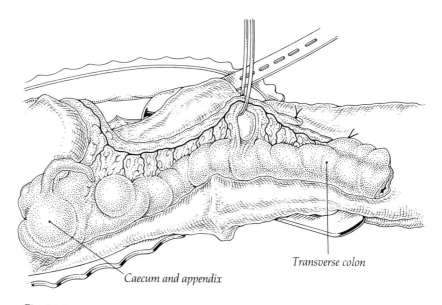

Transverse colon

Caecum and appendix

Fig. 8.28

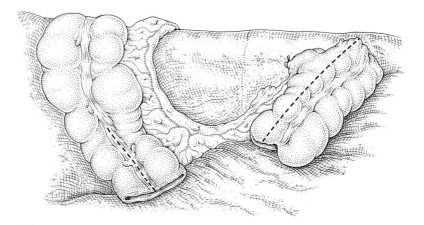

Fig. 8.29

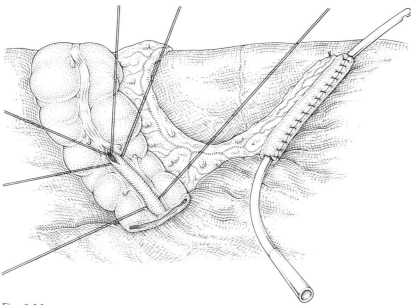

Fig. 8.30

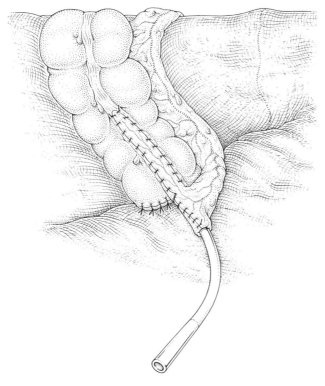

Fig. 8.31

to correct problems now than later. A trench is then formed in a taenia coli (Fig. 8.30) and the neourethra is anastomosed to the cystoplasty (Fig. 8.31) as described above.

Likewise the neourethra is anastomosed to the perineum to form a neomeatus, the ureters are implanted into the cystoplasty and the cystoplasty is then closed with a 22 F suprapubic catheter to provide urinary drainage.

Postoperative management

Both catheters are left in place for about 2 weeks. At that time a cystogram through the suprapubic catheter will show whether or not the anastomoses have healed. If healing is satisfactory as judged by the absence of extravasation and if the neomeatus looks healthy, the urethral catheter is removed, the suprapubic catheter is clamped and the patient starts self catheterisation. When self catheterisation is obviously satisfactory the suprapubic catheter is removed.

Complications

Other than the complications of any cystoplasty (discussed earlier) and the problem of meatal stenosis (avoided by anastomosing the neourethra to the perineum rather than to a stump of natural urethra) the main problems are difficulty with catheterisation and incontinence. Difficulty with catheterisation is quite common when the urethral catheter is first removed, when everything is still a bit inflamed and sore. As long as the neourethra was made easily catheterisable and checked peroperatively this problem should not persist.

Incontinence will be due to failure or breakdown of the tunnelled anastomosis of the neourethra to the cystoplasty, usually because of distal ischaemia in the appendix. This should not occur if the appendicular mesentery is carefully looked after.

With either problem it may be possible to revise the neourethra or its anastomosis to the cystoplasty but limitations of access make it unlikely to succeed. The only alternative is to close off the neourethra if it is incontinent and convert the cystoplasty into a surface diversion.

The use of this technique for continent diversion

As discussed below and in other chapters later on in this book, this technique can be used just as easily for continent diversion as for substitution cystourethroplasty. The only difference between the two is the site of the external meatus.

Alternative techniques of continent diversion are discussed from a practical point of view in Chapter 10 with reference to the treatment of neuropathic bladder problems in children with spina bifida and there is a more theoretical discussion of the 'concepts' of continent diversion in Chapter 15 in relation to undiversion.

POST-RADIOTHERAPY PROBLEMS

Post-radiotherapy problems are of two main types: irradiation cystitis in either sex following radiotherapy to the pelvis for whatever reason and the combined effects of irradiation and a hysterectomy in women with carcinoma of the cervix.

Irradiation cystitis

Severe irradiation cystitis can only really be treated by cystectomy and substitution cystoplasty. Lesser procedures have no effect on the 'cystitis' symptoms although haematuria as an isolated symptom may be controlled. The only real problem, having decided that the symptoms are severe enough to warrant surgery, is to decide whether to remove the whole bladder (and prostate in men) which more or less guarantees relief of

symptoms but risks incontinence or to leave the trigone which risks persistence of symptoms but with less likelihood of incontinence. My approach depends on whether the problem is mainly one of 'cystitis' or one of reduced bladder capacity assuming that it is possible to make such a decision. If gross reduction of bladder capacity is the problem I would advise total cystoprostatectomy, as for bladder cancer, in men but a subtotal cystectomy, as for interstitial cystitis, in women, with substitution cystoplasty in both sexes.

As with interstitial cystitis, the results of substitution cystoplasty in those patients with a grossly reduced bladder capacity are good. Because of the risks of surgery in the heavily irradiated pelvis this sort of surgery should only be considered in younger and fitter patients who are well motivated. For the remainder and for those whose problem is active pancystitis, a continent diversion using either of the techniques described in the last section for substitution cystourethroplasty but bringing the meatus of the neourethra out as a stoma on the abdominal wall or preferably in the umbilicus, where it is concealed, is a simpler and safer solution to the problem. This, in my opinion, is one of the best indications for continent diversion, the particular advantage being that all of the surgery is kept out of the irradiated area. Obviously for the more fragile patient or those who want the simplest solution to their problem an ileal conduit urinary diversion would be best, leaving the bladder behind. As with interstitial cystitis diversion of the urine stops the bladder pain.

Post-radiotherapy/hysterectomy problems

There are three main types of problem — irradiation cystitis, stress incontinence and fistulae. Whenever a patient presents with any symptom after radiotherapy and a hysterectomy it is wise to bear all three in mind both as potential diagnoses and as potential

complications of subsequent treatment. Thus, for example, irradiation cystitis may restrict bladder capacity and thereby compromise the results of the treatment of stress incontinence (if that is the presenting problem) and simple closure of a fistula (if that is the presenting problem) may give an unsatisfactory result because of a small capacity, poorly compliant bladder and sphincter weakness.

That aside, generalised irradiation cystitis is managed as described above. Fistulae are described in Chapter 12.

A major problem is that irradiation cystitis in some patients is sharply circumscribed (perhaps not surprisingly after radiotherapy for carcinoma of the cervix particularly). A common finding is of a sloughing ulcerated area over the trigone with surrounding oedema and erythema and often an adherent stone or calcified 'mush'. There is a strong urge to biopsy such lesions but this should be done very carefully because there is a high risk of a fistula developing and one which will be very difficult to treat. A biopsy should therefore be taken with great care.

Removal of stone material often helps symptoms considerably. Cystectomy and cystoplasty should only be performed in patients with incapacitating symptoms because the involvement of the bladder neck area makes reconstructive surgery fraught with problems (see Ch. 12). As always in difficult situations, when surgery is discussed the discussion should include the alternatives of continent or ileal conduit urinary diversion.

Stress incontinence after radiotherapy and hysterectomy can be a big problem. It is not clear whether it is due to surgical damage to the pelvic plexuses during excision of the upper vagina or due to radiotherapy, and, if it is the radiotherapy, whether it is a direct effect on the urethra or a more remote effect

Chapter 9

Non-neuropathic urodynamic problems in children

Interest in the urodynamic problems of children has developed relatively recently as compared with adults, and these problems are less well understood as a result. Only where urodynamics and reconstruction meet, as in epispadias, is there a 'history' of interest in surgical intervention.

Most urodynamic problems in children are similar in cause or type to those seen in adults and most do not require surgical treatment. The pattern is different — detrusor instability is much more common and sphincter weakness much less so than in adults — and the approach is different, mainly because there is a natural tendency for improvement during puberty, particularly with detrusor instability.

If the major congenital structural abnormalities considered in Chapter 14 are excluded, the non-neuropathic problems that need to be considered are:

— detrusor instability
— sphincer weakness incontinence
— the 'post-valve bladder' seen after treatment for posterior urethral valves
— the 'bad bladder' of indeterminate cause.

Other conditions are occasionally seen. Bladder neck obstruction (in boys) and distal urethral obstruction (in girls) do occur in children and have been dealt with briefly in Chapter 4. Interstitial cystitis (Ch. 8) is another rare occurrence in childhood. Voiding inefficiency is seen in the prune belly syndrome and in children with lazy bladders who consciously void as infrequently as possible. When treatment is required then, as in adults with severe voiding inefficiency, CISC is the treatment of choice.

DETRUSOR INSTABILITY

In the majority of children the symptoms are the same as in adults — frequency, urgency and urge incontinence — but bedwetting is much more common. Impaired development of bowel control is also fairly common but not commonly volunteered. Some children attempt, consciously or unconsciously — it is difficult to tell — to resist unstable detrusor contractions by contraction of the distal sphincter mechanism and this contraction sometimes occurs during voiding as well as when the child is attempting to hold. Obstructed voiding results and, when this is longstanding, produces the appearance of a much more aggressive bladder than usual. This pattern is called the 'occult neuropathic bladder' or 'non-neuropathic neuropathic bladder' by some but the postulated 'neuropathic' aetiology is purely conjectural and in my view the condition simply represents the end result of voluntary sphincteric obstruction attempting to contain an extreme form of detrusor instability. It may be that this can go on, as in longstanding obstruction in adults, to give detrusor decompensation and poor compliance. This problem is certainly seen in boys and girls, often with hydroureteronephrosis and impaired renal function, for no apparent reason and it is tempting to ascribe this to a pathological progression similar to that seen in adult males with bladder neck or prostatic obstruction.

Outflow obstruction is indeed an occasional cause of detrusor instability in boys although rarely so. The three conditions to consider are dyssynergic bladder neck obstruction, previously unsuspected posterior urethral valves and anterior urethral 'valves'. All of these are rare causes of otherwise apparently uncomplicated detrusor instability in childhood: firstly because they are uncommon problems in any case whereas detrusor instability is very common; secondly because obstructions commonly cause poor bladder emptying which more commonly causes a palpable bladder and recurrent urinary infection; and thirdly because obstructions more often present earlier in childhood (age 2–3 years if not earlier) than does detrusor instability (age 7 or thereabouts).

Milder obstructions may however be overlooked in early life if the bladder is still capable of reasonable emptying.

Dyssynergic bladder neck obstruction and posterior urethral valves are easily diagnosed video-urodynamically if the diagnoses are considered but anterior urethral valves may be missed because the anterior urethra is not usually within the radiological field of a video study. The clue therefore is the peak pressure of the unstable detrusor contractions. If these are in excess of $70\,cmH_2O$ and particularly if they are in excess of $100\,cmH_2O$, and therefore in the 'obstructed' range, outflow obstruction should be suspected and the full length of the urethra should be screened radiologically.

Usually the symptoms of detrusor instability in childhood are life-long but there is a group of children, usually aged 9 or 10, who present with a much more acute onset and often much more severe incapacitation. In both groups the symptoms tend to improve during later childhood and it is this fact that tends to colour the approach to treatment more than anything else.

Fortunately most children respond to treatment with anticholinergic drugs such as oxybutynin (or improve coincidentally but spontaneously). Supportive measures such as bladder training and the use of enuresis alarms are also important, indeed for many paediatricians they are the principal lines of treatment. Not only is the response rate to drugs higher than in adults but the side-effects in children are less. The dry mouth that plagues adults on anticholinergic drugs is rarely seen in children, even on an adult dosage.

Some children do not respond to medication and it is difficult to know what to do with them. On the one hand we have a treatment modality in 'clam' ileocystoplasty which we know will work and on the other hand we know that the problem will often clear up spontaneously by the end of the teens (even if we also know it will recur in later life in many). In my view an ileocystoplasty is rarely if ever warranted in childhood, however apparently incapacitating the symptoms, because of the unknown long-term side-effects of incorporating bowel segments into the urinary tract. It seems unacceptable to risk even a theoretical possibility of tumour in the long term to treat a problem that in the short term will usually resolve spontaneously.

This approach begs the question 'When is the end of childhood and when therefore would one suggest surgical treatment and its potential risks?'. The time, in my view, is when the individual has made the break with home. It is at this time (again a strictly personal view) that two things happen. Firstly there is the social impact of taking responsibility for oneself — the ultimate in 'bladder training in childhood'. Having to stick to a timetable of work, take care of one's own washing and bedclothes (perhaps sharing the bed with someone else) and the general culture-shock of striking out on one's own are the factors that often seem to reverse a previously intractable bladder. If the problem persists despite all of this then it seems likely to stay. Secondly the patient is more likely to understand the implications and risks of surgical intervention and is also more likely to comply with follow up to ensure thereby that those risks are reduced to a minimum.

In summary then, my view is that at the present time detrusor instability is a condition that should not be treated

surgically in children except in unusual circumstances.

STRESS INCONTINENCE

Compared to detrusor instability and consequent urge incontinence, this is uncommon in girls and very rare in boys in the absence of surgical damage to the distal sphincter mechanism or a major structural abnormality.

The two main causes in girls are a congenitally incompetent bladder neck and a congenitally short urethra (also associated with bladder neck incompetence). In neither does urethral sphincteric incompetence necessarily occur but when it does, and particularly when detrusor instability coexists, sphincter weakness incontinence can and does occur. It is worth emphasising that in both conditions when severe symptoms do occur, detrusor instability, overt or occult, almost invariably coexists. Occult in this context means that the instability may be masked on urodynamic investigation by sphincter weakness and a consequent limitation of bladder capacity.

Symptoms usually include frequency and urgency as well as daytime and sometimes night-time wetting even in the absence of coexisting instability. In such circumstances this may be a reflection of a reduced bladder capacity and a reduced ability to hold, in some it may be an indication of hypersensitivity (some attribute this to the presence of urine in the proximal urethra but this is unproven) or it may simply be due to the fact that the history is usually given by the mother who interprets the child's symptoms in her own words and in the light of her own experience.

Urodynamic investigation may be confusing or inconclusive. In some, bladder neck incompetence alone is shown with no overt sphincter weakness incontinence because the child is able to

hold for the short duration of the study. In some, detrusor instability and bladder neck incompetence coexist without leakage. In the remainder leakage occurs either because of instability or sphincter weakness. The study must therefore be evaluated cautiously and carefully.

The distinction between a congenitally incompetent bladder neck (urodynamic bladder neck incompetence with an endoscopically normal urethral length) and a congenitally short urethra (both investigations abnormal) is purely academic. The treatment is the same for both. Indeed they may both be manifestations of the same condition with the short urethra being the more extreme form.

In theory the treatment of both should be by reconstruction of the bladder neck as for epispadias (Ch. 14). Unfortunately, in my experience this is rarely effective on its own unless a frankly obstructive bladder neck is produced making the child dependent on CISC thereafter. The reason is that bladder neck reconstruction does nothing to improve the function of the distal sphincter mechanism. Improvement in sphincter function is best achieved by colposuspension and this is the procedure of choice unless the urethra is so short that a bladder neck reconstruction is necessary in order to achieve a satisfactory colposuspension.

The other reason why bladder neck reconstruction is rarely helpful is that most girls with symptoms severe enough for surgical intervention to be considered often have overt or covert detrusor instability as well. As I have said before in this book (and will say again) it has always been my experience that when detrusor instability and sphincter weakness coexist, the detrusor instability is always the most significant problem no matter how minor it appears urodynamically, unless the sphincter weakness is extreme.

For pure sphincter weakness incontinence the results of surgery are acceptably good but not as good as in adult women with 'simple' stress incontinence. Because of this it is best to defer surgery until puberty, firstly in the hope that symptoms improve as the urethra becomes thicker and more vascular and secondly because this gives the vagina a chance to mature which makes colposuspension easier and more effective.

When there is overt instability or there are marked symptoms of frequency and urgency suggesting 'occult' instability, the results of colposuspension with or without bladder neck reconstruction are poor. Surgery should therefore be avoided if at all possible until simultaneous clam ileocystoplasty is justifiable along the lines outlined in the last section. This assumes of course that the problem does not respond to anticholinergic medication.

THE POST-VALVE BLADDER

The bladder in posterior urethral valves is potentially dangerous to renal function even after elimination of the obstructing valves themselves. Upper urinary tract obstruction may persist and progress either because of 'obstruction' to the intramural ureters by the thick-walled bladder or, more commonly, because of urodynamic dysfunction of the bladder as a whole.

The serious urodynamic dysfunction in the post-valve bladder is poor bladder compliance causing persistently raised intravesical pressures. The exact cut-off point between a safe bladder pressure and a dangerous one has not been clearly established and may well vary according to the degree of renal impairment or, to be more exact, the renal filtration pressure. As a guide, pressures below 25 cmH$_2$O seem to be safe, pressures above 40 cmH$_2$O are certainly dangerous and pressures

between 25 and 40 cmH$_2$O should be watched carefully.

The pressures that matter are the pressures that are normally present in the bladder which are not necessarily the same as those found on urodynamic study if the bladder is first emptied and then filled thereafter. It is important to study the pressures over the volume range that the child's bladder carries under usual circumstances of filling and emptying. Other abnormalities such as detrusor instability and vesico-ureteric reflux act to compound the problem but poor compliance and consequent persistent elevation of intravesical pressure is the main problem.

Occasionally the bladder after posterior urethral valves becomes decompensated and chronic retention develops. This is also associated with poor compliance and elevated intravesical pressures but the pressures in such cases tend to be lower than when detrusor contractile activity is preserved.

Another cause of dangerous urodynamic dysfunction is the development of a urethral stricture at the site of the valve resection. Obviously, persistent valvular obstruction should also be excluded. By contrast, bladder neck obstruction does not occur although the bladder neck may look very prominent radiologically. This prominence is due to a combination of generalised thickening of the detrusor, of which the bladder neck is part (albeit with differences of structure histologically), and excavation of the prostatic urethra between the bladder neck and the valves because the tissue in this area is less resilient than the bladder neck itself.

A final urodynamic problem to consider is sphincter weakness incontinence due to damage at the time of valve resection.

A careful video-urodynamic evaluation should give an exact diagnosis as far as

the lower urinary tract is concerned and may explain persistent and progressive upper urinary tract dysfunction but is often inconclusive on its own in this respect. Persistent and progressive upper urinary tract dysfunction is usually diagnosed on the basis of deteriorating renal function combined with obstructive changes on ^{99m}Tc-DTPA renal scanning but unfortunately the scan is often inconclusive particularly when renal function is severely impaired. In such circumstances percutaneous upper tract pressure studies (Whittaker testing) may (but do not usually) help. An alternative if investigations thus far are inconclusive is DTPA scanning or even just simple estimation of the serum creatinine before and after 2–3 months of indwelling urethral catheterisation (or vesicostomy in small children). If either of these parameters improves with a period of indwelling catheterisation then it is safe to infer that there is a persistent and progressive upper tract problem and that the urodynamic dysfunction is the cause. It should be stressed that this discussion is concerned with persistent and progressive renal deterioration due to active lower urinary tract dysfunction as distinct from persistence or deterioration of any intrinsic renal disease that developed as a consequence. It is the distinction between these two that is all important.

Treatment
Treatment is primarily concerned with preservation of renal function. Incontinence alone is only a relative indication for surgical treatment although many if not most of those with progressive renal impairment will also be incontinent. If incontinence is the only problem then detrusor instability is usually the cause and this is treated as described in the first section of this chapter.

Mild sphincter damage is sometimes compensated for by prostatic growth at puberty. Severe sphincter damage, which is rare these days, may require implantation of an artificial sphincter, as described in Chapter 6 in general and in Chapter 10 with particular reference to retropubic implantation of the cuff. For reasons of growth this is best deferred until 10–12 years of age but this is not an absolute rule.

Other than detrusor instability and sphincter weakness, the other problem that is sometimes seen, although less commonly, is poor bladder emptying. This may be due to residual valve tissue or to a stricture at the site of previous valve resection and these should obviously be excluded by endoscopy. Otherwise poor emptying is due to ineffective detrusor contractile activity as a result of decompensation. This is best treated by clean intermittent self catheterisation (CISC) but this may be impossible in practice because the catheter gets caught up in the prostatic urethra below the posterior lip of the bladder neck. If this occurs it might seem tempting to resect the lip of the bladder neck but this should not be done because the bladder neck may well be the only effective sphincter mechanism that the child has. The alternatives are either a vesicostomy or an indwelling suprapubic catheter in younger children or a Mitrofanoff procedure (Ch. 10) in older children. The Mitrofanoff procedure is also useful if there is a difficult stricture causing chronic retention. It has the advantage of giving continued and regular bladder filling and emptying as well as continence and is a useful temporising measure in this situation until either the lower urinary tract improves spontaneously or the child is in better shape for definitive treatment. In general poor bladder emptying only needs surgical treatment if it is causing secondary upper tract changes or recurrent urinary infection. Otherwise it is best left alone.

Surgical treatment of the post-valve bladder is necessary when poor compliance and detrusor instability are causing persistent and progressive upper tract problems in which case a clam cystoplasty is performed as described in Chapter 7. If there is vesico-ureteric reflux or proven vesico-ureteric junction obstruction (which is rare), ureteric reimplantation using the Cohen technique may be performed simultaneously. Substitution cystoplasty is rarely necessary.

In those patients who are likely to require renal transplantation it is important to get the lower urinary tract right before transplantation if at all possible. The post-valve bladder destroys transplanted kidneys just as effectively as it does native kidneys. All too often one sees children who lose their transplanted kidneys for just this reason. The most important point is to do the cystoplasty when there is a good urine throughput. 'Dry' cystoplasties are difficult to manage because of the mucus accumulation that occurs. If absolutely necessary this can be dealt with by twice daily acetylcysteine washouts using 30 ml of a 20% solution instilled either by CISC or through an indwelling catheter but this is often unsuccessful at dealing with the problem and it is much better, if at all possible, to plan the child's management to include the cystoplasty before end-stage renal failure is reached and to transplant the child without an intervening period on dialysis. If this is not possible it is best to do the cystoplasty some months after transplantation when renal function has stabilised and the future of the transplanted kidney looks promising. Until then the bladder should be kept on free drainage with either an indwelling catheter or a vesicostomy.

THE 'BAD BLADDER' OF INDETERMINATE CAUSE

If you work in conjunction with a busy paediatric renal unit you will regularly come across children with renal failure of variable degree who have dilated upper tracts but no evidence of vesico-ureteric reflux or outflow obstruction who are nonetheless abnormal. The bladder is often thick-walled and poorly compliant, often with a significant residual urine, sometimes with detrusor instability but more commonly with no evidence of instability and no evidence of voluntary detrusor contractile activity either. The sphincter mechanisms may appear normally functioning; more commonly they appear to open inadequately during voiding but there is no conclusive abnormality.

If outflow obstruction can be excluded urodynamically and endoscopically then an exact diagnosis will be impossible but, as indicated above, I believe that many if not all of these children will have developed this urodynamic pattern as a result of longstanding detrusor instability with voluntary sphincteric 'obstruction' in an attempt to resist incontinence. My experience is that by the time these children have developed an acontractile or decompensated detrusor with secondary upper tract changes the abnormality has become irreversible and surgical intervention will be required to prevent further deterioration of the upper tracts. The situation is therefore the same as in the post-valve bladder and is treated along the same lines.

REFERENCES

The articles by Borzyskowski & Mundy and Mundy et al refer to
non-neuropathic urodynamic problems in children in general and to the
congenital wide bladder neck anomaly respectively. Unfortunately there
is little in the way of high quality publications in this field — not that
either of these two articles would qualify for that distinction. Hopefully this
defect will be corrected before long.

Borzyskowski M, Mundy A R 1986 Videourodynamic assessment of diurnal
urinary incontinence. Archives of Diseases in Childhood 62: 128–131
Mundy A R, Murray K, Nurse D, Borzyskowski M 1988 The 'congenital'
wide bladder neck anomaly: a common cause of incontinence in children.
British Journal of Urology 59: 533–538

Chapter 10

Neuropathic vesicourethral dysfunction

For descriptive purposes it is convenient to consider neuropathic problems as having three anatomical and three urodynamic subgroups:

The anatomical sub-groups are:
    Suprapontine lesions
    Suprasacral cord lesions
    Sacral and peripheral lesions

The urodynamic subgroups are:
    Contractile
    Intermediate
    Acontractile.

There are occasional exceptions and variations but in general this theme works very well in clinical practice for all types of neuropathic problems, congenital and acquired.

The categorisation is simplified because suprapontine lesions generally cause contractile dysfunction and peripheral lesions generally cause acontractile dysfunction; only cord lesions cause all three.

There are other factors that influence the presentation and management of neuropathic bladder problems apart from the behaviour of the detrusor and the sphincter mechanism and these may be at least as important as the urodynamic abnormality if not more so.

These other factors include vesicourethral sensation, the presence or absence of voluntary control of voiding or of the pelvic floor musculature, the general neurological status especially affecting the abdomen and lower limbs, the state of the anorectum, sexual function, general intelligence and manipulative skills. Thus normal sensation in a male may (but does not usually) preclude intermittent self catheterisation as a treatment option; residual sensation and pelvic floor control means that the patient may present with frequency, urgency and possibly urge incontinence rather than just insensible incontinence; those with

abdominal muscle activity can strain to void, those without cannot; the greater the lower limb disability the larger the interval between voids must be for continence to be a worthwhile goal — controlled incontinence (indwelling catheter, sphincterotomy and condom drainage device, urinary diversion) is generally preferable to hourly frequency in a wheelchair-bound patient; constipation makes all bladder problems worse; patients have to be intelligent enough to comply with some types of treatment or the treatment may not work; certain treatment options such as CISC and the use of an artificial sphincter require intelligence and manipulative skills. These are but a few examples.

Contractile bladders
A contractile bladder (Fig. 10.1) is one that is capable of contracting with sufficient strength and duration to produce a useful degree of bladder emptying assuming that there is no associated outflow obstruction to restrict emptying or that any obstruction has been, or can be, eliminated. In patients with suprapontine lesions there is no associated outflow obstruction, because the lesion is above the level in the pons

where detrusor contraction and sphincter relaxation are coordinated, unless of course the patient has coincidental benign prostatic hyperplasia or some other unrelated condition. In patients with cord lesions detrusor-sphincter coordination is often damaged by the lesion and outflow obstruction occurs due to detrusor-sphincter dyssynergia. In addition, 50% of patients have bladder neck incompetence for reasons which are not clear.

Persistent untreated outflow obstruction may lead to poor compliance but this is unusual; compliance otherwise is normal.

Patients with residual sensation will have frequency, urgency and urge incontinence. If sensation is absent the incontinence will be the only symptom.

If there is residual control of the pelvic floor musculature then the patient may be able to resist incontinence but pelvic floor control does not mean that the patient does not have detrusor-sphincter dyssynergia, indeed the reverse is more likely to be the case.

In summary then, patients with contractile bladders and suprapontine

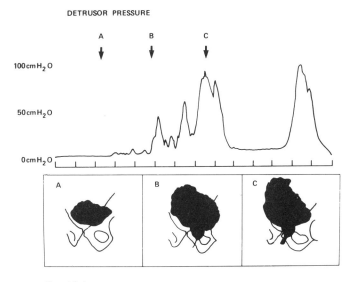

Fig. 10.1

lesions have detrusor hyperreflexia but no detrusor-sphincter dyssynergia whereas those with cord lesions may have both. This means that those with suprapontine lesions are not at risk of upper tract problems whereas those with suprasacral cord lesions are because of the sphincteric obstruction.

Intermediate bladders
Intermediate type bladders (Fig. 10.2) are only found in patients with cord lesions, usually those with extensive cord injuries or spina bifida in the thoracolumbar region. In this group detrusor activity is present but it does not cause discrete bladder contractions that give a useful degree of emptying. Indeed the contractile activity is more a constant writhing or fibrillation when looking at the detrusor pressure trace. Bladder compliance is reduced; whether or not the detrusor activity is the cause of the poor compliance is not known but in my opinion it probably is although undoubtedly secondary fibrotic changes develop in the bladder with time which make compliance worse.

The bladder neck is always incompetent unless the bladder is emptied to less than its usual residual volume when bladder neck closure may occur.

The distal sphincter mechanism tends to be of fixed resistance, or functioning in a way similar to the bladder but with the same end result. Thus, above a certain bladder pressure, overflow incontinence occurs and below that pressure retention occurs. Thus the distal sphincter is both incompetent, causing sphincter weakness incontinence, and obstructive (called static distal sphincter obstruction — SDSO — to distinguish it from the DSD seen in the contractile group), causing a high intravesical pressure and residual urine. This high intravesical pressure is a potent cause of upper urinary tract obstruction.

A degree of sensation is occasionally retained in these patients but pelvic floor control rarely, if ever, is.

Acontractile bladders
This pattern may be seen in cord lesions or peripheral lesions (Fig. 10.3). Here there is little or no detrusor activity. If there is then a low-pressure form of the intermediate type should be suspected. This is important because if sphincter weakness incontinence is corrected, an acontractile bladder remains acontractile whereas a low-pressure intermediate type develops high pressures with all the attendant complications.

Acontractile bladders due to cord lesions often have normal compliance whereas in those due to peripheral lesions compliance is usually reduced, possibly due to a higher degree of outflow resistance in the latter group.

Like an intermediate bladder, an acontractile bladder has bladder neck incompetence and a distal sphincter that is both incompetent and obstructive. However, as the levels of urethral resistance are lower than in the intermediate group, at least in patients with cord lesions, sphincter weakness incontinence predominates and tends to mask the degree (often very mild) of outflow obstruction. In peripheral lesions urethral resistance tends to be higher

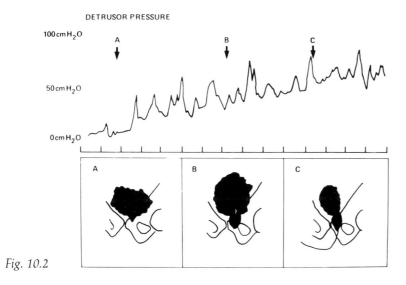

Fig. 10.2

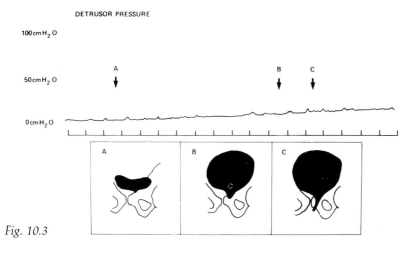

Fig. 10.3

than that seen in cord lesions and so a degree of residual urine, often quite large, is common.

In practice the bulk of patients with neuropathy requiring urological intervention have either congenital cord lesions or spinal cord injuries. Patients with acquired non-traumatic neurological problems rarely require surgical intervention although some patients with multiple sclerosis (or similar spastic paraplegias) require a clam ileocystoplasty for uncontrollable detrusor hyperreflexia or, in a few men, a sphincterotomy for detrusor-sphincter dyssynergia. In some patients surgery should be strenuously avoided, notably men with Parkinson's disease who are only helped surgically by a transurethral resection of the prostate for acute retention.

ASSESSMENT

Although it is obviously important to get a full investigation of all patients, one can, with practice, make a good guess as to the pattern of abnormality from one feature alone. Thus an average patient with multiple sclerosis would be expected to have an incomplete suprasacral cord lesion causing detrusor hyperreflexia and detrusor-sphincter dyssynergia. The main variable will be the competence or otherwise of the bladder neck. This has obvious therapeutic considerations because if a sphincterotomy is deemed necessary for DSD a patient with a competent bladder neck will be unchanged postoperatively, whereas a patient with an incompetent bladder neck will be rendered totally incontinent.

Similarly the finding of a detrusor pressure trace showing poor compliance and high frequency, short duration, low amplitude detrusor activity in a patient with an extensive thoracolumbar cord lesion would lead one to expect to find an incompetent bladder neck, sphincter

weakness incontinence, static distal sphincter obstruction and residual urine on the video study.

The importance of this anticipatory 'guesswork' is not so as to avoid the need for more detailed study but because it makes the surgeon more likely to spot odd findings which do not fit the usual pattern. An example might be the observation of sphincteric obstruction in a patient with a suprapontine lesion. In fact this may be seen with cerebral palsy and with Parkinson's disease and related conditions, but it is nonetheless unusual. Equally it is most unusual to see bladder neck obstruction in neuropathy and rare to see sphincter weakness with a contractile bladder. The latter is very suggestive of previous surgical intervention.

Assessment involves:

1.	Assessment of the urinary tract problem,
2.	Assessment of the general neurological problem,
3.	Assessment of the urinary tract problem in relation to the overall neurological problem,
4.	Assessment of the prognosis for both the urinary tract problem and the neurological disease,
5.	Assessment of the patient as an individual.

It is important to consider all these factors because in neurological disease it is common to find differences between different patients in their assessment of the importance of their urological problem in relation to their other disabilities and in relation to their age and experience. These in turn alter the surgeon's approach to treatment.

Thus it is common to find in transverse myelitis (for example) in a young teenage girl that initially the patient is paraplegic and emotionally devastated and that the bladder is hyperreflexic. Six

months later, perhaps, the paraplegia is considerably improved and she is at home. Back with her friends she is severely embarrassed by urge incontinence. This she finds more of a disability than a bit of residual leg weakness. Six months later her legs are entirely normal for all practical purposes and she now has a large capacity acontractile bladder because the pattern of bladder behaviour in transverse myelitis tends to change with time. She is now wet because she is disinclined to use CISC properly except when she goes out with her boyfriend when her main worry is incontinence during intercourse. Her parents' main worry is the bedwetting. Her teachers' main worry is that she smells at school and her family doctor's main worry is recurrent bacteriuria. A year later, having previously been apathetic, she has learnt to empty well by straining because she is going to get married and she is effectively asymptomatic, essentially without any specific treatment. The urological surgeon may have been tempted to intervene at any of the earlier stages in response to any of the individual's pressures and the end result may not have been so good.

Assessment of the urinary tract problem

Although clinical features give some guide, video-urodynamic studies are the basis for lower urinary tract assessment. If there is perineal sensation there may be urethral sensation, if there is an anocutaneous reflex there is likely to be detrusor contractility, and if the anal sphincter is lax, the urethral sphincter is likely to be 'lax' as well, but this is not sufficient for deciding on treatment. (These are however very useful diagnostic and prognostic clinical signs in the very young and should not be overlooked.)

An IVU is a useful screening investigation for the upper urinary tract, but a good quality ultrasound study is perfectly adequate for routine follow up or as a first time study if reflux is shown on video-urodynamics to be absent.

If the IVU or ultrasound are abnormal, a ^{99m}Tc-DTPA scan should be the next step if obstruction is suspected. A measurement of GFR and a ^{99m}Tc-DMSA scan to look at total and differential renal function should be organised if there is a suggestion of impaired renal function.

Assessment of the general neurological problem

The important points are: the severity of the neurological dysfunction; the time since onset of the problem (or the last attack with diseases such as multiple sclerosis); whether the neurological deficit is static and likely to remain so or, alternatively, chronically deteriorating or remitting and relapsing; are the hands impaired or likely to be so; is the patient mobile and if so how does he or she get around; is the brain affected or likely to be so?

Obviously if the hands or brain are likely to be affected any form of treatment requiring intelligence, cooperation or manipulative skills, such as the use of intermittent self catheterisation or an artifical sphincter will be contraindicated. The question of mobility is discussed below under 'Assessment of the individual'.

The relationship of the bladder problem to the overall neurological deficit

This concerns the relative importance of incontinence (or recurrent retention due to DSD in MS or related problems) in relation to impotence, bowel problems, flexor spasms, autonomic dysreflexia and the like. Many patients get referred because they have a bladder problem regardless of whether or not they may want treatment. There is no point in treating an incontinence problem just because it is there (the Everest syndrome), particularly when the

patient's main concern lies elsewhere.

Assessment of the prognosis

Here it is important to pick out those who are at risk of upper tract problems by virtue of outflow obstruction or poor compliance or a combination of the two.

As far as the underlying neurological disease is concerned the main prognostic points are whether or not the hands and brain are likely to be involved, thereby influencing manipulation, motivation, intelligence and cooperation, and whether or not further loss of mobility is anticipated. Obviously the likelihood of improvement is also important to note but neurological diseases are not renowned for their tendency to improve.

Assessment of the individual

Everybody wants normality for themselves and their children. It is all too common to be referred hopelessly 'windswept' patients with urinary incontinence in the hope that they might be made dry and therefore more normal.

With few exceptions surgery for neurological problems tends to be fairly major surgery with a fairly high incidence of niggling postoperative problems requiring minor secondary procedures or supplementary therapy for their correction. A common example is voiding dysfunction after cystoplasty which may require CISC. If disappointment and upset is to be avoided this requires intelligence, understanding, motivation and manipulative skills on the patient's part. Such attributes are often lacking, particularly in spina bifida patients who form one of the largest groups (if not the largest) for whom such treatment may be considered. Many spina bifida patients, particularly with controlled hydrocephalus, appear to be bright, but they often lack manipulative skills, motivation and the general ability to maintain a sustained interest and approach to a problem. This has obvious

implications when it comes to a consideration of major surgery, particularly if there is going to be an interval period in a multi-stage procedure, when acute depression and anxiety states are common, or when compliance with CISC or the use of an artificial sphincter is necessary.

I am always cautious about operating on wheelchair-bound patients, particularly males. There is no great advantage in continence in the wheelchair-bound as the time involved in finding a disabled-person's toilet and transferring from wheelchair to toilet and back again will take up a substantial part of anyone's day if there is any degree of frequency. Males are often perfectly adequately controlled with a condom collecting device and patients of either sex may be kept dry with the use of an indwelling catheter. Females are more difficult to keep dry and implantation of an artificial sphincter, if that is all that is required, is, in my opinion, reasonable and can be justifiable even, occasionally, in men. But when cystoplasty, sphincter ablation and an AUS would be necessary then a simpler alternative such as a continent or conduit urinary diversion would seem to be preferable. Best of all the patient may be a candidate for implantation of a Brindley sacral anterior root stimulator, but this applies almost exclusively to patients with complete spinal cord transections with preservation of an intact cord below the level of the lesion.

On the other hand, confinement to a wheelchair should not, in my view, be regarded as an absolute contraindication to reconstructive surgery. Many such patients are intelligent, happy individuals with a useful contribution to make and should not be denied surgical treatment on the basis of one parameter alone. Each patient should be assessed as an individual and their problems assessed in the light of *all* the relevant considerations of which lack of mobility is but one.

Finally one should remember the special problems of patients who get around on crutches with or without the use of calipers as well. The effort that this involves causes very considerable surges in intra-abdominal pressure with each step that are often so high that no artificial or surgically reconstructed sphincter can resist. This is an important factor to consider when faced with a patient with a naturally obstructive sphincter mechanism. Preservation of the natural sphincter with CISC may leave the patient a lot drier than sphincter ablation and an AUS.

Equally there are some patients who use crutches and calipers or wheelchairs who could be dry theoretically with CISC but in whom the circumstances of life in calipers or a wheelchair make CISC impracticable. In these circumstances a continent diversion with an abdominal stoma through which they can easily do CISC may be an ideal solution.

The obvious point is that there is more to the assessment of a patient than just the urodynamic assessment.

TREATMENT OPTIONS

After a full investigation and assuming that all non-surgical methods have failed to help or are inappropriate, the procedures that might be necessary are:

Corrective treatment of sphincter obstruction
— sphincterotomy

Corrective treatment of sphincter weakness
— implantation of artificial sphincter

Corrective treatment of detrusor dysfunction
— the phenol technique
— augmentation cystoplasty
— substitution cystoplasty

Palliative treatment
— suprapubic catheterisation with or without urethral closure
— the Mitrofanoff procedure
— other forms of continent urinary diversion
— conduit urinary diversion.

Several of these procedures (the phenol technique, implantation of an AUS in a female and around the bulbar urethra in a male, and augmentation cystoplasty) have been described in previous chapters. The others will be described here and the remainder will be discussed where there are special considerations or variations in technique which apply to this particular group of patients. Otherwise the reader is referred to the descriptions in earlier chapters.

It is important to remember that patients with neuropathic dysfunction usually have multiple urodynamic abnormalities and so are likely to need more than one treatment modality, although not necessarily surgical.

SPHINCTEROTOMY

Throughout most of urological training one works in fear and trepidation of damaging the distal sphincter mechanism. I always therefore feel somewhat guilty when performing a sphincterotomy. Perhaps other surgeons do as well. In many ways this is probably a good thing because few procedures are so (theoretically) quick and simple and yet have such a profound effect.

The procedure is rarely required except in some male patients with multiple sclerosis, spinal cord injury or a congenital cord lesion. In a patient with a contractile bladder who has a competent bladder neck, continence should be (theoretically) unchanged afterwards. If the bladder neck is incompetent or the patient has an intermediate type of bladder then the patient will become totally incontinent. This is obviously not a problem for a male patient if it is intended that he uses a condom drainage system thereafter, but otherwise some consideration must be given to the means of maintaining social continence postoperatively. It is therefore always important in all patients, before undertaking a sphincterotomy, to reconsider alternative methods of treatment namely intermittent or permanent catheterisation. In most patients CISC is a much better option than sphincterotomy and should be tried first, reserving sphincterotomy for failures. In female patients sphincterotomy is rarely indicated. CISC is infinitely preferable.

Technique
There is no special preparation other than to ensure that the urine is sterile. If not, the procedure should be performed under antibiotic cover.

A resectoscope with a diathermy point is used. A loop resection of the sphincter often leads to heavy bleeding. If the bladder neck is competent and it is intended that it should remain so, care should be taken not to damage it. If a bladder neck incision is planned then a bilateral incision at 5 o'clock and 7 o'clock, or an incision at either of these points and then in the anterior midline, is usually more effective than a single incision as is normally used for simple dyssynergic bladder neck obstruction.

Using the diathermy point, the incision runs from just below the bladder neck (Fig. 10.4) through the remainder of the prostatic and the membranous urethra down into the bulbar urethra. The cutting mode will be necessary to breach the urothelium but once through the urothelium the coagulation mode gives a more gentle incision and therefore better control.

The aim of the incision is to divide the full thickness of the sphincter throughout its length. The incision must therefore be at least 5 mm deep (in an adult) throughout the extent from bladder neck to bulbar urethra. At this depth the adequacy of the incision is usually shown by the change in appearance of the tissue from homogeneous to flimsy (as with a resection of the prostate that has gone right out to the capsule) and by bleeding.

At the end of the procedure the lower limit of the incision should be seen to be well below the level of the verumontanum (Fig. 10.5). When the procedure is finished a urethral catheter is passed and left in for 48 hours.

The paucity of landmarks means that a sphincterotomy is often incomplete and it is commonly necessary to repeat the sphincterotomy to divide any remaining sphincter-active tissue, particularly distally. This residual tissue has the appearance of a stricture at the site of the sphincterotomy when seen radiologically at about three months from the time of the procedure. (It is surprising, in fact, when one considers how easy it is to damage the sphincter

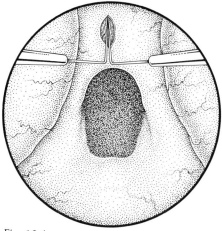

Fig. 10.4

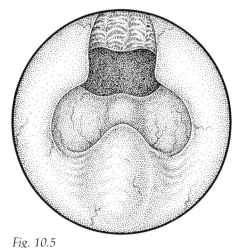

Fig. 10.5

unintentionally during a transurethral resection of the prostate, with disastrous incontinence as a result, how difficult it is to damage the sphincter mechanism intentionally during a sphincterotomy. Perhaps neurological disease alters the morphology of the sphincter mechanism as well as its function.)

Sphincterotomy, it should be stressed, is rarely required in female patients except sometimes as a preliminary to implantation of an artificial sphincter because the alternatives of intermittent or indwelling catheterisation are usually preferable. When required it is usually best performed with a nasal speculum and a hand-held, angled diathermy needle incising the distal half of the urethra to a depth of about 5 mm under direct vision. The technique is similar to that described and illustrated in Chapter 4 for bladder neck incision in women.

IMPLANTATION OF AN ARTIFICIAL SPHINCTER

Implantation of an artificial sphincter has already been described in general and for bulbar urethral cuff placement in male patients in Chapter 5 and for female patients in Chapter 6. The technique of implantation of an AUS in females is the same irrespective of the cause of the incontinence and need not be described again here — if anything it is easier in females with neuropathic sphincter weakness because they have usually not had all the previous retropubic surgery that other groups have had.

In general, retropubic cuff placement is preferred in younger male patients with neuropathic sphincter weakness for four reasons:

1. In children and younger adolescents the bulbar urethra is smaller than the smallest available cuff.
2. Positioning the cuff above the level of the ejaculatory ducts in those with preserved sexual function will allow antegrade ejaculation while continence is maintained.
3. The tissues of the bladder neck area seem to tolerate a higher pressure than the bulbar urethra.
4. Continence appears to be controlled more effectively.

On the other hand:

a.   Further bladder neck, prostate or sphincter surgery is hazardous once a retropubic cuff has been implanted, whereas it is easy with a bulbar urethral cuff. Given the high incidence of prostate disease secondary to sphincter obstruction, this is an important consideration.

b.   Revision of a retropubic cuff is more difficult than revision of a bulbar urethral cuff, particularly if the patient has also had a cystoplasty.

c.   Implantation of a retropubic cuff after a previous cystoplasty is also difficult irrespective of the question of revision.

Thus each case needs to be decided on its merits although obviously the size of the bulbar urethra is an absolute consideration. In general, however, I prefer a retropubic cuff placement if possible.

Retropubic placement of an AUS cuff in a male

The preoperative preparation is as for all patients having an artificial sphincter and is described in Chapter 2. The patient is placed supine on the operating table and prepared and draped for a Cherney/Pfannenstiel incision.

There are two sites where the cuff might be placed:

1.   Above the level of the ejaculatory ducts, around the bladder neck in patients where the preservation of antegrade ejaculation is desirable, when AUS placement is the only procedure being undertaken.

2.   Around the membranous urethra when antegrade ejaculation is not an important consideration and when a cystoplasty is being performed at the same time or is likely to be performed at some stage in the future. The more distal site keeps the cuff away from the cystoplasty suture line through which it would otherwise tend to erode. Because

of the common need for a cystoplasty in patients with neuropathy I prefer the membranous urethra site for most patients.

Either way the first step is to open the retropubic space widely to expose the bladder, the prostate and endopelvic fascia of the pelvic floor. The endopelvic fascia and pubourethral ligaments are then incised (Fig. 10.6) to expose the prostate and the subprostatic urethra lying in the sling of the levator ani, as described in detail in Chapter 3.

For a membranous urethral cuff placement, a pair of curved forceps such as a Lahey forceps or a Satinsky clamp are passed around the subprostatic urethra. The calibre of the urethra is then measured and a cuff of the appropriate size is pulled through into place (Fig. 10.7). If the correct plane has been found there is only slight resistance to the Lahey forceps in the posterior midline in the region of the rectourethralis. No other resistance should be found.

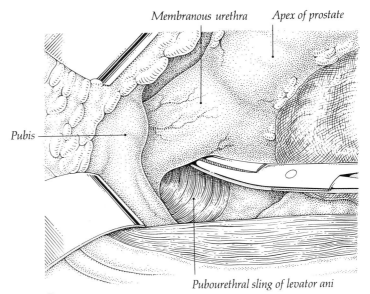

Membranous urethra   *Apex of prostate*

Pubis

Pubourethral sling of levator ani

Fig. 10.6

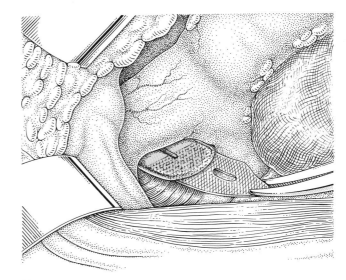

Fig. 10.7

For a bladder neck placement the layer of fascia that encloses the bladder neck, prostate and genital structures must be broken through to allow the cuff to be passed between the bladder neck anteriorly and the ejaculatory ducts, ampullae and vesicles posteriorly. With practice and with a balloon catheter in the bladder it is usually possible to feel a gap between the urinary and genital structures once the endopelvic fascia has been incised and a pair of Lahey forceps can then be insinuated through into this plane. When performing this manoeuvre for the first time it is sensible to open the bladder to allow the bladder neck and trigone to be seen and palpated whilst the Lahey forceps or Satinsky clamp are being manipulated through.

When the forceps have been passed round it is useful to pull a sling through to hold the plane open. This passageway must be stretched up to accommodate the width of the cuff, a measuring tape must then be passed and finally the cuff itself. The sling will make sure that all further manipulations take place in the plane already dissected without causing further trauma.

The main problem arises when the bladder or urethra (or both) have been damaged. The presence of a cuff will cause failure of healing and a persistent hole in the bladder or urethra. Even if the hole is repaired the presence of a cuff close by, let alone in direct contact, always seems to prevent normal healing. It is therefore essential to interpose tissue between the cuff and the damaged zone and omentum is best used for this purpose. Obviously, in the male, another solution is to site the cuff in a different place, either at the membranous urethra, if the bladder neck has been damaged, or vice versa, or alternatively, if the patient is large enough, to abandon a retropubic cuff site and place the cuff around the bulbar urethra.

The rest of the procedure and the subsequent management of the patient

are as for all other patients with artificial sphincters, as described in Chapters 5 and 6.

Much the most common and important complication of AUS implantation in patients with neuropathy is infection. This occurs in about 15%, which is much higher than in post-prostatectomy or female stress incontinence where the incidence is only about 2%. Why this should be so is not clear but it may be related to skin changes secondary to incontinence that many neuropathic patients have. Chronic ammoniacal dermatitis (nappy rash) is common in this group and this leads to an altered and more pathogenic bacterial flora and fungal overgrowth as well. Many patients also have appliances or catheters to control their incontinence which act as foci or reservoirs of infection. Faecal incontinence and immobility add to these problems.

Preoperative preparation must seek to neutralise these problems as far as possible, cleaning the patient up outside and in, to keep the infection rate down. Skin problems must be healed, if necessary with a period of indwelling catheterisation to allow the skin to dry up although the catheter must be removed a few days before surgery so that the urine can be sterilised.

In the long run 1 in 3 patients with neuropathy require a reoperation after AUS implantation. Half of these are for the same problems that affect all patients, particularly the requirement to change the pressure-regulating balloon for one with a higher range. The other half will be for infection. In these patients the device must be removed before infection leads to erosion, particularly in female patients, because erosion significantly reduces the chances of implanting another device at a later date. To keep the plane open to facilitate reimplantation an omental wrap should be performed — a tongue of omentum is mobilised and pulled into

the space previously filled by the cuff. In women labial fat pads serve the same purpose. Three to six months later another device is implanted. Unfortunately the same statistics apply so ultimately about 3% will develop repeated infections and after three attempts I give up — if the patient hasn't already given up.

The question of simultaneous bowel surgery and its effect on the risk of infection of an AUS is discussed below. Essentially, it makes no difference.

THE PHENOL TECHNIQUE

This has already been described in detail in Chapter 7. There are no special variations in technique for patients with neuropathy. The main use for this procedure is in women with multiple sclerosis and drug-resistant detrusor hyperreflexia, particularly those more debilitated patients with indwelling catheters who are leaking around their catheters. Most of these ladies will be helped by the phenol technique although in many the benefit is only short lived.

AUGMENTATION CYSTOPLASTY

If a cystoplasty is required and an augmentation cystoplasty is possible then this is the procedure of choice. Again the reader is referred to Chapter 7 for details of this technique. If the bladder is unusually small or thick-walled or causing secondary vesico-ureteric junction obstruction then substitution cystoplasty will be required but this is not very common.

For most patients with neuropathic bladder problems for whom reconstructive surgery is indicated, augmentation ('clam') cystoplasty is likely to be the procedure they require because bladder dysfunction is much the commonest urodynamic problem.

Surgery is rarely indicated in high cord lesions because most patients in the category respond to anticholinergic medication. The patients in this category most likely to require a cystoplasty are women with multiple sclerosis. Most patients with lumbar, lumbosacral or sacral cord lesions will have either a spinal cord injury or spina bifida. With complete spinal cord transection the Brindley sacral anterior root stimulator should be considered. Cystoplasty is therefore mainly indicated for mobile patients with either incomplete spinal cord injuries or spina bifida. Most such patients have a degree of detrusor hyperreflexia or autonomous contractile

activity or poor compliance or a combination, and a degree of sphincter weakness as well. Only an occasional patient has pure sphincter weakness for which an AUS alone would be appropriate. In the remainder a 'clam' cystoplasty is necessary, often with an AUS as well to correct sphincter weakness (Fig. 10.8 — note the irregularity of the bladder outline due to the ileocystoplasty). Unfortunately the requirement for an AUS is not always predictable so we have adopted a policy of implanting the cuff alone at the time of the 'clam' whenever an AUS seems likely to be necessary, leaving the cuff tubing plugged off in the inguinal canal

where it can be found at a later date if necessary to connect to the rest of the components.

If a policy of using a 'clam and a cuff' procedure is followed about one third will be continent thereafter without the need for implantation of the remainder of the AUS. In the remaining two thirds of patients a degree of incontinence will remain which will require implantation of the rest of the device at a later date. Because one third is a significant percentage of patients cured with one procedure alone and because implantation of the remainder of the AUS is a relatively minor subcutaneous

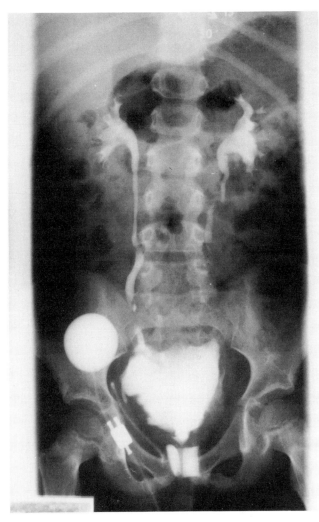 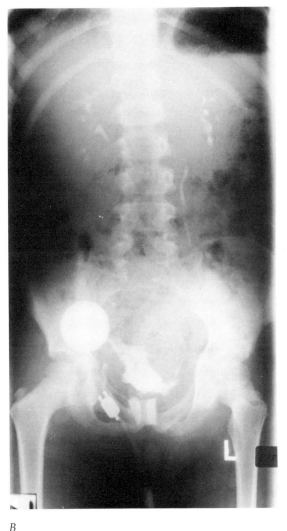

Fig. 10.8   A   B

procedure, having done the difficult part — implanting the cuff — previously, this seems a reasonable approach to adopt. To a certain extent the need for an AUS at all can be anticipated by the degree of sphincteric obstruction seen on preoperative video-urodynamic studies. If there is significant sphincteric obstruction giving a fair-sized residual urine volume, especially in the face of high intravesical pressures, then an AUS will probably not be necessary, and a cuff is not implanted. A cystoplasty alone should suffice with CISC to provide bladder emptying thereafter. A relatively weaker sphincter with no substantial residual urine despite low intravesical pressures, on the other hand, will almost certainly require an AUS as well as a cystoplasty and the entire device is implanted. Unfortunately most patients are not as clear cut as this and fall in between these two groups. Furthermore sphincter behaviour sometimes seems to change after a cystoplasty for reasons which, as with so many things, are not clear. It is for this 'in between' group — which is the majority — that the clam and a cuff approach is indicated.

In theory, simultaneous cystoplasty and AUS implantation would be expected to lead to a high incidence of infection of the AUS but this does not seem to be the case, although this is not everybody's experience. In my own experience the incidence of infection is the same with simultaneous cystoplasty as with implantation of an AUS alone, assuming that an ileal segment is used for the cystoplasty and that there has been a satisfactory preoperative bowel preparation. Interestingly, in the few device infections that have occurred, most patients who were using CISC and were continent before removal of the infected AUS have remained continent afterwards. The reason for this is, again, not clear but it seems likely that the cuff caused the development of a restrictive sheath around the urethra that remained

as a sort of obstructive 'sphincter mechanism' thereafter.

Sphincter weakness is of course only one aspect of sphincteric dysfunction in neuropathy. The other consideration is sphincteric obstruction and its effect on bladder emptying, particularly in patients with intermediate type bladders who are the largest group for whom surgery is considered and in whom sphincter weakness and sphincteric obstruction commonly coexist. This sphincteric obstruction means that intermittent self catheterisation is commonly required and all patients must expect to have to self catheterise and prove preoperatively that they are willing and able to do so. If they are unwilling or unable to self catheterise they should not be considered for this type of surgery whatever the reason. It is important to stress that a requirement for self catheterisation in this group of patients is not a complication of cystoplasty, it is a necessary result of reducing intravesical pressure and abolishing involuntary contractile activity in patients who coincidentally have sphincteric obstruction as part of their urodynamic abnormality.

SUBSTITUTION CYSTOPLASTY

In general this is indicated when a cystoplasty is required but when the bladder is so abnormal that a 'clam' is impossible. Thus when the bladder is more than usually thick-walled, when the bladder capacity is more than usually reduced, or when there is vesico-ureteric junction obstruction and most commonly when all three of these criteria apply, a substitution cystoplasty is preferred to a 'clam'. Since the introduction and widespread use of the clam procedure, substitution has been required only rarely.

When used for patients with neuropathic bladder dysfunction, the technique of substitution cystoplasty has to be varied

from that described in Chapter 8 for interstitial cystitis because of the increased contractile activity of the colonic segment used for the substitution in neuropathy. Whereas a substitution cystoplasty in a neurologically normal individual may generate no pressure at all worth mentioning or at worst may generate pressures of up to 50 or 60 cmH$_2$O, pressures in neuropathy are regularly in excess of 100 cmH$_2$O. As most patients with neuropathy also have sphincteric incompetence or an artificial sphincter, which makes them unable to resist these contractions even in the lower pressure range, or loss of sensation, which makes them unable to sense them and therefore unable to resist them, these involuntary cystoplasty contractions may cause a severe degree of incontinence. Accordingly, the cystoplasty technique has to be modified to reduce colonic contractile activity as far as possible. This is achieved by opening up the cystoplasty segment to disrupt the continuity of the smooth muscle and then reconstituting it in some other way, usually to form a pouch shape. This is certainly effective in reducing the risk of postoperative incontinence but it must be emphasised that although pressures are considerably reduced they are not abolished altogether. These questions are discussed in more detail in Chapter 8. The principle of the procedure is much the same as for clam cystoplasty in that a patch is incorporated into the colonic bladder by mobilisation of part of the terminal ileum with the right colonic segment, then opening the ileum and colon along the antimesenteric border and then sewing them both together to form an ileo-colonic pouch. In this way the cystoplasty is said to be 'detubularised'. Certainly it looks more like a bladder radiologically (Fig. 10.9 — here combined with an AUS although in this view only the pressure-regulating balloon is visible) than does a straight cystoplasty.

Technique

The operation begins with a subureteric subtotal cystectomy. It is important to remove as much as possible of the bladder to prevent diverticularisation of the cystoplasty segment. If any bladder is left above the level of the trigone and ureteric orifices, there is always far more left than anticipated. Leaving just the trigone avoids this problem and leaves quite enough for anastomosis to the cystoplasty segment. The theoretical advantage of leaving the ureters and ureteric orifices intact — to avoid the need to reimplant them into the cystoplasty — is offset by the two disadvantages of leaving too much bladder behind and of almost inevitable reflux if the bladder is excised close to the ureteric orifices. There is therefore no advantage in leaving the ureters in place and three potential disadvantages:

— diverticularisation of the cystoplasty segment
— contractile activity from the residual bladder
— vesico-ureteric reflux.

For the cystoplasty itself I prefer to use the ileocaecal segment (many surgeons prefer a long section of ileum) because colon forms the bulk of the cystoplasty and colon is physiologically more expendable than ileum and, more importantly, the mobilised colon will predictably reach into the pelvis for anastomosis to the bladder remnant without tension which is not the case with ileum.

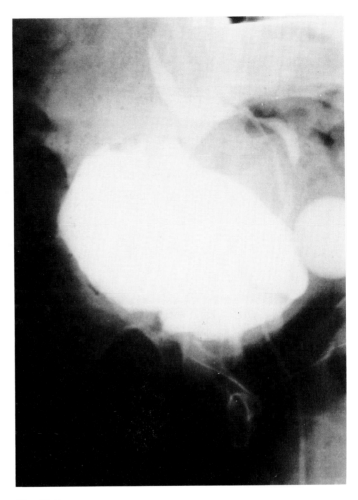

Fig. 10.9

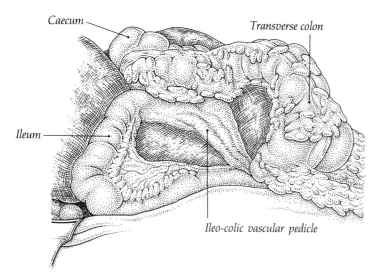

Fig. 10.10

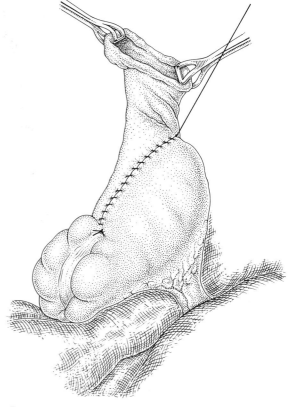

Fig. 10.13

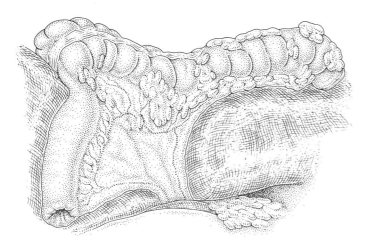

Fig. 10.11

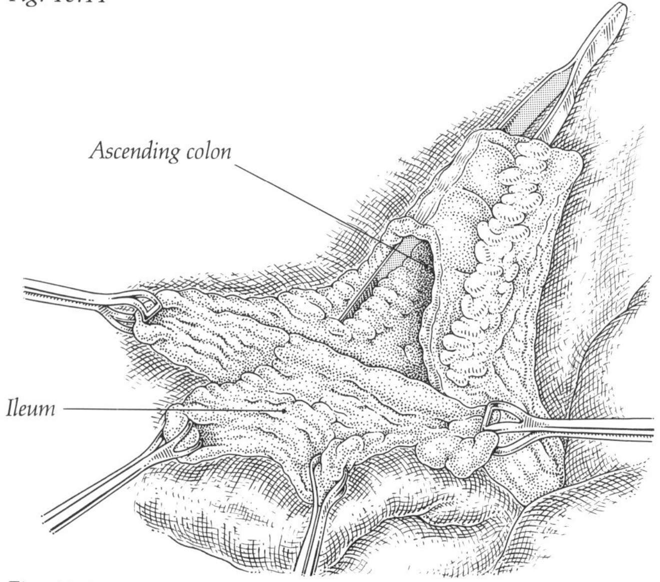

Fig. 10.12

In practice the procedure is almost exactly the same as that described for a 'straight' substitution cystoplasty except that a slightly longer ileal segment is mobilised with the colon (Fig. 10.10). When the cystoplasty segment has been isolated on its vascular pedicle (Fig. 10.11), the ileum is split along its antimesenteric border and this division is continued along a taenia coli into the caecum and then the colon (Fig. 10.12) leaving 2–3 cm at the distal end for anastomosis to the bladder neck. The ileum is then sewn into the colon to form the ileo-colonic pouch (Fig. 10.13) and the segment is then rotated through 180° in the usual way to anastomose to the bladder base. Before complete closure of the 'pouch' the ureters are implanted into the colonic segment at a convenient point using a tunnel technique to provide an anti-reflux mechanism.

Postoperative management is as for a 'straight' substitution cystoplasty (see Ch. 8) except that when the suprapubic catheter is clamped a trial of voiding self catheterisation is begun rather than spontaneous voiding.

More complicated 'pouch' procedures have been described; indeed it seems that there is hardly a city left in the western world that does not have a pouch named after it, either for substitution cystoplasty or for continent diversions. The majority of them seem to be unnecessarily complicated and the one described here seems to work perfectly well.

PALLIATIVE SURGERY

Suprapubic catheterisation — with or without urethral closure

Essentially this is an alternative to a conduit urinary diversion. The most suitable patients are those who are wheelchair-bound, particularly women for whom a urethral catheter either does not contain sphincter weakness incontinence or in whom complications of indwelling catheterisation have occurred or are likely to occur. The typical suitable patient will have severe multiple sclerosis or a spinal cord injury with a docile bladder; not, unfortunately, a common combination.

In the first instance it is always worth trying simple percutaneous suprapubic catheterisation as this is the least invasive option. If urinary incontinence persists there are two possibilities. Firstly, there may be persistent sphincter weakness incontinence in which case urethral closure is likely to produce a satisfactory resolution of the problem. Secondly, incontinence may be due to detrusor hyperreflexia in which case urethral closure may well be followed by suprapubic leakage around the catheter as a result of persistence of the hyperreflexic contractions. If hyperreflexia does not respond to anticholinergic drugs it is wiser to consider an alternative technique such as an ileal conduit urinary diversion, rather than proceed to urethral closure.

It is surprising how often a division of the urethra and two-layer closure of the bladder neck from above, even with separation of the divided ends, is followed by recanalisation, either in the early postoperative period or three to six months later. It is this problem of urethral closure that has plagued the procedure more than anything else.

I am indebted to Peter Worth of University College Hospital, London and the Institute of Urology for the technique of urethral closure described below which appears to work better than most.

Preoperative preparation. Blood loss is occasionally troublesome so blood should be available. Any urinary infection should be treated. There is no other special preparation.

Technique. This is a synchronous abdomino-perineal procedure involving mobilisation of the urethra from the perineum and then inversion of the urethra up into the bladder from above. The patient is therefore placed in the lithotomy position and draped appropriately.

A horizontal incision about 2 cm long is made in the first instance between the meatus and the introitus. This incision is deepened as for a Stamey-type procedure (Ch. 6) to separate the urethra from the anterior vaginal wall. Through the suprapubic incision (a Pfannenstiel incision is adequate) the retropubic space is opened widely to expose the urethra and bladder neck from above. A stout nylon thread with its needle attached is then passed from the bladder down the urethra and out of the meatus. The perineal incision is then extended around the urethra, so that the meatus is circumcised (Fig. 10.14) and the urethral meatus is then transfixed with the nylon suture (Fig. 10.15). Traction on the suture from above will tend to invert the urethra into the bladder (Fig. 10.16).

Progressive dissection around the superior aspect and both sides of the urethra, initially from below and then subsequently retropubically will allow progressive inversion of the urethra into the bladder until the whole urethra has been pulled through in this way. The bulk of the urethra can then be amputated and the stump transfixed and ligated with an absorbable suture material such as Vicryl (Fig. 10.17). Haemostasis is then secured in the retropubic space.

Whether or not a formal anastomosis of the bladder to the skin is desirable is a matter of debate. In time any track between the bladder and the skin will tend to epithelialise, but it seems sensible having exposed the bladder to perform a direct anastomosis. In the chronically inflamed, thick-walled neuropathic bladder this is not always possible, but it usually is in the type of bladder for which this procedure is most appropriate, as thick-walled trabeculated bladders are most commonly associated with a degree of hyperreflexia that will, of itself, prevent a satisfactory result from this procedure. It is my practice to raise a flap from the anterior bladder wall up to the dome, like a Boari flap (Fig. 10.18), and then to convert this into a tube (Fig. 10.19) which is then anastomosed to the skin above the level of the Pfannenstiel incision.

Complications. The only specific complication of this procedure is breakdown of the bladder neck closure which ultimately leads to a perineal urinary fistula. Revising the bladder neck closure is almost certainly doomed to failure and may damage the intramural ureters by virtue of their proximity to the suture line. The safest way out is an ileal conduit urinary diversion.

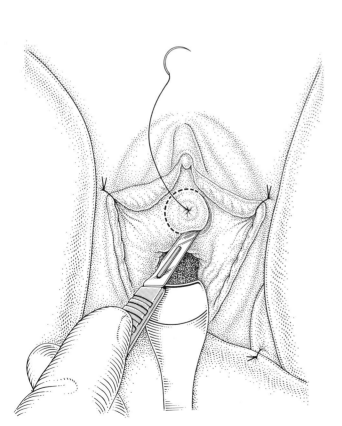

Fig. 10.14

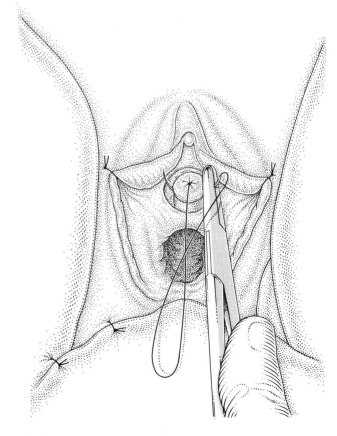

Fig. 10.15

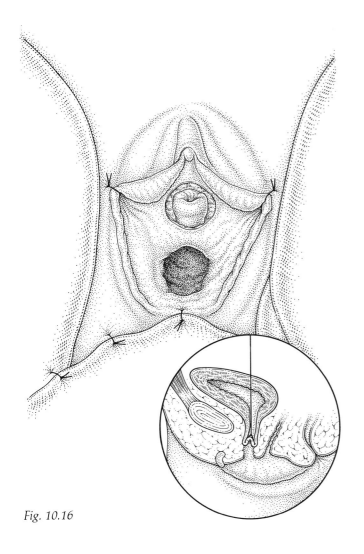

Fig. 10.16

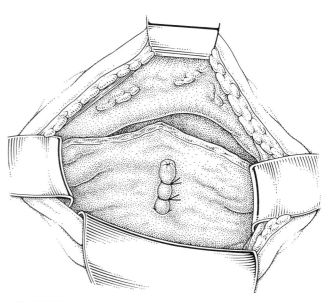

Fig. 10.17
The view from within the bladder.

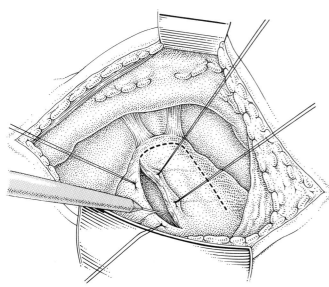

Fig. 10.18

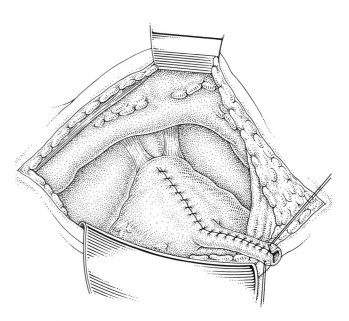

Fig. 10.19

The Mitrofanoff procedure

This procedure was described originally using the appendix to provide a catheterisable suprapubic track between the skin and the bladder (Fig. 10.20). Since then there have been a number of descriptions of variations in technique that have extended the indications for the procedure. Unfortunately the appendix is only really usable in children with any regularity. In adults the alternative is to perform a transureteroureterostomy to drain both kidneys through one distal ureter and then to bring the residual distal ureteric stump out to skin level to provide a catheterisable tract. In such a situation the natural vesico-ureteric junction provides continence by virtue of its anti-reflux mechanism (Fig. 10.21).

The ideal patient is a patient with chronic retention of urine with a large capacity, low-pressure bladder and bladder outflow obstruction who for whatever reason is unable to self catheterise urethrally. The best examples of suitable patients are those with a peripheral autonomic neuropathy, most commonly women with diabetes or post-radical hysterectomy, who for one reason or another are unable to self catheterise urethrally, but some children with spina bifida and low-pressure intermediate type bladders are also suitable. An important feature of such patients is that they are almost totally unable to void urethrally so bladder neck closure is not required. In many respects the procedure suits the same type of 'bladder' as does a permanent indwelling suprapubic catheter but whereas that will often suit the needs of the more severely handicapped patient, the Mitrofanoff procedure is more appropriate to the needs of a more mobile patient.

One of the great advantages of this procedure is that it is a comparatively minor procedure and it doesn't involve irreversible surgery to the urinary tract, particularly when the appendix is used as the catheterisable tract. Thus a Mitrofanoff procedure may be used in a number of situations to temporise until a definitive reconstruction at a later date.

Preparation. The patient should be admitted to hospital two days preoperatively for a short bowel preparation (Ch. 2). The urine should be sterile. There is not usually much blood loss but blood should be cross matched and available if necessary. A recent cystogram should be available proving that vesico-ureteric reflux is absent in case (and particularly if) the ureter is necessary to provide the catheterisable track.

Position. The patient should be supine and draped for a lower midline incision with the right iliac fossa exposed for placing of the stoma.

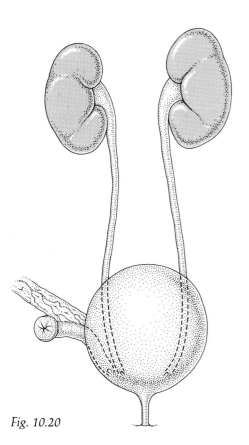

Fig. 10.20

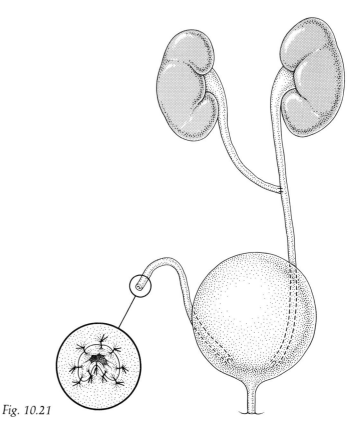

Fig. 10.21

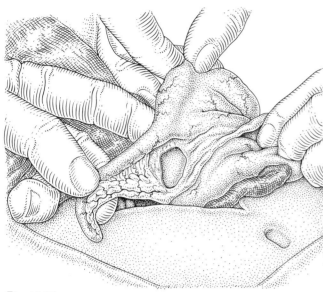

Fig. 10.22

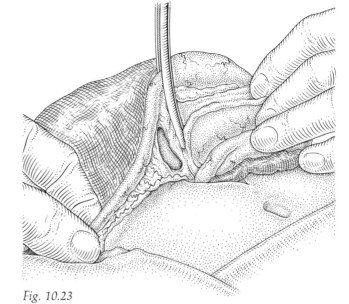

Fig. 10.23

Technique. The first step is to open the retropubic space and divide the peritoneum and underlying fascia (the superior hypogastric wing) lateral to the obliterated umbilical artery back to the lateral pedicle on each side, in order to mobilise the bladder sufficiently to allow it to be tacked to the psoas on the side of the proposed stoma later on in the procedure.

The next step is to find the appendix and see if it is suitable for the proposed procedure. If not the ureter will have to be used as described below. If the appendix is not scarred, can be brought down to the groin and is long enough to reach from the surface of the abdominal wall, through the abdominal wall, through the bladder wall and with enough residual length for an adequate suburothelial tunnel then it is suitable. For an average patient who is not too fat, 5 cm of length is adequate, reckoning that some extra length can be gained by taking a cuff of caecum with the appendix.

It is important to be able to get the appendix comfortably down to the inner aspect of the inguinal ligament so that when it is mobilised on its vascular

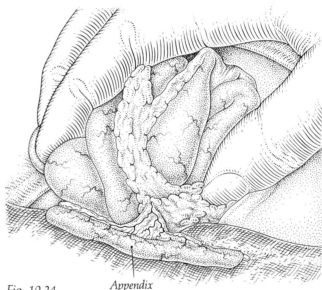

Fig. 10.24   *Appendix*

pedicle it is under no tension. This may require full mobilisation of the caecum, ascending colon and hepatic flexure. When sufficient mobility has been achieved, the appendix is mobilised carefully on its vascular pedicle preserving as many branches as possible of the vascular arcade of the appendicular artery (Fig. 10.22) including any branches running onto the adjacent wall of the caecum.

Whether or not it seems necessary it is a good idea to take a generous cuff of the adjacent caecal wall (Fig. 10.23) with the appendix in case it turns out that more length is required than was initially thought. If extra intra-abdominal length is necessary the caecal cuff can be formed into a tubular extension of the appendix around a catheter in the lumen of the appendix. When the appendix has been mobilised there should be 2–3 cm of appendix on either side of the attachment of its mesentery (Fig. 10.24).

The bladder is then opened by an incision on its anterior wall to allow a finger to lift the right side of the bladder up to the abdominal wall just above the inguinal canal. The bladder is then tacked by 3 or 4 absorbable sutures to the underlying psoas to hold it in place and the adjacent surfaces of the bladder and the abdominal wall are opened to allow the appendix to run through both (Fig. 10.25).

The skin incision at the site where the caecal end of the appendix will emerge should be stellate so that the subsequent suture is less liable to stenosis (Fig. 10.26).

The bladder is then opened widely to give a clear view of the posterolateral wall where the 'anti-reflux' anastomosis

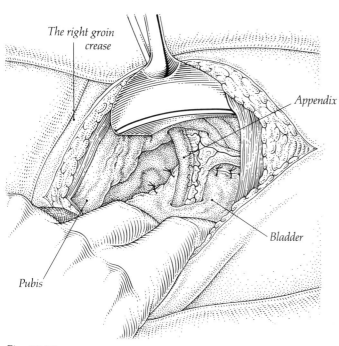

Fig. 10.25

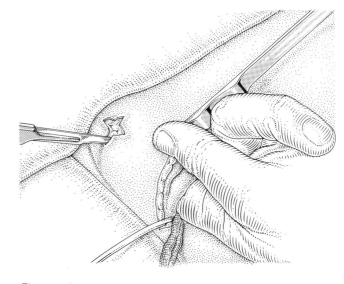

Fig. 10.26

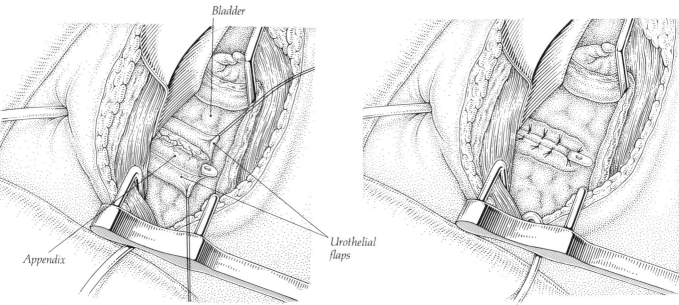

Fig. 10.27

Fig. 10.28

of the appendix to the bladder will be formed. With the tip of the appendix spatulated open a fairly stiff catheter of an appropriate calibre, 12 F or thereabouts, will straighten it out to show the best lie within the bladder. The urothelium along this line from the point where the appendix enters the bladder to its tip is then incised and raised as two flaps (Fig. 10.27). These flaps should be wide enough to cover the appendix and its mesentery comfortably. The appendix is then tacked to the underlying muscle and the urothelial flaps are sutured over the appendix and its mesentery so that when complete healing has occurred they will be in a suburothelial tunnel (Fig. 10.28). At the spatulated tip of the appendix three sutures should be placed, picking up the full thickness of the wall of the appendix and a good bite of the bladder wall as well as urothelium to fix the tip and to ensure epithelial apposition.

The skin edges are then sutured to the caecal end of the appendix and a soft catheter is left running through it and into the bladder (Fig. 10.29). The bladder is closed around a suprapubic Foley catheter of appropriate calibre.

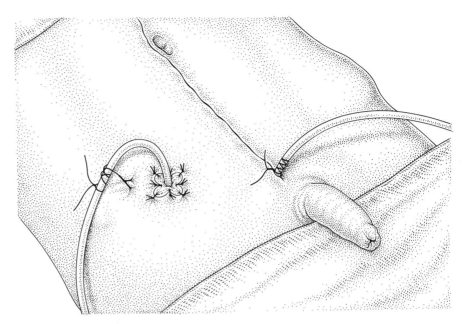

Fig. 10.29

If the appendix is unavailable or unsuitable for any reason and the ureters are very tortuous (Fig. 10.30) then the distal ureter on one side should be used as the catheterisable track. The distal half or more of the ureter is mobilised with a generous amount of the surrounding 'mesentery' to ensure good vascularity (Fig. 10.31). The bladder is then mobilised as described above and hitched up to the psoas, only in this instance the hitch is up superiorly to the psoas above the common iliac vessels (i.e. towards the kidney) rather than up laterally to the area of the inguinal ligament as it would be for an appendix-type of Mitrofanoff.

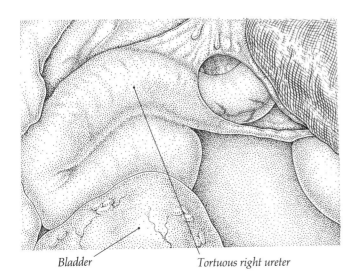

Bladder   Tortuous right ureter

Fig. 10.30

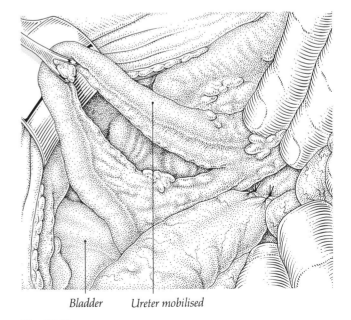

Bladder   Ureter mobilised

Fig. 10.31

The ureter is then divided at a point to give enough length proximally for a tunnelled or trench-type ureteric reimplantation as described above for the appendix (Fig. 10.32) and enough length distally for the cut end of the distal ureter to be brought out through the abdominal wall to be sutured to the skin (Fig. 10.33). As for the appendix the skin incision and closure should be stellate to prevent stenosis.

If the ureter is not long enough for both exteriorisation of the distal end and reimplantation of the proximal end into a psoas hitch or if the bladder is not capable of sufficient mobilisation of the hitch then it is obviously necessary to give priority of length to the distal end. It is vitally important that this should reach comfortably to the skin without tension. The divided proximal ureter is

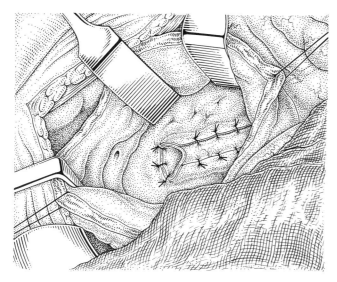

Fig. 10.32

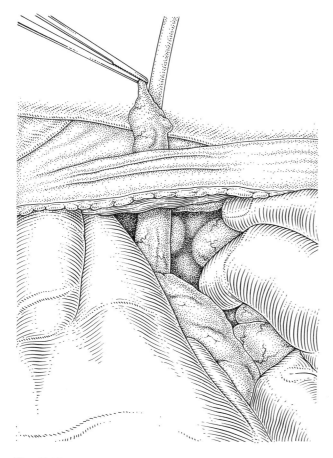

Fig. 10.33

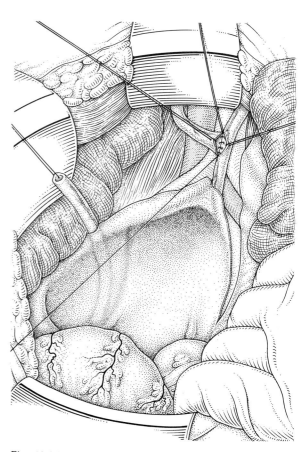

Fig. 10.34

then mobilised for a transureteroureterostomy (TUU) to the contralateral ureter (Fig. 10.21).

To achieve this the ureter on the side of the proposed stoma must be divided well above the pelvic brim and common iliac vessels to ensure that the divided end of the distal part will reach up comfortably to the lower abdominal wall to form the stoma. This leaves rather a short length of proximal ureter for the TUU. To allow a TUU without tension the full length of the contralateral ureter may need to be mobilised, from the renal pelvis to the bladder, to allow it to be tented medially to lie across the great vessels above the inferior mesenteric artery where the TUU anastomosis will be (Fig. 10.34).

Whether the appendix or the ureter is used it is important to ensure that the track is easily catheterisable before the operation is completed. Any difficulties with catheterisation should be sorted out there and then rather than risk reoperation at a later date.

Postoperative care. The anastomoses should be sufficiently well healed at 2 weeks to remove the appendicular/ureteric catheter and begin self catheterisation. The suprapubic catheter should be clamped but kept in for a day or two to be sure that there are no problems with bladder emptying.

If a TUU was performed a one-shot 20 minute IVU film should be taken at about 6 weeks to ensure satisfactory drainage of both upper tracts past the TUU anastomosis.

Complications. The two main complications are difficulty with catheterisation or incontinence through the stoma. Difficulty with catheterisation should not occur if catheterisability has been unequivocally proven at the time of operation unless an ischaemic or traumatic stricture develops somewhere along the appendix/ureter. Incontinence

should not occur if the distal ureter has been used, assuming of course that the vesico-ureteric junction was not refluxing on the preoperative cystogram. If the appendix was used, incontinence through the stoma means that either the suburothelial tunnel was of inadequate length or the distal appendix has become ischaemic and has sloughed. Whatever the complication the Mitrofanoff must be revised or the situation must be rectified in some other way. The obvious solution if the appendix was used and has failed is to convert the patient to a ureteric type of Mitrofanoff.

Other types of urinary diversion
There are two types of urinary diversion, a continent urinary diversion and a conduit urinary diversion. Continent diversion involves creating an intra-abdominal reservoir for the urine which is then emptied by intermittent catheterisation of an otherwise continent channel through from the abdominal wall to the reservoir. The best form of reservoir is the natural bladder and the simplest form of continent diversion is the Mitrofanoff procedure described above in which the appendix or ureter is used as the catheterisable channel with a flap valve type of continence mechanism where the appendix or ureter runs into the bladder.

Alternative methods of continent diversion vary in whether the reservoir is made of bladder or bowel or a combination of the two and whether the continence mechanism is a flap valve or a nipple valve. The most widely used type of continent diversion is a gut pouch with a nipple valve based on the Kock pouch model. This is commonly modified to use the ileocaecal segment rather than the ileum as originally described by Kock. Whatever the gut segment used the main problem with this type of operation is the high failure rate of the nipple valve and high incidence of reoperation to correct it. Flap valves are inherently much more

stable and reliable. The use of long segments of ileum is also disadvantageous because of the important absorptive role of ileum, particularly in growing children. For these reasons I prefer to use a colonic or ileocolonic segment to form the reservoir and a flap valve to form the continence mechanism with either the appendix or a colonic tube, if the appendix is not available or not suitable, to form the catheterisable channel. Either of the techniques described in Chapter 8 for substitution cystourethroplasty is suitable, only bringing the external meatus to the anterior abdominal wall, preferably to the umbilicus where it is concealed.

There is a theoretical advantage in preserving the bladder and incorporating it into the reservoir because the trigone can then be preserved and ureteric reimplantation into the reservoir will not be needed. This advantage is offset in most instances by the consequent need to close off the bladder neck with its relatively high failure rate. It also means that undiversion may be compromised as a future option should some new treatment be developed in years to come. It is easy to forget that in 20 years time some of the treatments we use at the moment will appear laughable to the urologists of that time, when we have retired but our patients are only just approaching their first mid-life crisis!

Ideal candidates for continent diversion in neuropathy are those who would be ideal candidates for urethral self catheterisation but who cannot self catheterise. Probably the best examples are those adolescents with spina bifida, mobile with calipers and strongly motivated, who find urethral self catheterisation impossible because of their calipers; and those who have repeatedly developed infection of an AUS in whom the urethra is no longer surgically approachable. More mobile and equally motivated patients would be better off with a 'clam and cuff' or otherwise appropriate corrective surgery as described above. Less mobile and less motivated patients would be better off with a conduit diversion. The theory of continent diversion is discussed further in Chapter 15.

Conduit urinary diversion needs no description as this is a standard urological technique. It might seem to some that a urinary diversion was the final admission of defeat to a reconstructive surgeon, but this is not really the case. Many patients, particularly those confined to a wheelchair existence, find continence no advantage because of the requirement for finding toilet facilities for disabled persons and because of the time taken to transfer on to the toilet and transfer off again afterwards. In such situations and particularly at night when sleep may otherwise be grossly disturbed, a conduit urinary diversion may be a blessing.

If it were possible to guarantee that an AUS or a cystoplasty, with or without an AUS or a continent diversion (or whatever), would give 4-hourly emptying with continence between times by day and an undisturbed night then we could afford to be less cautious in considering corrective surgery in wheelchair-bound patients. Unfortunately these requirements cannot be guaranteed and although less stringent requirements may be perfectly satisfactory for a fully mobile patient with no need of special facilities they will not usually be satisfactory for those confined to wheelchairs. So for the meantime we must continue to be more conservative in this group.

Vesico ureteric reflux in neuropathy
Vesico-ureteric reflux is fairly common in the neuropathic bladder and obviously undesirable, particularly in the presence of high bladder pressures, outflow obstruction and recurrent urinary tract infection. Unfortunately, surgical correction of the reflux is less

successful than usual in the neuropathic bladder, not least because of the technical difficulties involved.

In general it is more important to correct the associated urodynamic abnormalities, either by catheterisation or surgically, or both (typically by a clam cystoplasty followed by CISC), and to keep the urine sterile, than it is to correct the reflux; if these goals can be achieved and if the kidneys stay normal on regular DMSA scanning then I tend not to reimplant refluxing ureters. If any of these goals cannot be achieved or if DMSA scanning shows renal scarring and significant impairment of total function then anti-reflux surgery is indicated using the Cohen technique — the Leadbetter–Politano technique seems prone to obstruction in the neuropathic bladder.

SPECIFIC NEUROLOGICAL PROBLEMS

Although the reader can probably extrapolate the surgical approach to most urodynamic problems seen in neuropathy from what has been said above, it may be useful to summarise the approach to the more common situations encountered with specific neurological disorders.

In each instance, whether explicitly stated or not, it is assumed that non-surgical methods of treatment have been tried but have failed to help. Specifically, detrusor overactivity in contractile and intermediate bladders is treated with oxybutynin in adequate doses and poor bladder emptying, whatever the cause, is treated with straining or expression, properly and appropriately performed, or with CISC. In general terms the aim of surgery for the neuropathic bladder is to help those who are capable of leading an independent existence but who are restricted by their urological problem to become more independent. For those

who are not capable of independent existence surgery has little to offer.

Spinal cord injury
Patients may be divided into two groups — those with complete cord transections and those with partial lesions. Those with complete lesions, with viable nerve roots and spinal cord below the lesion, are best treated by implantation of a Brindley sacral anterior root stimulator assuming that the relevant neurological criteria are satisfied. For the remainder the only absolute indication for treatment is the presence of secondary upper tract problems. These are usually the result of severe obstruction due either to detrusor-sphincter dyssynergia in those with contractile bladders or to the combination of poor compliance and static distal sphincter obstruction in those with intermediate bladders. If a condom drainage device is acceptable then sphincterotomy is the treatment of choice in males; secondary upper tract problems are very rare in females. If a condom drainage device is unacceptable or inappropriate then intermittent catheterisation should be used although this will often need to be combined with anticholinergic medication or, if that fails, a 'clam' cystoplasty for coincidental detrusor hyperreflexia or poor compliance. This group is easy to treat because the upper tract problem forces the surgeon to intervene and the almost inevitable severe degree of obstruction almost guarantees the success of CISC if the attendant bladder problem is corrected.

Patients of either sex with a marked degree of sphincter weakness incontinence are also easy to treat because implantation of an artificial sphincter is the only viable option other than the use of condom drainage devices in men or indwelling catheters in either sex. Many patients are quite happy with catheters; a sphincter prosthesis should never be forced on them. It is important before implanting an artificial sphincter to be quite sure that there is no sign of detrusor overactivity in addition to the sphincter weakness because if there is detrusor behaviour always becomes more aggressive once an artificial sphincter has been implanted and a cystoplasty will then be necessary unless the bladder responds to oxybutynin.

Such situations are not difficult to manage because the urodynamic problems are clear cut. The patients with whom it is more difficult to know what to do are those with multiple and more complicated urodynamic problems, those with the problems of a wheelchair existence, and those who do not have secondary upper tract problems to force the issue. Generally speaking all these go together.

1.   Patients with intermediate type bladders who require both a cystoplasty and something for sphincter weakness: should it be an artificial sphincter with an endoscopic sphincterotomy, hoping that they will then be able to void spontaneously; should it be an artificial sphincter without a sphincterotomy; or should it be to wait and see, hoping that with a low-pressure bladder as a result of the cystoplasty the distal sphincter mechanism will be sufficient to maintain continence with CISC providing bladder emptying if necessary? In general I have moved away from sphincterotomy in favour of CISC because sphincterotomy is not always reliable and because with an AUS it may be necessary to use CISC even when it was unnecessary beforehand. My approach now is based on the presence or absence of residual urine as an indirect measure of sphincteric obstruction. If there is no residual urine (low sphincter resistance) then an AUS cuff is implanted at the time of cystoplasty. If there is a significant residual urine (high sphincter resistance) then a wait and see policy is adopted as far as an AUS is concerned and I just do the cystoplasty. In less clear cut

situations a cuff is implanted in females; the option of the easier bulbar urethral implantation of an AUS at a later date in males inclines me towards a more conservative approach in men.

2.   Wheelchair-bound patients with severe hyperreflexia unresponsive to drugs, extruding catheters and unable to fit an external appliance: here the question is — is cystoplasty plus probable sphincter surgery justified or would a continent or conduit urinary diversion be more appropriate? This is a philosophical as much as a surgical question but my inclination as a general (but not universal) rule is in favour of some sort of diversion as the simplest way out, because this approach avoids the infective risks of an AUS and the practical problems of finding toilet facilities that continence imposes on those who lead a wheelchair existence (as discussed above).

3.   Wheelchair-bound women with totally patulous urethras. One would hope that such patients had acontractile bladders, in which case an AUS or a suprapubic catheter with urethral closure would be the best bet, but the bladders are often hyperreflexic and so a conduit or continent diversion is safest.

In general terms I am surgically aggressive with mobile patients but much more conservative with those confined to wheelchairs.

Spina bifida and related conditions
This is essentially the same in urodynamic terms as incomplete spinal cord injury. Patients with cervical and upper thoracic cord lesions usually have contractile bladders and rarely require surgery other than endoscopic sphincterotomy in very carefully selected cases, because they usually respond to anticholinergic medication with or without CISC to improve bladder emptying. Patients with lumbar or lumbosacral lesions usually have intermediate bladders, in which case the

'clam and cuff' approach described in the last section is indicated. Acontractile bladders are much less common and are treated by implantation of an AUS if there is severe sphincter weakness incontinence. Patients with thoracolumbar lesions or low sacral lesions generally have the worst bladders, requiring both a 'clam' cystoplasty and an AUS. Why low sacral lesions should have such bad bladders is not clear.

As a general rule, in female and young male patients, as with spinal cord injury patients, I tend to put in an AUS cuff at the time of a 'clam' cystoplasty unless there is a marked degree of sphincteric obstruction on preoperative urodynamic testing, so that it is there if the patient has persistent sphincter weakness incontinence postoperatively. This means that implantation of the rest of the device is a simple subcutaneous procedure rather than a major intrapelvic undertaking as it would be to implant the whole device. Adult male patients who seem likely to be dry with the cystoplasty alone do not have the cuff as well, as they can always have a bulbar urethral AUS implantation at a later date — which is a much more minor procedure than a retropubic AUS implantation in someone who has had a cystoplasty if the hunch proves to be wrong. Having said that, Tony Rickwood at the Children's Hospital in Liverpool has recently been using colposuspension rather than AUS, combined with cystoplasty in female children and has been getting good results. I see no reason why a cystoplasty with colposuspension should not be as good as a cystoplasty with an AUS and have used this approach successfully on several occasions. The three main advantages of this are firstly that it avoids the expense of an AUS, secondly it avoids the short-term complication of infection/erosion and thirdly because it avoids the anxiety associated with any prosthesis in childhood as to the long-term problems of a prosthesis when considered in decades rather than years.

All patients are warned that they must expect to self catheterise afterwards, at least temporarily. If this is a problem for them the operation is deferred. Many patients will not need to do so and some will only require it for a month or so until they learn to empty by straining but some will need to self catheterise permanently and with the best will in the world this is not always possible to predict.

Those patients willing and able to self catheterise but in whom there are problems because of calipers or something of that nature should be considered for continent diversion.

Those patients in whom any form of corrective surgery is unrealistic because the severity of the neurological deficit has left them with insufficient intelligence, motivation, mobility and manipulative skills to cooperate in their treatment and lead an independent existence are best treated by ileal conduit diversion if appliances or indwelling catheterisation prove unsuccessful in containing their incontinence.

Multiple sclerosis
In men the problem is either urge incontinence which usually responds to oxybutynin or recurrent acute retention for which endoscopic sphincterotomy is occasionally required. For detrusor hyperreflexia phenol is contraindicated unless the patient is impotent beyond any shadow of a doubt. In practice surgery of any sort is rarely required.

In women surgery is required more commonly, mainly because the disease is more common in women. Detrusor hyperreflexia is the main problem; when drugs fail the phenol technique is used. When this fails a 'clam' cystoplasty is advised for those with good legs and hands (CISC is often necessary in these women) and no cerebral dysfunction. A conduit diversion is advised for those with bad legs or hands, or cerebral dysfunction.

Parkinson's disease
There are few things in urological life more unrewarding than treating dysfunction in Parkinson's disease. Most patients have symptoms of detrusor instability and of outflow obstruction although the latter symptom(s) is more commonly due to detrusor failure with or without a failure of normal sphincter relaxation than to bona fide obstruction. My experience is that the only patients who respond to surgical treatment are those who have a transurethral resection of the prostate for acute retention. The rest are uniformly unresponsive to any treatment, medical or surgical, whatever the urodynamic problem.

Cerebrovascular accidents (CVA)
Surgical treatment of CVA-related urodynamic dysfunction has never been indicated in my experience.

Transverse myelitis
The clinical picture tends to change during the two years or so following the initial lesion so it is best to do nothing. The pattern is variable in both time and type but most commonly starts as detrusor hyperreflexia followed in time by an acontractile bladder. These patients require CISC not surgery.

Pelvic autonomic nerve lesions
There are two common patterns — the first is with low sphincter resistance leading to sphincter weakness incontinence which can be treated as for stress incontinence although surgery has a higher failure rate in this group than in patients with 'simple' stress incontinence. Nonetheless a Stamey-type bladder neck suspension would be my first choice for these patients assuming they accept the need for CISC afterwards as this is commonly necessary. The second pattern is with high sphincter resistance leading to chronic retention with either overflow or stress incontinence or both. The group should respond to CISC or a Mitrofanoff procedure if a gynaecologist has wrecked the urethra, making it uncatheterisable.

REFERENCES

The neuropathic bladder is a huge subject although in purely surgical terms it really boils down to cystoplasty, artificial sphincter, a combination of the two, sphincterotomy or conduit or continent diversion, with other procedures used occasionally. Spina bifida and spinal cord injury patients get considered for surgery most frequently because patients with other neurological problems usually respond satisfactorily to drugs and other non-surgical measures or are otherwise unsuitable for surgical intervention. For a general review of spinal cord injury Thomas (1984) is recommended, as is Rickwood (1984) for spina bifida. Mundy (1987) has reviewed the neuropathic bladder in children and Mundy & Blaivas (1984) have reviewed non-traumatic neurological disorders.

For a discussion of the Brindley sacral anterior root stimulator the man himself should be consulted (Brindley et al 1986) and the interested reader should also consult Tanagho's work although his results with his stimulator in humans have not yet been published.

In relation to Brindley's work it is worth noting that he performs a posterior rhizotomy of S2, 3, 4 bilaterally at the time of implantation of his stimulator to abolish detrusor hyperreflexia in contractile bladders or the poor compliance due to autonomous detrusor contractile activity seen in intermediate bladders. This 'deafferentation' of the bladder, but without implantation of the sacral anterior root stimulator, may eventually come to replace 'clam' ileocystoplasty as a means of producing a docile low-pressure bladder (which can then be combined with CISC, for bladder emptying) in selected patients with spinal cord injury.

McCrae et al (1987) have reviewed their experience of the clam cystoplasty in neuropathy, and the review by Stephenson & Mundy (1985) includes the role of the AUS in such patients.

The greatest protagonists of the Mitrofanoff procedure are (at present) Duckett & Snyder (1986); Skinner et al (1987) are firmly in the Kock pouch camp (although neither specifically for the treatment of the neuropathic bladder).

Brindley G S, Polkey C E, Rushton D N, Cardozo L 1986 Sacral anterior root stimulators for bladder control in paraplegia: the first 50 cases. Journal of Neurology, Neurosurgery and Psychiatry 49: 1104–1114

Duckett J W, Snyder H M 1986 Continent urinary diversion: variations on the Mitrofanoff principle. Journal of Urology 135: 58–62

McCrae P, Nurse D E, Stephenson T P, Mundy A R 1988 Clam ileocystoplasty in the neuropathic bladder. British Journal of Urology 61: 523–526

Mundy A R 1987 The neuropathic bladder. In: Postlethwaite R J (ed) Clinical paediatric nephrology. John Wright & Sons, Bristol, pp 312–328

Mundy A R, Blaivas J G 1984 Non traumatic neurological disorders. In: Mundy A R, Stephenson T P, Wein A J (eds) Urodynamics: principles, practice and application. Churchill Livingstone, Edinburgh, pp 278–287

Rickwood A M K 1984 The neuropathic bladder in children. In: Mundy A R, Stephenson T P, Wein A J (eds) Urodynamics: principles, practice and application. Churchill Livingstone, Edinburgh, pp 326–384

Skinner D G, Lieskovsky G, Boyd S D 1987 Continuing experience with the continent ileal reservoir (Kock Pouch) as an alternative to cutaneous urinary diversion: an update after 250 cases. Journal of Urology 137: 1140–1145

Stephenson T P, Mundy A R 1985 Treatment of the neuropathic bladder by enterocystoplasty and selective sphincterotomy or sphincter ablation and replacement. British Journal of Urology 57: 27–31

Thomas D G 1984 Spinal cord injury. In: Mundy A R, Stephenson T P, Wein A J (eds) Urodynamics: principles, practice and application. Churchill Livingstone, Edinburgh, pp 259–272

RECONSTRUCTIVE PROBLEMS

Introduction

The main difference between the problems described in this section and those described in the last section is that the treatment of a urodynamic problem is dictated, more or less, by the findings of a properly performed, accurately evaluated urodynamic study whereas with a reconstructive problem, urodynamic studies are usually unhelpful in deciding treatment although the end result of that treatment should be a urinary tract that is urodynamically satisfactory.

In other words reconstructive problems require a urodynamic approach to treatment in order to get the best results but preoperative urodynamic testing is not usually helpful, if indeed it is possible, in deciding which surgical procedure to perform. A good example is that it is usually pointless simply to close a complex vesico-vaginal fistula following radiotherapy and hysterectomy for carcinoma of the cervix. Although this is sometimes sufficient, it is more likely to leave a small capacity, poorly compliant hypersensitive bladder with sphincter weakness incontinence, to say nothing of residual vaginal and rectal problems. The 'urodynamic approach' anticipates these problems and modifies the approach to treatment accordingly, beyond what is required simply to correct the obvious abnormality. The urodynamic principles developed in the last section that are applicable to the resolution of most of the reconstructive problems described in this section are that the bladder should be of good capacity and low pressure, with a competent and easily catheterisable outflow and that, when a high-pressure bladder and a weak bladder outflow coexist, correction of the bladder problem is usually more important than correction of the outflow problem. The techniques of augmentation and substitution cystoplasty have been described and their problems discussed. The technique of implantation of an artificial sphincter has been described (and the problems discussed) and the concept of urethroplasty (in females) to produce a competent bladder outflow has been introduced.

Another much more debatable point that has been alluded to is the question of whether, when attempting surgically to construct or repair the bladder outflow, to err on the side of incompetence and ease of bladder emptying, relying on an AUS to produce continence if necessary, or on the other hand to attempt to produce an obstructive bladder outflow which is thereby continent, relying on CISC to achieve bladder emptying. In general the tendency is to lean towards obstruction and CISC particularly in females.

In this section other principles are introduced — this time more practical than theoretical. The major principle is the repair or reconstruction of the lower urinary tract by the mobilisation and deployment of tissue from elsewhere. An example is the use of pedicled preputial skin for the repair of urethral strictures in men. It is important to realise that this is a principle and not just an isolated technique — by the same principle, for example, pedicled labial skin can be used for urethral substitution in women. Another principle is the mobilisation of a structure to bridge a gap and produce a tension-free anastomosis as in anastomotic urethroplasty and the psoas hitch technique. A third is the principle of keeping suture lines separated as in the closure and prevention of fistulae and, in the same vein, of using omental wrapping, the closure of mesenteric defects (to prevent internal herniae) and other points of technique that reduce the incidence of postoperative complications to a minimum.

The problems discussed in this section are urethral strictures, urinary fistulae, bladder cancer and related problems, congenital problems and urinary undiversion. The treatment of strictures is discussed in particular detail because the surgical procedures described all illustrate the important principles mentioned in the last paragraph. The surgical treatment of complex fistulae also involves points of principle and, additionally, introduces a philosophy of aggressive surgical intervention for the correction of major structural defects rather than relying on diversion as a safe 'opt out'. This theme is continued in the remaining chapters which also introduce the concept of pelvic surgery as a field of practice in its own right, involving gynaecological and colorectal surgery as well as urology. Although some would argue with the aggressive surgical approach to major problems and with the concept of pelvic surgery performed by a dedicated individual rather than a group of specialists in each particular field, there are considerable advantages to the patient from both these approaches.

Undiversion has a chapter of its own although the treatment of most of the conditions that lead to diversion in the first place have already been covered. This is because undiversion has to take account of several factors simultaneously, each of which may interfere with another.

Chapter 11

Urethral strictures

Strictures have plagued mankind for thousands of years and the treatment of strictures has a history that is longer than history itself. Times have changed, however, and strictures and their treatment have changed with it. The gonococcus is no longer the commonest cause and wax bougies are no longer used for treatment. Although it is generally realised that strictures may be a cause of major disability and that inappropriate treatment may make this disability worse, it is not always easy to decide which of the several currently available treatment options is most appropriate for an individual stricture. Nor is it easy to decide when or how to modify treatment in a previously treated patient. The crucial factor in deciding the most appropriate form of treatment for a stricture is an understanding of the pathology of the stricture process and the attendant natural or iatrogenic complications. The pathology of strictures is rarely covered in standard texts and it therefore seems appropriate to give some consideration to this first.

PATHOLOGY

The urethra consists of a layer of urothelium pitted by mucous glands and surrounded by the prostate initially, by the distal sphincter mechanism in its membranous part, and by the corpus spongiosum throughout the rest of its length. The mucous glands are predominantly in the proximal bulbar and distal penile sections of the urethra. The reaction of the urethra to a traumatic or infective insult is determined to a large extent by its relation to these glands and to the corpus spongiosum.

Minor urothelial trauma within the lumen of the urethra exposes the delicate vascular erectile tissue of the corpus spongiosum, leading to local fibrosis. Passage of urine over the exposed spongy tissue tends to

exacerbate this 'spongiofibrosis' (as Turner Warwick calls it) and passage of infected urine makes matters worse. Healing of the traumatised area is the result of a balance between urothelial regeneration on the one hand, which tends to restore the urethra to its original state, and the combination of cross-adhesion of the inflamed urothelium and contracture due to spongiofibrosis on the other hand, which tends to cause stricturing.

Greater degrees of urothelial injury cause full thickness 'spongiofibrosis', and if the urethral wall is disrupted, this will be compounded by periurethral haematoma formation, which in turn causes periurethral fibrosis. Again extravasation of urine and particularly of infected urine will exacerbate the reaction.

Similarly, infection of the urethral mucous glands will lead to fibrosis of the spongy tissue surrounding them, and inflammation of the overlying urothelium, and if pockets of pus form and rupture through to the surrounding tissue, this will lead to periurethral fibrosis and provide a route for urinary extravasation which will extend and exacerbate the inflammatory reaction around the urethra.

Complete urethral disruption additionally causes loss of urothelial continuity, the gap between the two ends filling with haematoma, and this will obviously be worsened if the two ends of the urethra are distracted from each other as in more severe types of pelvic fracture injury of the membranous urethra. In such a situation, urethral continuity can only be restored by development of a passage through the haematoma cavity, which at best will be an epithelialised passage through an area of fibrosis.

Thus, following any urethral insult, there are several different factors acting simultaneously, but at varying rates and to varying degrees, the balance of which

determines the final outcome. The favourable factors are:

— minimal urothelial damage and complete urothelial regeneration
— minimal exposure of the spongy tissue and therefore minimal spongiofibrosis
— absence of infection
— no local haematoma
— no periurethral extension of the inflammatory reaction
— no loss of urethral continuity.

The unfavourable factors are:

— urothelial cross-adhesion
— loss of urothelial continuity
— spongiofibrosis
— infection
— periurethral extension or haematoma formation with periurethral fibrosis.

In addition, there are several other secondary factors that act to compound the problem. These are the secondary obstructive effects, the presence of associated injuries and the effects of surgical intervention.

Secondary obstructive effects
As with all obstructions, the bladder compensates by raising voiding pressure to maintain flow rate and to attain complete emptying. In time the bladder becomes thick-walled, trabeculated and sacculated, and later still obstructive changes develop in the upper tracts as well.

At the same time, the raised voiding pressures are transmitted to the urethra proximal to the stricture, causing dilatation of the urethra and blowing open of the mucous glands. If there is already transmural and periurethral pathology as described above, this will be accentuated, tending to cause diverticula and, with extension of infection, urethro-cutaneous fistula formation.

If urethral disruption has occurred and there is therefore a haematoma-filled gap in the urethra, the raised voiding pressure leads to tracking and excavation within the haematoma, and these tracks and cavities are foci for persistent infection and stone formation.

Associated injuries

These relate principally to pelvic fracture injuries of the membranous urethra, and include bladder injuries, rectal injuries and damage to the intra-abdominal viscera. Damage to the neurovascular bundles innervating the corpora cavernosa (and thereby responsible for potency) is also common. Occasionally the bladder neck or its innervation is damaged with important consequences for continence and this is particularly common in children. Another cause of bladder neck incompetence in adults, excluding iatrogenic damage, is encasement of the bladder neck in haematoma–fibrosis from spread of a perimembranous urethral haematoma, secondary to rupture of the pubourethral ligaments and the dorsal vein complex. Associated rectal injury is a potent cause of recto-urethral fistula formation.

The effects of surgical intervention

These are of three types. Firstly, indelicate instrumentation of the urethra either with a catheter or an endoscope may introduce infection or may convert a partial thickness rupture to a full thickness rupture.

Secondly, instrumentation of the urethra at a later stage after a urethral injury may create problems in various ways. Blind forceful instrumentation with a urethral sound may cause a false passage whilst the bladder and urethra are softened by the inflammatory response to injury and the urethra is surrounded by haematoma. In this way, for example, a false passage might be created through the bulbar urethra just distal to the rupture or stricture, across the front of the prostate and into the bladder in front of the bladder neck. With lesser degrees of forceful instrumentation a comparatively minor injury may be made considerably worse. The use of balloon catheter traction in an attempt to approximate a bulboprostatic urethral distraction may damage the bladder neck. Equally misguided endoscopic surgery of the bladder neck may also impair its competence. All of these are avoidable.

Thirdly there are the effects of instrumental or surgical treatment of an established stricture. Even excluding potential complications such as those just described, urethrotomy and dilatation are themselves urothelial injuries. By incising or disrupting the stricture they are treating, they expose the underlying spongy tissue and may cause extension of spongiofibrosis. With a long stricture or a very short and flimsy stricture, this may not be important, but with a 0.5–1 cm post-traumatic stricture with normal urothelium on either side, this extension of spongiofibrosis may convert a stricture which would be eminently suitable for excision and anastomotic repair, with a success rate of almost 100%, to a longer stricture, which is no longer amenable to such definitive repair. Still more important is the risk, with urethrotomy for proximal bulbar strictures, of damaging the distal sphincter mechanism by inadvertent incision.

All these factors must be taken into account when considering the best form of treatment for an individual stricture. Thus post-prostatectomy sphincter strictures are best treated by dilatation because it is fibrosis and therefore impaired function of the distal sphincter that is the most important consideration. Short post-traumatic strictures (Fig. 11.1) are best treated by excision and end-to-end anastomosis because the long-term success rate is higher than

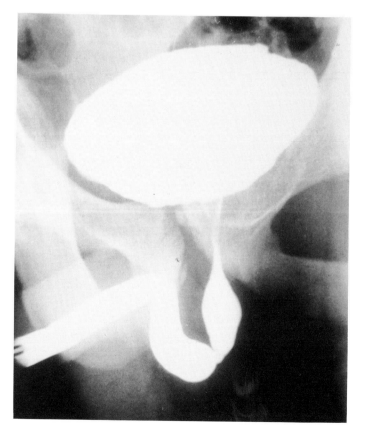

Fig. 11.1

with dilatation or urethrotomy which additionally run the risk of precluding a later anastomotic repair by extending spongiofibrosis. On the other hand urethrotomy is more appropriate for the first-time treatment of ischaemic or infective strictures (Fig. 11.2) because the length of involved urethra will almost invariably preclude an excision and end-to-end anastomosis. These factors will be discussed in more detail below.

ASSESSMENT

With or without an appropriate history, most patients present with symptoms of obstructed voiding. In the absence of gross periurethral fibrosis or other major complications, physical examination is unrewarding. A low peak flow rate and obstructed voiding pattern give the diagnosis of outflow obstruction, but the definitive diagnosis of stricture, its site and complicating factors are made by radiological and endoscopic investigation.

Radiological assessment is not essential before instrumental treatment but is mandatory before urethroplasty. Having said that, it is extremely difficult to resist the temptation to perform a visual internal urethrotomy having seen a stricture endoscopically even when one is aware that urethroplasty may be a better form of treatment if the stricture is short. As most of the short strictures best treated by urethroplasty are post-traumatic, it is wise to arrange the appropriate X-rays before endoscopy if the history is suggestive, so that urethroplasty can be discussed with the patient and appropriate operating time allocated.

Adequate radiological assessment requires both an ascending urethrogram and a micturating cystogram: the former to show the urethra distal to the stricture and the distal part of the stricture (Fig. 11.3) and the latter to show the bladder, the bladder neck and

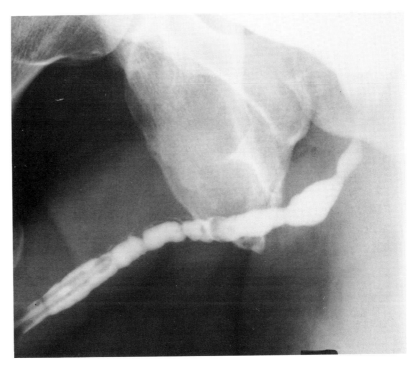

Fig. 11.2

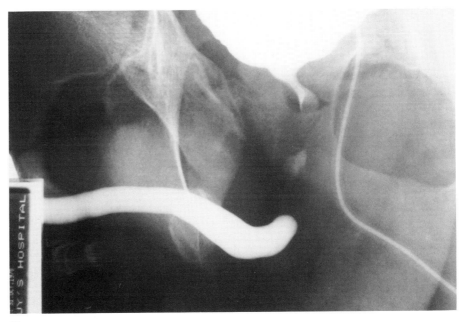

Fig. 11.3

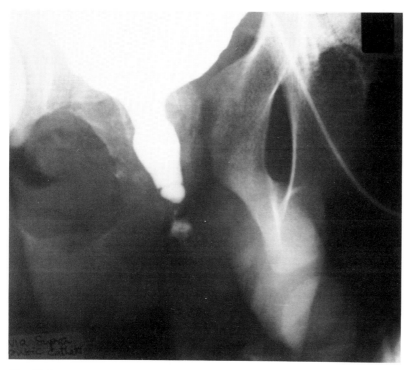

Fig. 11.4

the urethra proximal to the stricture (Fig. 11.4). As can be seen from the Figures, either investigation on its own would be inadequate. Many of the complicating factors of a stricture are only shown on the micturating cystogram (Figs 11.5, 11.6).

Endoscopy gives very little information about the complicating factors and adds little to the radiological assessment of the stricture itself, but is helpful in the further assessment of those areas of the urethra that appear radiologically normal or equivocal. In other words, it is a useful guide to the longitudinal extent of the urothelial damage and underlying spongiofibrosis on either side of the radiologically overt stricture.

If there is a totally obliterative stricture of the urethra and the patient has a competent bladder neck it may be impossible to assess the urethra between the bladder neck and the stricture either

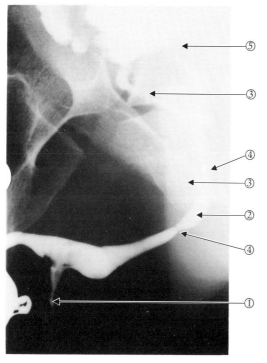

Fig. 11.5

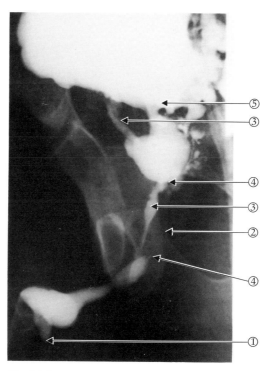

Fig. 11.6

① = Fistula
② = Bulbar urethra
③ = False passage
④ = Stricture
⑤ = Bladder neck

radiologically, because the bladder is unable to expel contrast material into the urethra when there is no way through, or by traditional retrograde endoscopy, because the stricture is impassable. In such a situation passage of a flexible endoscope through the inevitable suprapubic cystostomy track can be very helpful to assess the state of the proximal urethra and the length of the stricture.

With longstanding strictures and those involving the sphincter mechanisms, it would seem a good idea to assess bladder behaviour urodynamically before operation, but in practice this is best left until after resolution of the stricture problem, so that the obstructive effect of the stricture is eliminated. The point that is important is to warn such patients than an underlying abnormality may be present and this may be a cause of persistent problems.

It is equally important to have the patient's potency documented before surgery, particularly in the region of the membranous urethra, so that 'postoperative' impotence cannot be attributed to the surgery by a litigation-conscious but previously impotent patient.

TREATMENT

There are basically three types of treatment that theoretically can be applied to any type of stricture at any site. These are dilatation, urethrotomy and urethroplasty. Until comparatively recently dilatation was the only option and it is therefore the yardstick by which the success of the other two are judged. Urethrotomy may be performed blindly with the Otis urethrotome or under direct vision with the optical urethrotome. The Otis urethrotome has had several decades of use with strictures, but with certain exceptions has never really superseded dilatation. The optical urethrotome has several

advantages over the Otis, and this, coupled with its recent introduction and general applicability, has generated a great enthusiasm for its use. The remaining advantage of the Otis urethrotome is that it is calibrated and is therefore capable of giving an even calibre to the full length of the strictured urethra, which is something that the visual urethrotome cannot do with accuracy.

Urethroplasty also has a short history of 25 years or so and was initially used only for impassable or complex strictures. The problem has always been that although reported to be very successful in the hands of its few pioneering exponents, it has not been generally favoured, partly because of poor results in the hands of others, partly because of the demanding nature of the techniques in terms of time and, to a lesser extent, surgical expertise and partly because of the sometimes catastrophic results of failed surgery. Finally the exact role of the various types of urethroplasty that have been described in relation to the different types of stricture that occur has never been clearly defined. Hence, in part, the enthusiasm for optical urethrotomy as a sort of halfway house between dilatation and urethroplasty.

In general it might reasonably be said that most urologists would regard optical urethrotomy as the first-line treatment option for most strictures, dilatation as best for sphincter strictures and for repeated out-patient instrumentation, and urethroplasty as best reserved for short traumatic strictures, recurrent strictures in young patients, strictures at any age that rapidly and regularly recur after dilatation or urethrotomy, and complex strictures, particularly of the membranous and proximal bulbar urethra. With this general approach in mind, various factors may of course act to alter the surgeon's approach under certain circumstances.

In recent years two other treatments have been developed. Firstly, lasers have been used as an alternative to a blade for optical urethrotomy and secondly various types of endoprosthetic stent have been developed for implantation into the stricture site to keep the urethra open. Lasers appear to be no more effective (at present) than standard optical urethrotomy but stents will undoubtedly prove to have an important role in the management of strictures (in my opinion). What that role might be is more difficult to define as they have only been in use for a very short time and experience is very limited but the potential role will be discussed at the end of this chapter.

It is perhaps easiest to discuss the treatment of strictures according to their site. Meatal and fossa navicularis strictures will not be discussed, as they are part of general urological practice. The types to be described are therefore:

1. Penile urethral strictures
2. Bulbar urethral strictures
3. Membranous urethral strictures
4. Bulbomembranous strictures.

PENILE STRICTURES (Table 11.1)

These are the easiest of all to deal with, whatever method is chosen, because it is the nearest part of the urethra to the meatus, because the full length of the penile urethra can be straightened out

Table 11.1 Penile strictures

1. Optical urethrotomy to open up the stricture followed by Otis urethrotomy to give an even calibre.
2. Consider urethroplasty if:
   — rapidly and repeatedly recurrent
   — complications
   — young man.
   a. pedicled preputial/penile skin patch
   b. Orandi
   c. urothelial free graft (tube graft for hypospadias cripples)

(excision and end-to-end anastomosis contraindicated).

for instrumentation and because, for urethroplasty, there is usually a ready supply of local skin which is suitable for reconstruction. Most strictures are secondary to instrumentation, ischaemia (a good example is prolonged catheterisation in a patient undergoing cardiopulmonary bypass surgery), infection, or a combination, and are long or are just the worst manifestation of a stricture-prone urethra. In younger patients penile strictures are frequently associated with balanitis xerotica et obliterans and it is common to find retrograde extension of the stricture up the penile urethra following an attempted meatoplasty.

The diagnosis is usually made endoscopically and anastomotic urethroplasty is contraindicated in the penile urethra (see below), so it is usual in the first instance to try urethrotomy.

URETHROTOMY

A Sachse or similar optical urethrotome is used with a 0° telescope. If the proximal urethra is clearly visible through the stricture, the stricture can be incised straight away. If not, a fine ureteric catheter or guidewire should first be passed through the stricture so that the correct line of incision can be determined. A stricture should never be cut through blindly with no sight of the way through — that is a sure way to lose the urethra at the other end. The best site for the urethrotomy incision is a matter of debate. Most surgeons incise at 12 o'clock or thereabouts because that is the way the blade is orientated when the urethrotome is held in its natural position. On the other hand Turner Warwick feels that the incision should be made inferolaterally at either 4 o'clock or 8 o'clock so that, should a deep incision be necessary, the incision can extend through to supple vascular tissue without risking damage to either the corpora cavernosa or the skin.

For a single short stricture this is all that is necessary. For a longer stricture or for multiple strictures, I incise sufficiently to allow onward passage of the endoscope and then perform an Otis urethrotomy to 24 F or thereabouts, to give an even urethral calibre. A catheter is left in place for 24 hours, until the patient is fully conscious and able to void in a normal position although for longer or more difficult strictures 5 days of catheterisation is more appropriate. The flow rate is checked at that time.

The flow rate is again checked at 3 months or thereabouts and compared with the flow rate study immediately after urethrotomy. If the flow rate is normal, it is checked again at 6-monthly intervals, until the patient has been free of trouble for 2 years. Thereafter he is discharged from further follow up, but warned that his problem may recur, in which case he should return for further assessment. If the flow rate is low, suggesting a recurrent stricture, the urethrotomy is repeated or, in elderly patients, the urethra is dilated under topical anaesthesia.

Unfortunately urethrotomy is only curative in about 50% of patients. Those with flimsier strictures and with lesser degrees of spongio-fibrosis tend to do well. The denser the stricture or the underlying fibrosis and the poorer the urethral blood supply the more likely the stricture is to recover.

If the stricture keeps recurring I would recommend urethroplasty using either the Orandi procedure or the pedicled preputial patch technique. An excision and end-to-end anastomosis should not be performed, however short the stricture, or chordee will result. Only patch urethroplasty is applicable to penile strictures.

PENILE URETHROPLASTY — THE ORANDI PROCEDURE

Preparation
No special preoperative preparation is required. An up-to-date urethrogram and micturating cystogram should be available to define the stricture and ensure the normality of the proximal urethra.

Technique
With the patient supine or in the lithotomy position, an incision is made on the ventral surface of the shaft of the penis to one side of the midline and curved over the urethra at each end (Fig. 11.7), and deepened through the subcutaneous tissue throughout its length. The length of the vertical limb of the incision should exceed the length of the stricture by 1 cm or so at each end.

The skin and the full thickness of the subcutaneous tissue are then reflected off the underlying corpus spongiosum, ensuring that the subcutaneous tissue is not damaged (Fig. 11.8). The corpus spongiosum is incised along the length of the stricture and this incision is then extended by 1 cm at each end into normal urethra as judged by a healthy looking pink urothelium and normal looking cut margins of the corpus spongiosum (Fig. 11.9).

There is usually some fairly brisk bleeding from the cut edges of the urethra/corpus spongiosum. This is controlled with a running stitch along each side which should tack the urethra laterally to flatten it and hold it open.

The skin flap created by the initial incision is then incised 1 cm (no more) in from its edge down to, but not into, the subcutaneous tissue (Fig. 11.10) which will now be used to create a vascular pedicle for the skin patch just created. To produce the vascular pedicle the rest of the skin of the flap is reflected off the subcutaneous tissue for a distance of

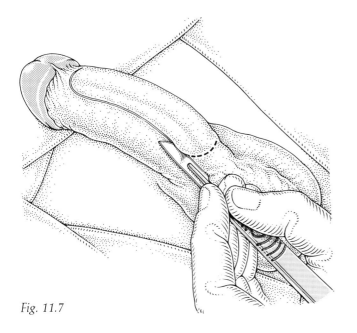

Fig. 11.7

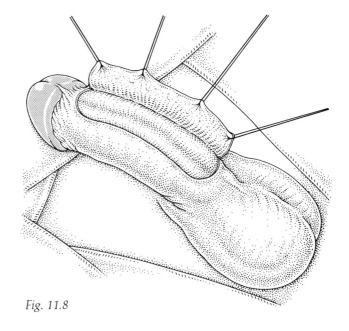

Fig. 11.8

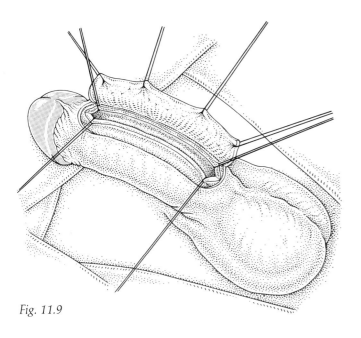

Fig. 11.9

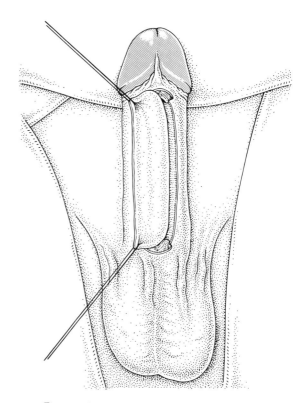

Fig. 11.10

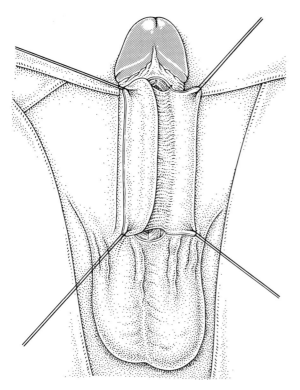

Fig. 11.11

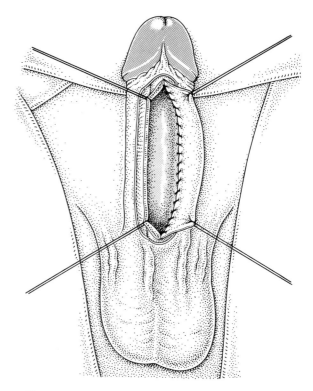

Fig. 11.12

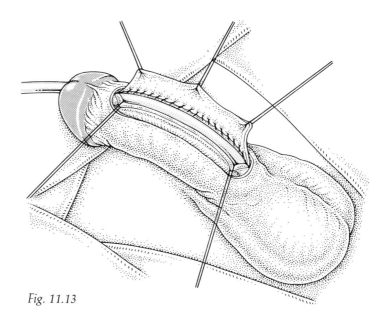

Fig. 11.13

1 cm or so, taking care not to damage either the skin or the subcutaneous tissue (Fig. 11.11).

It is important to recognise that there are in fact two quite distinct layers of subcutaneous tissue deep to the skin of the penis. There is the thin superficial layer immediately under the skin and from which the skin gets its blood supply and there is the thicker so-called 'dartos layer' beneath that. There is a definite plane between these two layers and it is this plane that the surgeon should identify to separate the skin with its own subcutaneous tissue from the 'dartos layer' below that will become the vascular pedicle for the skin patch. If *all* the subcutaneous tissue is dissected from the undersurface of the skin then the skin will be devascularised.

The patch is now ready to sew in place to close the urethral defect. This is done with a 4/0 Vicryl stitch running from the proximal apex to the distal apex, suturing from inside to invert the sutured margins (Fig. 11.12). A 16 F silicone Foley catheter is then passed up the urethra from the meatus to the bladder (Fig. 11.13) and the other side of the patch is sewn in place.

The final step is to cover the otherwise exposed suture line by tacking the subcutaneous vascular tissue over it to the fascia of the corpus cavernosum (Fig. 11.14). This will keep the patch suture line separated from the skin closure thereby reducing the risk of fistula formation. The skin is then closed (Fig. 11.15). Any tension in the skin suture line is readily eliminated by a dorsal relaxing skin incision but this is not usually necessary.

Postoperative management
The catheter is left in for 2–3 weeks. As it is being removed a 'catheter-gram' is performed by instilling water-soluble contrast up the drainage channel of the catheter. Contrast will then pass out of the tip and back around the catheter in the region of the patch, ensuring that the repair is sound.

A check flow rate and urethrogram are then performed 6 months later to confirm that the satisfactory result has been maintained.

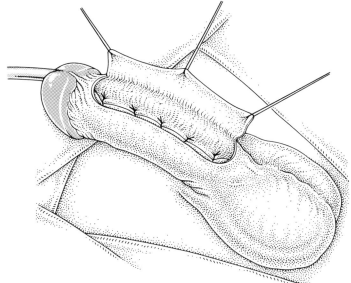

Fig. 11.14

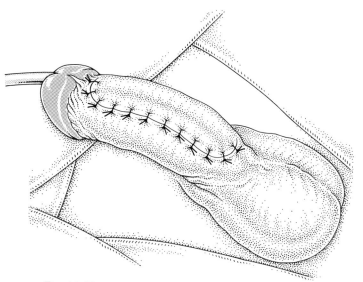

Fig. 11.15

Complications

The problem with the Orandi procedure is that despite tacking subcutaneous tissue over the urethroplasty suture line, the latter is still very closely related to the skin closure line which itself is a bit tight (and also uncomfortable) postoperatively. These factors predispose to fistula formation. The Orandi procedure is usually perfectly adequate for a fairly short uncomplicated penile urethral stricture in a young man but in those older patients with long strictures or with urethro-cutaneous fistulae or periurethral inflammation which is affecting the overlying skin, a better procedure, in my opinion, is a modification of this technique and of the transverse preputial island flap technique described by Duckett for the treatment of hypospadias. This has the advantage of preserving intact the skin over the urethroplasty patch, thereby minimising the risk of skin necrosis and fistula formation. The technique is illustrated here in Figures 11.16–11.23 and described in detail below under

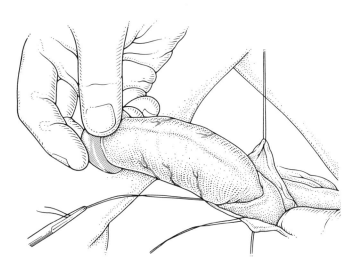

Fig. 11.16

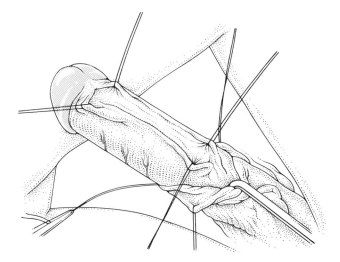

Fig. 11.17

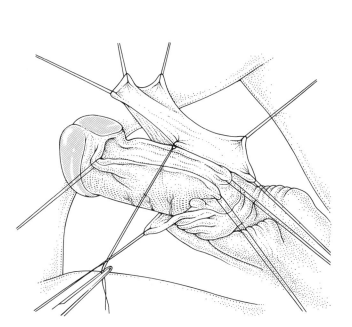

Fig. 11.18

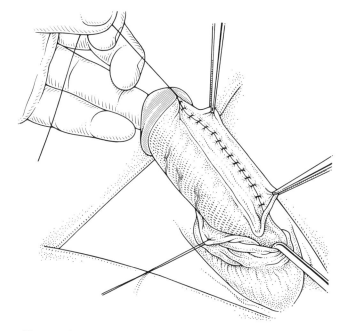

Fig. 11.19

one-stage patch bulbar urethroplasty. Briefly, the penis is degloved of both skin and subcutaneous tissue (Fig. 11.16) and the urethra is opened into healthy tissue at each end (Fig. 11.17). A preputial skin patch is mobilised on a subcutaneous vascular pedicle and laid alongside the 'stricturotomy' (Fig. 11.18). It is then trimmed to size and sewn in place (Figs 11.19, 11.20). The subcutaneous tissue of the pedicle is then tacked over the suture line to the fascia of the corpus cavernosum (Fig. 11.21) to provide a second layer of closure (Fig. 11.22). The penile skin is rolled back over the penis and the wound is closed as for a circumcision (Fig. 11.23). The preoperative and postoperative appearances are shown in Figure 11.24 and Figure 11.25 respectively.

Most patients who come to penile urethroplasty have either multiple strictures or a 'rifled' urethra that is prone to stricture formation. For this reason most patients need a full length

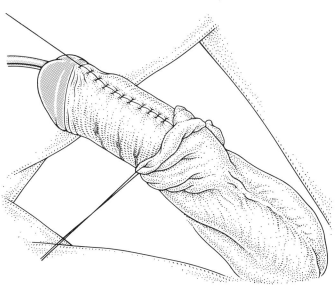

Fig. 11.20

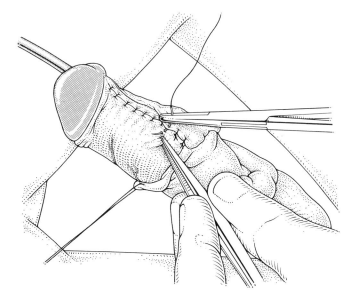

Fig. 11.21

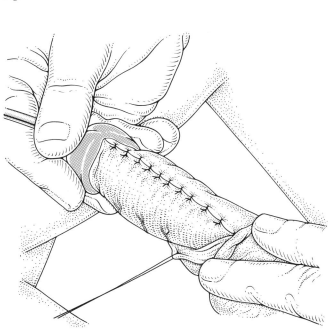

Fig. 11.22

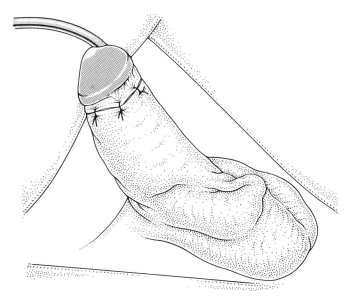

Fig. 11.23

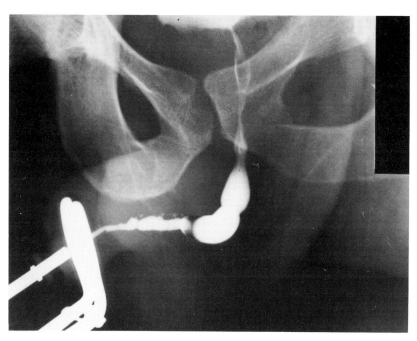

Fig. 11.24

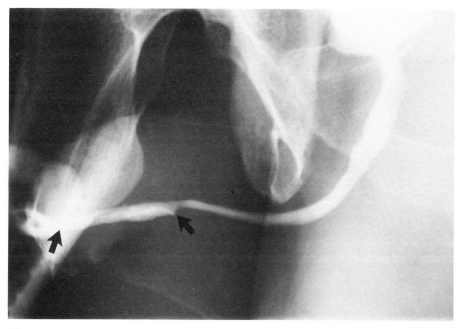

Fig. 11.25

The arrows show the proximal and distal extent of the skin inlay.

penile urethroplasty even if the calibre in much of the penile urethra is fairly well preserved. For the same reason patients are prone to recurrent stricture formation. Indeed any patient who has had a stricture anywhere in the urethra other than a simple short post-traumatic stricture should be regarded as having a stricture-prone urethra thereafter.

Penile strictures in hypospadias 'cripples'

The problems here (assuming that any chordee has been adequately corrected) are that good quality penile skin is in short supply, there is scarring from previous surgery, tissue planes have been obliterated and there is tethering of the skin or subcutaneous tissue to the corpora. Nonetheless it is often possible to mobilise a skin patch of adequate size to use for urethroplasty although a bit of imagination might be required to achieve this. If skin is not available a urothelial graft or buccal mucosa should be used. This is described later in this chapter.

BULBAR URETHRAL STRICTURES
(Table 11.2)

These are more difficult to treat than penile strictures because the natural curve of the bulbar urethra makes instrumentation more difficult, because they are more prone to complications, because of the close proximity to the distal sphincter mechanism of proximal bulbar strictures and because the more restricted access makes urethroplasty at this site technically more demanding.

As with penile strictures, the diagnosis is usually made endoscopically and so optical urethrotomy is often the first line of treatment, although with short tight post-traumatic strictures of 2 cm or less in length, primary excision and end-to-end anastomosis is preferable because the cure rate is higher and because incision may make the stricture longer and no longer amenable to an

Table 11.2 Bulbar strictures

A. Short post-traumatic strictures (<2 cm):
— excision and end-to-end-anastomosis
— avoid urethrotomy unless the stricture is very flimsy.

B. Long strictures:
1. Optical urethrotomy to open up the stricture followed by Otis urethrotomy to give an even calibre.
2. Consider urethroplasty if:
— rapidly and repeatedly recurrent
— complications
— young man.
a. Unusual local pathology 2–4 cm long, excise the segment, tack the urethral ends together dorsally, one-stage pedicled skin patch to close the ventral defect.
b. Stricture any length
i. Uncomplicated — stricturotomy, one-stage pedicled skin patch to close
ii. Complicated — excise or stricturotomy, two-stage reconstruction with interval scroto-urethral inlay.

In the elderly with ischaemic strictures:
— avoid urethroplasty
— persevere with endoscopy or dilatation (?CISC)
— consider an endoprosthetic stent.

Patches:
— pedicled preputial/penile skin the best
— pedicled scrotal skin second best in an adult
— urothelial free graft, second best in a child; otherwise if no alternative or if a tube graft is required.
— buccal mucosa graft

Tube grafts:
— hypospadias cripples
— tumours ⎫ when too long for
— vascular malformations ⎭ an excision as in 2a.

anastomotic urethroplasty. I should perhaps emphasise that by short tight stricture I mean just that — a short tight tough fibrous occlusion — not the more common but flimsy superficial web that a cystoscope or dilator will almost fall through which is decidedly unsuitable for urethroplasty.

The technique of urethrotomy for longer, usually post-infective or ischaemic, strictures and the subsequent follow up (and success rate) is as for penile strictures.

BULBAR URETHROPLASTY

Bulbar strictures which keep recurring, especially in young men, strictures complicated by refractory infection in pockets or false passages or by urethro-cutaneous fistulae, and short tight post-traumatic strictures are treated by urethroplasty, of which there are three types in my repertoire:

1. Excision and end-to-end anastomosis
2. One-stage patch urethroplasty
3. Two-stage urethroplasty.

The basic principles of the bulbar urethroplasty techniques described here are those established over the years by Richard Turner Warwick. The technique of patch urethroplasty that I prefer to use is derived from the transverse preputial island flap procedure for the treatment of hypospadias developed by John Duckett, although the late Ronald Yaxley seems to have been the first to describe the technique for the treatment of strictures. To these surgeons should go the credit for their pioneering work in these fields.

1. EXCISION AND END-TO-END ANASTOMOSIS

This is applicable to short tight post-traumatic strictures. The crucial factor here is the elastic lengthening of the urethra that can be obtained by full mobilisation of the bulbar urethra, bearing in mind that 1 cm of normal urethra on either side of the stricture will be required for an adequately spatulated anastomosis. As a general rule 4 cm of elastic lengthening can be achieved, which means that the technique is suitable for strictures which are less than 2 cm long. Most strictures that are suitable for this type of repair are post-traumatic because most post-infective strictures of the bulbar urethra are either longer or have a length of abnormal urethra (spongiofibrosis) on either side which is liable to restenosis. Whatever the type of stricture and its apparent suitability for excision and primary anastomosis, it is wise to begin the reconstructive procedure in such a way that an alternative procedure can be used if the urethra proves, on direct inspection, to be unsuitable for excision and primary anastomosis.

Preparation and position
No special preoperative preparation is required other than to ensure that the urine is sterile. The patient is placed on the operating table in the low lithotomy position. Blood loss is not usually significant and transfusion will not usually be required.

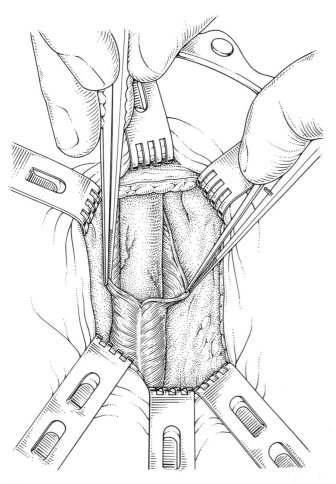

Fig. 11.26

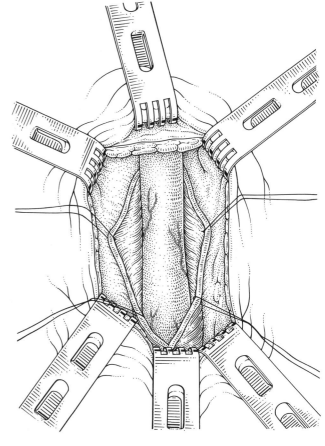

Fig. 11.27

Technique

A midline perineal incision is made over the bulbar urethra and deepened down to the bulbospongiosus muscle (Fig. 11.26), which is divided in the midline and reflected laterally on each side (Fig. 11.27). A perineal ring retractor is placed to hold the wound open and the small vessels that run at about 1 cm intervals from the corpus cavernosum to the spongiosum on each side are coagulated and divided. A bougie is then passed down from the meatus to define the distal end of the stricture and the urethra is opened by a longitudinal midline incision at this point and extended proximally to open the full length of the stricture (Fig. 11.28).

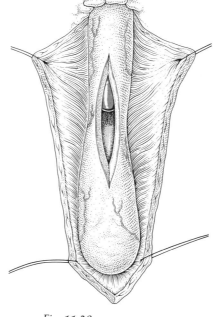

Fig. 11.28

Having opened the stricture itself, the urethral incision is extended a little way on either side to inspect the urothelium and surrounding spongy tissue and see if they are normal. If the length of the stricture is less than 2 cm and the urethra on either side is normal then the procedure can proceed as planned; normality is judged by a normal pink colour of the urothelium and absence of fibrosis in the surrounding spongy tissue. If there is any doubt about the normality of the urethra on either side of the stricture or if the stricture is longer than it was thought to be, then an alternative procedure will have to be used — usually a one-stage patch urethroplasty.

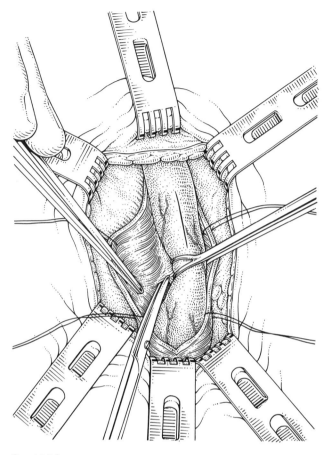

Fig. 11.29

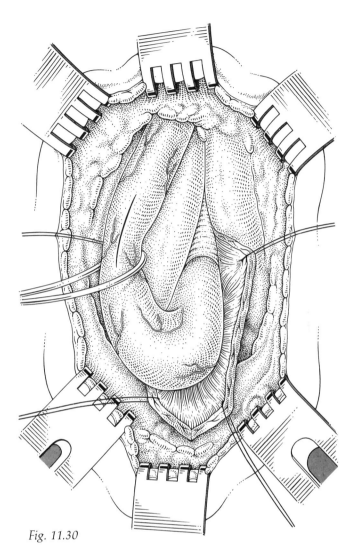

Fig. 11.30

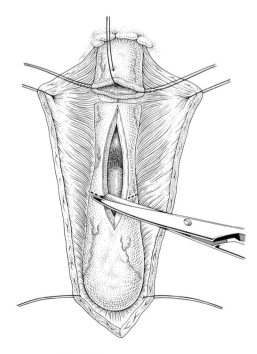

Fig. 11.31

Having decided to proceed, the next step is to mobilise the full length of the bulbar urethra by dividing the fibrous septum that tethers it between 11 o'clock and 1 o'clock (Fig. 11.29), all the way up to the membranous urethra (Fig. 11.30). The stricture is then excised (Fig. 11.31).

Before performing the bulbo-bulbar anastomosis, I usually put a suprapubic catheter as a precaution to provide urinary drainage in case the urethral catheter gets blocked and because I regard the urethral catheter more as a stent than as a drainage channel. One of the several percutaneous suprapubic catheters that are available as kits would probably be satisfactory but I prefer to use a suprapubic 16 F Foley catheter which is placed by passing a Hey-Groves staff, with a hole just before its tip, up the proximal bulbar urethra and into the bladder, tenting the bladder wall up to the anterior abdominal wall. A scalpel then makes a stab incision down onto the tip of the Hey-Groves staff (Fig. 11.32) allowing it to protrude through the abdominal wall. A length of nylon is threaded through the hole and tied to the eye of the Foley catheter (Fig. 11.33), which is then pulled through the bladder and proximal urethra by withdrawing the Hey-Groves staff (Fig. 11.34). The nylon loop is then cut, the tip of the catheter is withdrawn or pushed into the bladder and the balloon is inflated to keep it in position. Another alternative is to use the trocar system devised by Will Lawrence when he was working in Nottingham, which is specifically designed to insert a suprapubic Foley catheter percutaneously.

The proximal free ends of the urethra are then spatulated (Fig. 11.35). If both ends have been fully mobilised, it should be possible to approximate them with ease and without tension, although they usually seem to spring a mile apart when the stricture is excised.

The distal end is now tacked down to the fascia of the corpora cavernosa at the site of the proposed anastomosis (Fig. 11.36). This has the double effect of stabilising the distal segment and of holding the spatulated cut end open. The proximal end of the urethra is then anastomosed to the distal end on their deep aspects, from within the lumen of

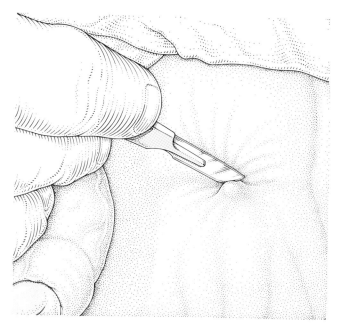

Fig. 11.32

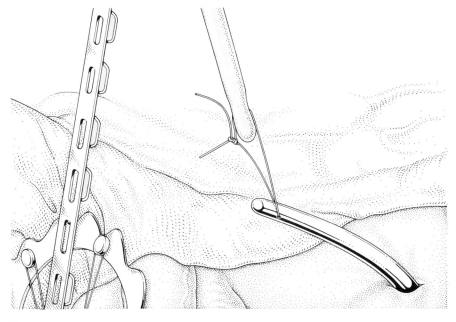

Fig. 11.33

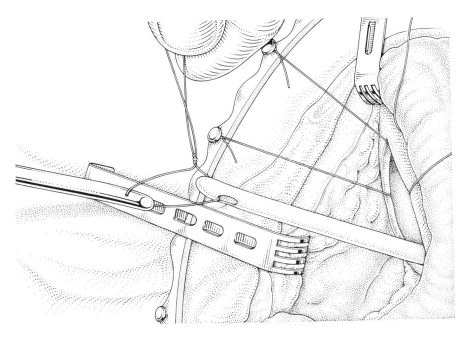

Fig. 11.34

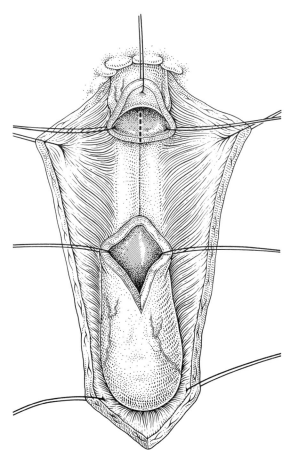

Fig. 11.35

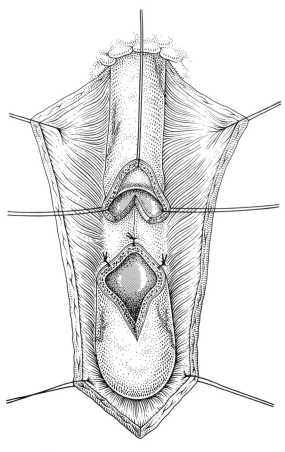

Fig. 11.36

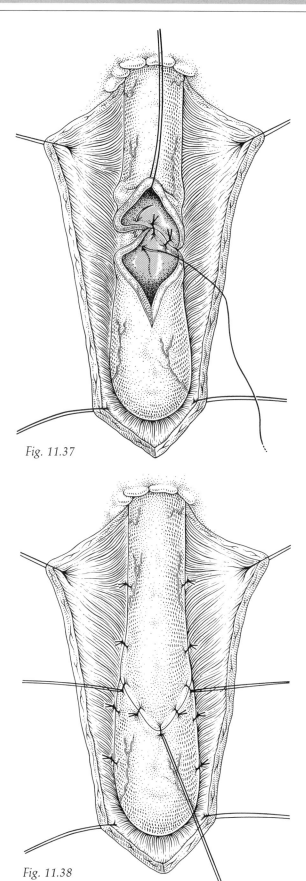

Fig. 11.37

Fig. 11.38

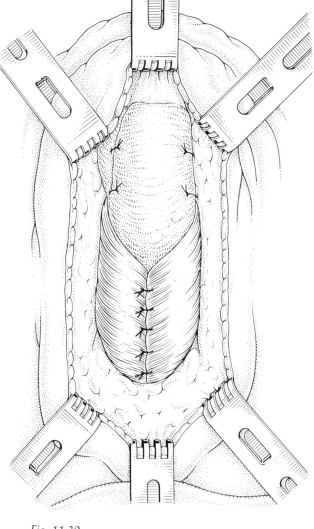

Fig. 11.39

the urethra by a series of interrupted
inverting 4/0 Vicryl sutures, knotted on
the inside, which also pick up the
underlying corporal fascia to stabilise the
anastomosis (Fig. 11.37).

When the deep half of the anastomosis
is complete, a 16 F silicone Foley
urethral catheter is passed up from the
meatus and into the bladder. The lateral
aspects of the corpus spongiosum are
then tacked to the corpora cavernosa on
either side of the anastomosis, again to
help stabilise the urethra and prevent
distraction of the anastomosis.

The anterior or superficial part of the
anastomosis is then closed by a further
series of interrupted 4/0 Vicryl sutures,
this time knotted on the outside (Fig.
11.38).

When the anastomosis is complete, the
bulbospongiosus muscle is closed over it
(Fig. 11.39) and the wound is closed
with interrupted 3/0 Vicryl mattress
sutures which pick up the full thickness
of the incision.

Postoperative management
The patient is kept in bed for the first
24 hours after operation and then
mobilised. He can usually be discharged
home at the end of 5–7 days, with both
catheters in situ, to return 2 weeks later
for a catheter-gram to check the
integrity of the anastomosis. This is
followed by removal of the urethral
catheter and a voiding cystogram
through the suprapubic catheter for final
confirmation of a satisfactory result (Fig.
11.40 — preoperative, Fig.
11.41 — postoperative, note the
dilatation at the site of the anastomosis).
The suprapubic catheter is then clamped
for 12–24 hours for a trial of voiding,
removing the catheter when satisfactory
voiding is established.

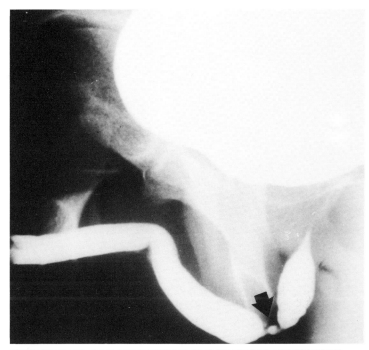

Fig. 11.40

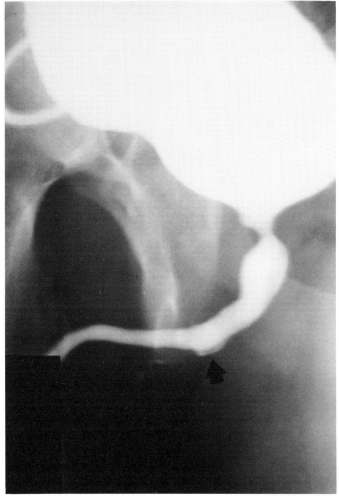

Fig. 11.41

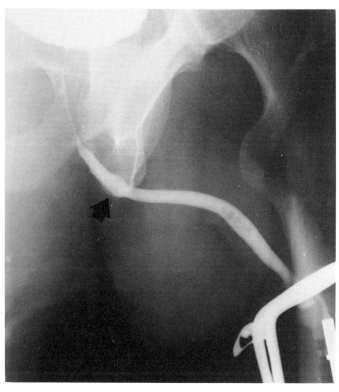

Fig. 11.42

The flow rate is checked on discharge and again in 6 months, at which time the urethrogram/cystogram is repeated to confirm that all is well (Fig. 11.42 —note the persisting dilatation as a result of the spatulation).

2. ONE-STAGE PATCH URETHROPLASTY

When the length of diseased urethra exceeds 2 cm or thereabouts an anastomotic urethroplasty is not possible because no more than about 2 cm of the urethra can be excised if the two ends are to be anastomosed without tension and because if the anastomosed ends are themselves affected by the stricturing process, the recurrence rate is high. Such strictures are treated by substitution urethroplasty using a patch technique.

Theoretically strictures that are 2—4 cm long could be excised completely; the two ends could then be spatulated, the two free edges could be sutured together leaving a ventral defect, and the defect could then be patched so that the entire repair involves healthy tissue. This should mean that the success rate would be high and the restricture rate low. Occasionally, in unusual circumstances, it is worth doing this but it is not generally worthwhile. Strictures longer than 4 cm cannot be excised and treated in this way as an excision of this length will leave a gap between the two cut ends. A tubed graft could be interposed (as described below) but unless the urethra *has* to be excised for some reason a better alternative is simply to open up the strictured urethra and patch it. This leaves the stricture-prone urethra in place and therefore carries a definite, albeit low, restricture rate. Although this makes it less than perfect it is nonetheless simple and is generally more applicable to the average patient.

Tube-graft procedures and two-stage urethroplasty are best reserved for more complicated problems and younger patients.

The principles of a one-stage patch urethroplasty are therefore to excise the stricture if necessary, and then to re-establish urethral continuity with either a patch or a tube graft, or otherwise to incise it and then patch it ventrally with suitable tissue to provide a repair of even calibre. The most suitable tissues for patching are a pedicled patch of penile skin, preferably the foreskin, or, if penile skin is not available, pedicled scrotal skin. If a pedicled skin graft is not possible, which is rare, then a free graft of buccal mucosa or bladder urothelium is the best option.

Preparation
No special preoperative preparation is required other than to ensure that the urine is sterile. The patient should have blood taken for grouping but transfusion is not usually required.

Position
The patient is placed in low lithotomy position with access to the lower abdomen for putting in a suprapubic catheter and in case bladder urothelium is required.

Technique
The urethra is exposed and opened as for an anastomotic repair, as it is often only after opening the stricture and exposing the urothelium and spongy tissue on either side that a final decision can be made as to the choice of procedure. If it is clear that an anastomotic repair is not going to be possible, each end of the stricturotomy incision is extended into healthy urothelium and spongy tissue so that healthy urethra is incised for 1 cm at each end. The next step is to decide whether:

— it is necessary or desirable to excise

the stricture (or other local pathology) and bring the two ends of the urethra together on their dorsal aspect to maintain urethral continuity with normal healthy tissue or,
— it is not necessary or desirable to excise the stricture but better just to incise the urethra and lay the urethra open.

Having made the decision as to how to deal with the stricture one must then decide how best to reconstitute the urethra. There are three alternatives:

1.   to sew in a pedicled skin patch (one-stage patch urethroplasty),
2.   to exteriorise the urethral defect for a few months and close it at a later date (two-stage urethroplasty), or
3.   when a long segment has been excised — to replace it with a tube graft.

As a general rule, option one — a one-stage patching — is best if only because it is easiest. Obviously, leaving the strictured urethra in place carries the risk of restricturing but the other two options have their own complications which at least balance this out. The tube-graft and two-stage procedures are therefore reserved for situations where a one-stage patch is contraindicated or impossible. Two-stage urethroplasties should always be considered when there is a lot of infection around or when a urethroplasty, particularly if it should be a tube graft, is likely to be less than perfect for any other reason. A one-stage tube graft is reserved for situations in which a substantial length of the urethra is more or less destroyed such as in some hypospadias cripples, or when it requires excision for unusual reasons such as a vascular malformation or a tumour but when the circumstances are otherwise right for a one-stage procedure and particularly when a urothelial tube graft is necessary.

Having decided to perform a one-stage patch urethroplasty the surgeon then has to decide whether:

— it will be possible to rotate in a pedicled preputial or penile skin patch or, alternatively,
— to use a pedicled patch of scrotal skin if a preputial/penile skin patch will not reach or is otherwise not practicable, usually because sufficient skin is unavailable, or
— to use a urothelial patch taken from the bladder or a buccal mucosa graft.

Preputial or penile skin is generally the best. When this is not available scrotal skin is usually preferable in an adult. A free graft of urothelium or buccal mucosa is preferable to scrotal skin in a child, is the best alternative in an adult when scrotal skin is also deficient, and is probably best at any age when a tube graft is required.

EXCISION OF THE STRICTURED (OR OTHERWISE DISEASED) URETHRA AND RESTORATION OF URETHRAL CONTINUITY

When the urethra is sufficiently deranged to warrant excision and the diseased segment is short enough to allow excision and then apposition of the two ends, then the segment is excised, the bulbar urethra is fully mobilised by division of the dorsal septum (as for an anastomotic urethroplasty), and the cut ends of the urethra are spatulated on their ventral aspects. The dorsal cut margins of the two ends are then sutured together with interrupted 3/0 and 4/0 Vicryl mattress sutures, picking up the underlying fascia of the corpora cavernosa (to stabilise the repair and prevent distraction) so that the dorsal half of the urethral circumference is reconstituted as a flat urethral plate (Fig. 11.43). The lateral

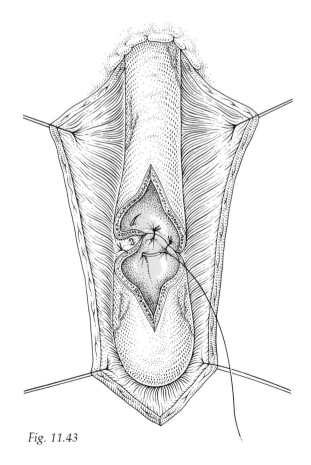

Fig. 11.43

aspects of the urethra on either side of this anastomosis are then tacked to the fascia of the corpora cavernosa to further reduce the risk of distraction of the anastomosis and suprapubic and urethral catheters are passed as for a simple bulbo-bulbar anastomosis. All that remains is to close the ventral urethral defect which will be a few centimetres only in length as described below.

When the diseased segment to be excised is too long to allow this the gap must either be bridged by a tube graft or exteriorised by sewing the two ends to the surrounding skin and then closed at a later date (see below).

Patch urethroplasty without excision of the stricture

For a patch urethroplasty urethral mobilisation is unnecessary. It is extremely important to be sure that the full length of the stricture is opened up and that this incision extends into healthy urethra at each end. The urethra is then tacked out laterally with a few stitches on each side. Any bleeding from the edges of the corpus spongiosum is controlled by a running stitch along the edges of the stricturotomy.

Use of a pedicled preputial/penile skin patch

However well or badly endowed the patient is, the length of the penis is almost always sufficient for it to be possible to raise a pedicled skin flap to rotate back comfortably to close the urethral defect created by one or other of the manoeuvres just described, particularly in an uncircumcised man, assuming that there has been no previous surgery to the penile skin.

The skin of the inner aspect of the prepuce is ideal. For a patch, a strip that is about 1 cm wide and equal in length to the length of the urethral defect will be necessary. For a skin tube, a skin strip 2.5 cm wide (and therefore 25 mm circumference or 25 F) will be necessary. In a circumcised man, a patch is almost

always still possible using the skin of the distal part of the penis, but there may be insufficient mobility for a tube graft, unless the penis is longer than average or the stricture is distally sited.

The aim of the procedure is to mobilise a patch of preputial or distal penile skin on a vascular pedicle created from the 'dartos' layer of the subcutaneous tissue of the shaft of the penis. In practice it doesn't matter where the skin patch is taken from as long as it is adequate in size for its purpose and has a sufficient vascular pedicle that will reach the urethral defect without tension. For the purposes of description I will describe the use of a preputial patch; obviously a patch taken from nearer the base of the penis is easier to raise.

To begin with, stay-stitches are placed around the margin of the prepuce (Fig. 11.44) and the foreskin is then incised in the ventral midline (6 o'clock) back to the coronal sulcus (Fig. 11.45). This incision is continued around the coronal sulcus (Fig. 11.46) incising both the preputial skin and the full thickness of the subcutaneous tissue, until the glans has been circumcised (Fig. 11.47). The penis is then degloved all the way round its circumference and all the way back to its base, carefully separating the skin (including the patch) and all the subcutaneous tissue together (including the dartos layer) off the underlying corpora cavernosa and corpus spongiosum (Fig. 11.48). If there has been no previous surgery this plane between the subcutaneous tissue and the

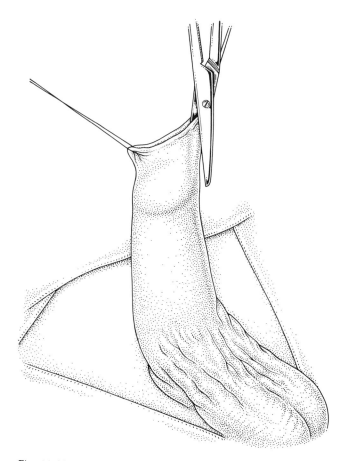

Fig. 11.44

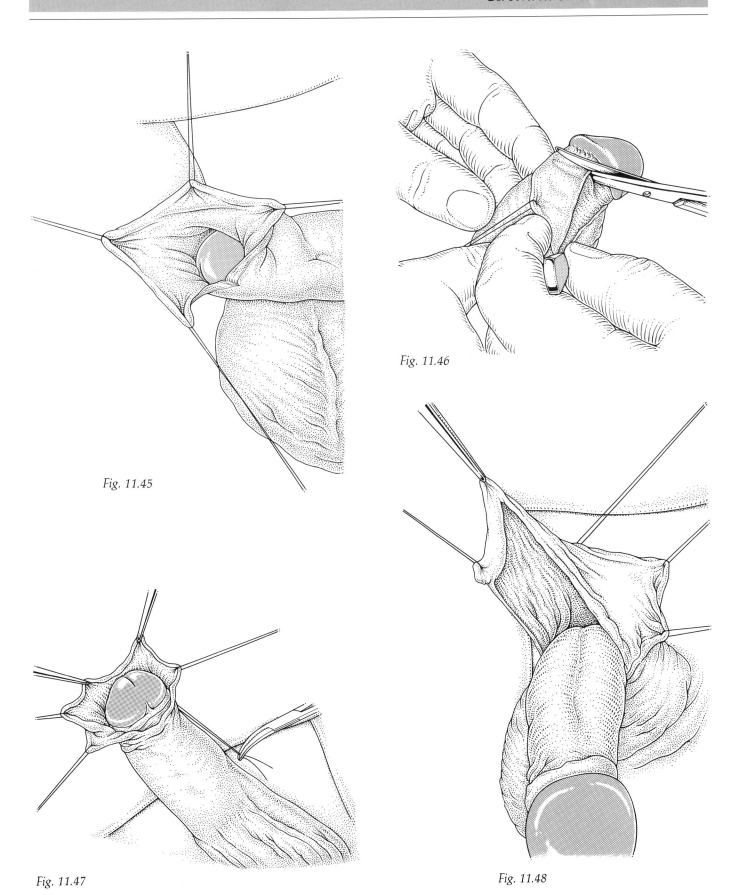

Fig. 11.45

Fig. 11.46

Fig. 11.47

Fig. 11.48

corpora is well defined and very easy to find. On the ventral aspect of the penis this dissection is continued proximally until space is opened up to communicate with the perineal dissection around the bulbar urethra. This space will form a tunnel so that the pedicled patch can be passed back to reach the strictured area later on.

The next step is to pull the skin back over the shaft of the penis and outline the proximal margin of the proposed skin patch. The skin alone is incised carefully, avoiding damage to the underlying dartos layer (Figs 11.49, 11.50). As with the plane deep to the dartos layer, there is a well defined and easily recognisable plane between the

skin of the penis with its own fine adherent layer of subcutaneous tissue, and the dartos layer (Figs 11.51, 11.52). This plane is widely opened, carefully separating the penile skin from the dartos layer all the way back to the base of the penis. By dissecting the penile skin off in this way, the dartos layer, previously separated from the corpora

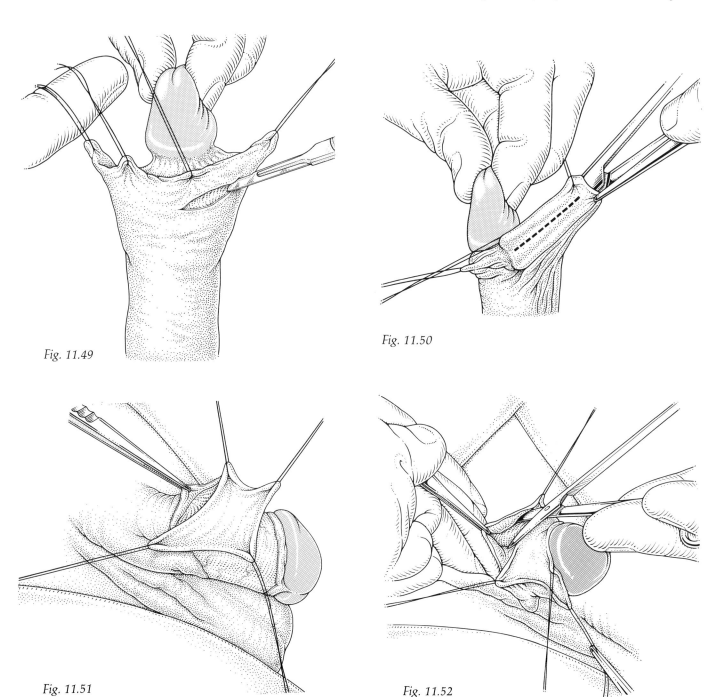

Fig. 11.49

Fig. 11.50

Fig. 11.51

Fig. 11.52

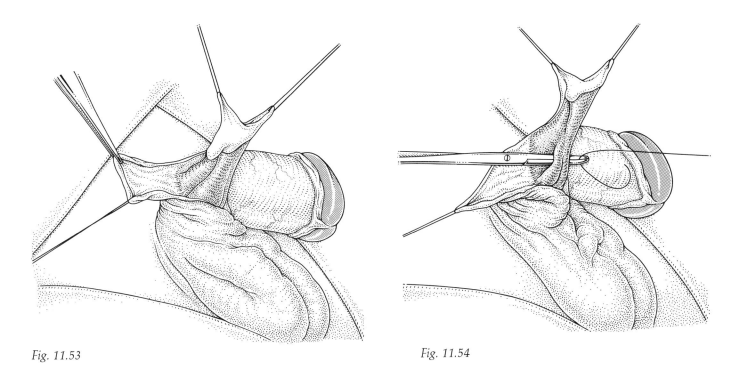

Fig. 11.53

Fig. 11.54

cavernosa on its deep aspect, is converted into a pedicle for the preputial skin patch (Fig. 11.53).

The lateral extent of this undermining of the penile skin is determined by the length of the skin patch itself. The width of the subcutaneous pedicle must be equal to the length of the skin patch and this in turn determines the degree of the undermining of the penile skin. If the whole of the circumference of the prepuce is required, to give a patch about 10–12 cm long, then the whole of the dartos layer will be required as its vascular pedicle and so the whole of the penile skin must be mobilised. For a smaller patch a correspondingly narrower pedicle and a correspondingly smaller skin reflection are required. Unless the entire prepuce and therefore the entire dartos layer is to be mobilised, the axis of dissection should be rotated through 90° as the undermining of the skin proceeds proximally so that the base of the pedicle comes to lie on one or other

side of the penis. This is important for two reasons. Firstly it is easier to rotate the patch and its pedicle back to the stricturotomy with the base of the pedicle on one side of the penis because the shaft of the penis does not get in the way. This is particularly important when dorsal penile rather than preputial skin is used or when the stricture is in the proximal part of the bulbar urethra. Secondly the main blood supply to the penile subcutaneous tissue, and therefore to the pedicle and the patch, is from a branch of the femoral artery that runs to the dorsolateral aspect of the penis on each side in a fairly definite palpable thickening of the subcutaneous tissue (Fig. 11.54 — here being ligated and divided on the right side so that the pedicle can be rotated round the left side of the penis). A laterally based pedicle therefore has better vascularity because it is centred around this point. If the whole of the dartos layer is used to support the maximum length of patch then both dorsolateral pedicles should be preserved unless this will prevent

adequate rotation of the patch back to the urethral defect. If both are preserved then the dorsal aspect of the dartos layer can be 'buttonholed' vertically so that the penis can be pulled through to bring the dartos layer and the preputial patch onto its ventral aspect.

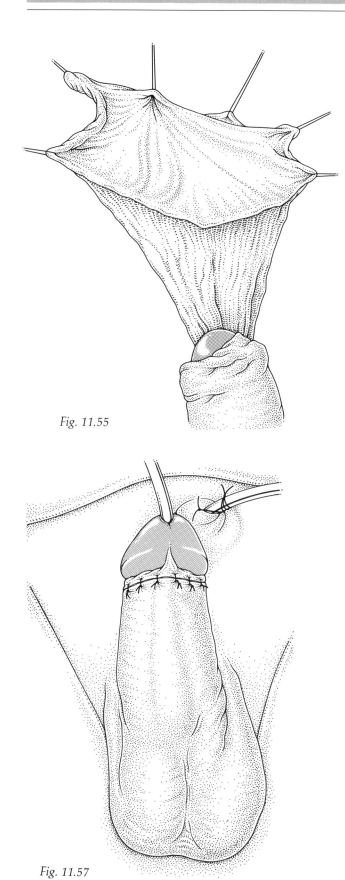

Fig. 11.55

Fig. 11.57

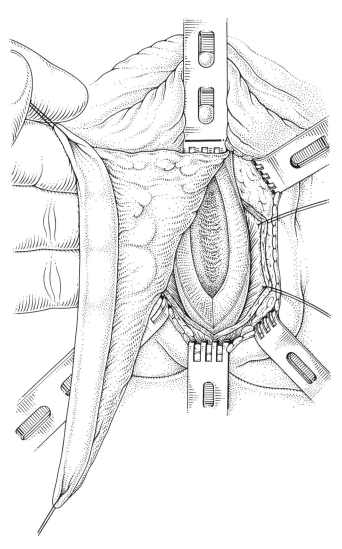

Fig. 11.56

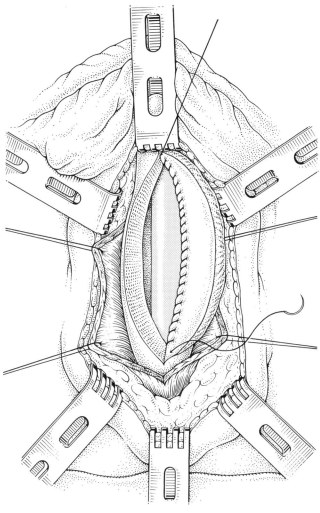

Fig. 11.58

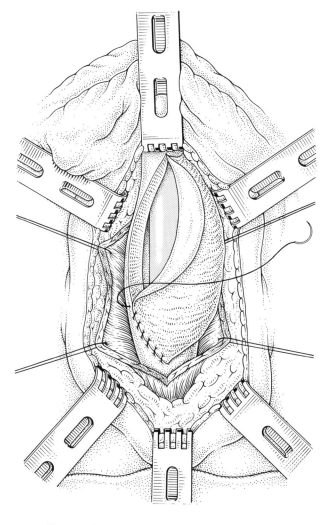

Fig. 11.59

At the end of this dissection the skin and subcutaneous tissue should have been dissected off the full length of the shaft of the penis. The proposed preputial/penile skin patch should have a dartos pedicle with a width that is at least equal to that of the patch itself (Fig. 11.55). During the course of the dissection of the penile skin from the dartos layer the feeder vessels from the superficial femoral artery on each dorsolateral aspect of the penis should have been carefully preserved, and for smaller patches the subcutaneous pedicle should have been developed on one side

of the base of the penis. Finally, at the end of this dissection the skin of the shaft of the penis should be intact to re-cover the penis.

The patch on its pedicle is then passed through the ventral subcutaneous tunnel at the root of the penis and scrotum to lie in the perineum alongside the urethra (Fig. 11.56) and the 'circumcised' skin margins at the coronal sulcus are trimmed and closed with interrupted 4/0 Vicryl (or similar) sutures (Fig. 11.57).

Before starting to sew the patch in to close the urethral defect suprapubic and urethral catheters are passed. Both should be 16 F silicone Foley catheters. The type and calibre of the urethral catheter is important but for the suprapubic it is not so important.

The patch is then trimmed to its exact size, excising only skin and leaving the subcutaneous pedicle intact (Fig. 11.58), and sewn in place with 4/0 Vicryl sutures (Fig. 11.59). The tissue of the pedicle is then tacked to the surrounding tissue to anchor it firmly in place and to

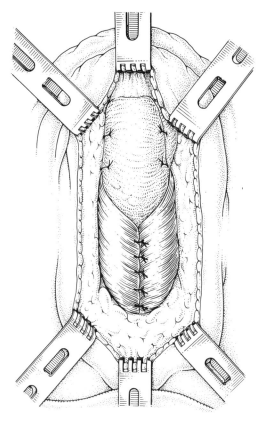

Fig. 11.61

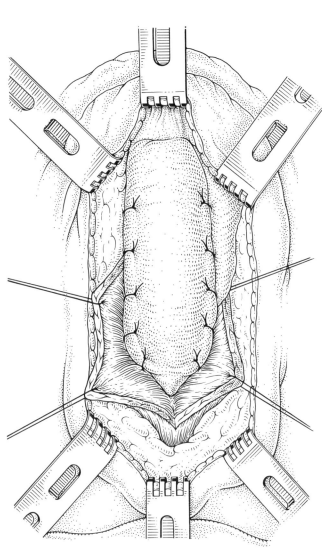

Fig. 11.60

cover the suture line (Fig. 11.60) and the bulbospongiosus muscle is closed (Fig. 11.61).

Postoperative management, as for other strictures, is 2—3 weeks of catheterisation and radiological proof of healing before removing the catheters. Six months later the X-rays are repeated to confirm a satisfactory result (Fig. 11.62 preoperative and 11.63 postoperative films).

On the rare occasions that a tube graft is required, there will be a defect where a segment of urethra has been excised for whatever reason. The cut ends of the urethra should be trimmed back to healthy tissue, spatulated and tacked down to fix them in place (Fig. 11.64). The preputial skin is cut accurately to size and then tubed with interrupted inverting mattress sutures of 4/0 Vicryl to fit snugly around a lubricated 20 or

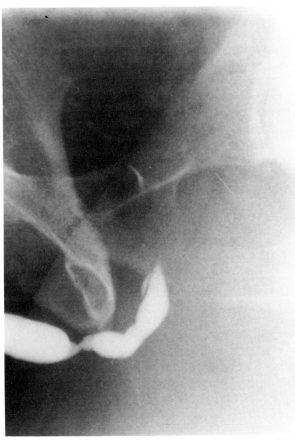

Fig. 11.62

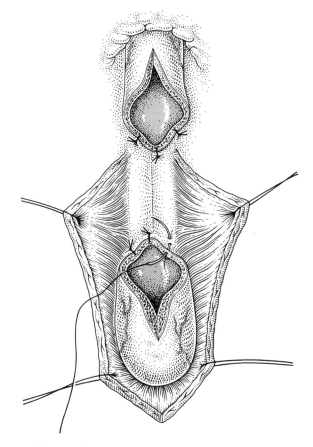

Fig. 11.64

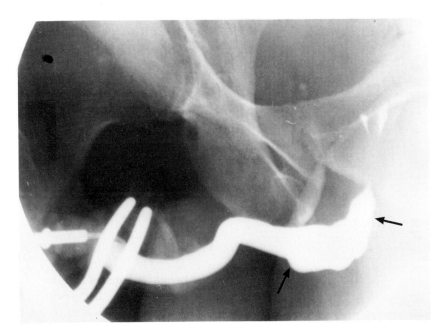

Fig. 11.63

22 F Neoplex bougie (or otherwise, of a calibre appropriate to the calibre of the rest of the urethra) (Fig. 11.65), which is then removed. The proximal end of the tube is then anastomosed to the proximal end of the urethra with 3/0 or 4/0 interrupted Vicryl mattress sutures (Fig. 11.66) and the repair is completed by a similar anastomosis of the distal end of the skin tube to the distal end of the urethra (Fig. 11.67). A 16 F silicone Foley urethral catheter is then passed through the urethra and into the bladder. The bulbocavernosus is then closed in the usual way (Fig. 11.68).

It is worth noting that although preputial skin is satisfactory for tube grafts penile skin is less satisfactory and scrotal skin is unsatisfactory and a urothelial or buccal mucosa free graft will usually be preferable.

Other tissues for urethroplasty
Other tissues can be and commonly are used for patching or replacing the urethra. The two most commonly used are free skin grafts and pedicled scrotal skin. Free urothelial or buccal mucosa grafts are a relatively recent introduction mainly used in paediatric practice for urethral substitution in difficult hypospadias problems. The principal protagonists for each claim good results with their technique in their own hands, as is usually the case with experts in any particular technique; but the principal arguments in favour of them are those of ease and speed. It is certainly quicker and easier to harvest a free graft than a pedicled graft and to prepare a pedicled scrotal skin patch than a preputial patch. Ease and speed are not however the main considerations in surgery.

There is no surgeon on earth who does not know from his earliest days of training that free grafts have a significant rate of failure to 'take' and that a significant degree of contraction of the graft is also common, although both problems seem to be less common with urothelium or buccal mucosa than with skin. Nonetheless, it seems pointless to accept these intrinsic complications when there is usually so much skin around that is suitable for a pedicled graft with a more or less guaranteed 'take' and no contraction thereafter.

As for the comparison between penile skin and scrotal skin: scrotal skin is hairy, it tolerates wetness poorly — sometimes becoming soggy and eczematous — but more importantly, it is thermolabile. Its thermolability makes it

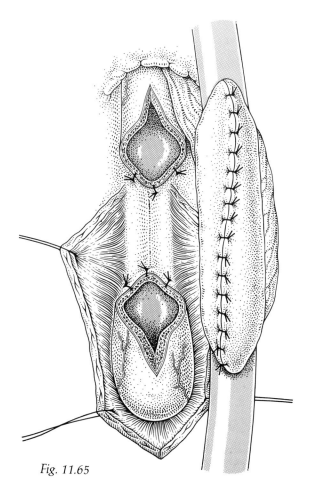

Fig. 11.65

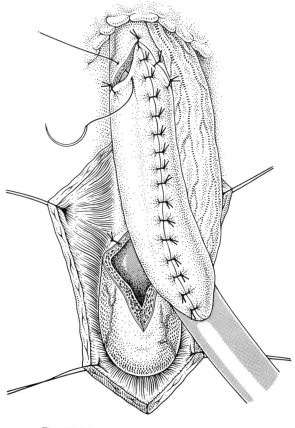

Fig. 11.66

difficult to size accurately — a scrotum that is a huge floppy bag under normal circumstances becomes a tightly wrinkled little walnut in the operating theatre, particularly after the skin has been 'prepped'. Then, after the patch has been laid into the urethra and has warmed up to body temperature, it relaxes again and is therefore oversized and baggy from the very beginning.

Sometimes one has to use scrotal skin for patching because an adequate amount of penile skin simply is not available but I prefer to use preputial or penile skin when I can. On the other hand, whereas I don't feel very strongly about the comparison between penile skin and scrotal skin because one can always warm up scrotal skin to size it properly and the other potential problems are rarely a problem in

practice, I do feel strongly that free grafts are definitely third best, with urothelium and buccal mucosa being the best free grafts currently available. Having said that, the scrotum in prepubertal children is less satisfactory than in adults so I would be inclined to recommend urothelial or buccal mucosa grafting in preference to pedicled scrotal skin in children when pedicled preputial/penile skin is unavailable.

Scrotal skin patch urethroplasty

Scrotal skin receives its blood supply in much the same way as penile skin. There is the dartos layer of well vascularised supporting tissue which feeds a distinct subcutaneous layer

beneath the scrotal skin which in turn supplies the skin itself. There are therefore two distinct layers of 'subcutaneous tissue' when scrotal skin is incised, with a distinct and readily identifiable plane in between. As with preputial/penile skin patch urethroplasty a scrotal skin patch is mobilised on an adequate vascular pedicle derived from the dartos layer which is created by dissecting off the overlying scrotal skin and subcutaneous tissue proper around the patch.

The principal protagonist of pedicled scrotal patch urethroplasty is John Blandy and the technique I use is derived from his. He prefers to begin his

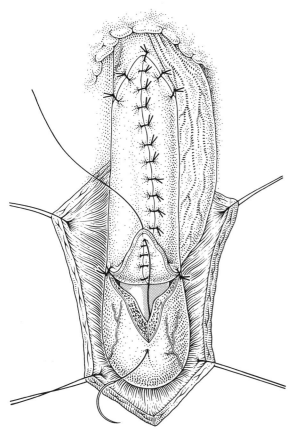

Fig. 11.67

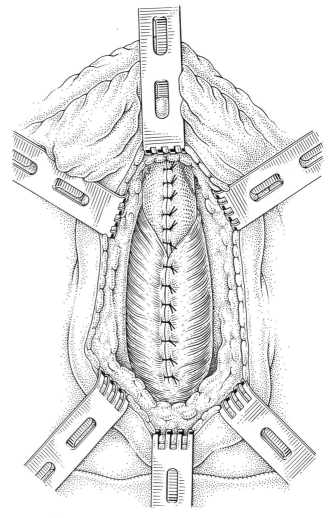

Fig. 11.68

procedure with an inverted 'U'-shaped incision extended onto the posterior aspect of the scrotum which is dropped back to expose the urethra. He then mobilises the skin patch from the apex of that flap. He does emphasise however that the incision and the mobilisation of the skin patch can be varied to suit the circumstances of the procedure because the blood supply to the scrotal skin is so good. I agree, but prefer to begin the procedure with the usual midline perineal incision, in most instances, because it is more extendable. I then take the skin patch from one edge of the extended incision and mobilise it on a laterally or posteriorly based dartos pedicle.

The two crucial factors for scrotal skin patch urethroplasty are the sizing of the patch and the creation of an adequate sized and adequately mobilised vascular pedicle. I have already mentioned that one of the main problems with scrotal skin is its thermolability. In order to ensure that the skin patch is going to be the right size when it is sewn into the urethra and therefore subject to body temperature, it is important to size the patch when the skin is fully relaxed, using hot packs if necessary to warm the skin in a cold operating theatre. I think that the other problems of scrotal skin are overstated when one considers the size of the piece of skin that is used for urethroplasty. Hair and the 'eczematous reaction' are indeed problems if an oversized piece of skin is used so that it becomes baggy but the problem here is the bagginess rather than the nature of the skin itself. In any case it is usually possible to avoid hair follicles when planning a scrotal skin patch. Sizing therefore is all-important and in the same vein it is also important to be prepared to trim further the size of the patch to fit the urethral defect when it is actually being sewn in.

As to the mobilisation of the dartos pedicle, the important point here is to make it long enough and wide enough.

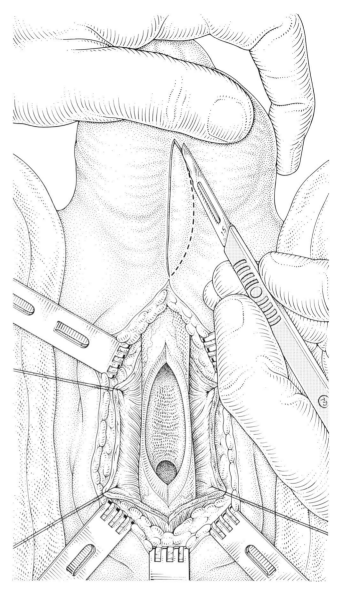

Fig. 11.69

It should be at least as wide as the length of the skin strip and long enough to reach comfortably down to the urethra and, just as important, to stay there when the scrotal skin is subsequently closed at the end of the procedure.

The pedicle itself can be formed either from the subcutaneous dartos layer deep to the scrotal skin or from the midline, inter-testicular dartos layer. The midline tissue is flimsier but can be mobilised without interfering with the position of

either testis. It can in any case be supplemented by including some of the subcutaneous dartos layer of the posterior aspect of the scrotum.

If the subcutaneous dartos layer is used and a wide pedicle has to be mobilised to support a fairly long skin strip (to repair a long stricture) then there may be problems posed by the position of the testis on that side. This doesn't usually present any difficulty with short patches but if the problem does occur it is readily overcome by 'buttonholing'

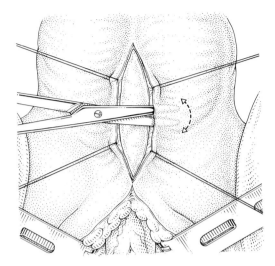

Fig. 11.70

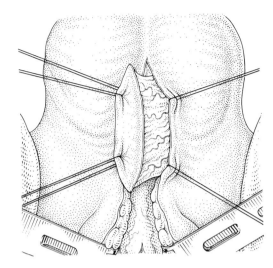

Fig. 11.71

the pedicle in the line of its fibres and pulling the testis through to be between the dartos and the skin as one would for a dartos pouch-orchidopexy.

Having considered these provisos the technique of mobilising a scrotal skin patch is straightforward. The urethra is prepared in the usual way by a 'stricturotomy' into healthy urethra at each end. The length of the defect is measured and a patch of the same length and a width of about 1 cm is outlined along the edge of the midline incision after extension of the incision along the raphe of the posterior aspect of the scrotum (Fig. 11.69). The scrotal skin should be warmed if necessary and put on the stretch to size the patch correctly; hair follicles should be avoided as far as possible in order to produce as hairless a patch as possible.

The lateral margin of the patch is then incised carefully through the skin and the immediately subadjacent connective tissue until the plane is reached between this subcutaneous layer and the dartos layer. This plane is then opened up to allow complete separation of the patch from the adjacent scrotal skin (Fig. 11.70) and then separation of the scrotal skin with its subcutaneous layer from the dartos layer (Fig. 11.71). This

separation should continue until a pedicle has been produced that is sufficiently long for the patch to reach down comfortably to the urethral defect. If the position of the testis proves to be a problem during positioning of the patch in the urethral defect it is repositioned between the mobilised dartos layer and the skin by pulling it through a dartos buttonhole as described above.

The rest of the procedure is as for a pedicled preputial patch urethroplasty.

The use of a urothelial patch (or tube)

In an uncircumcised man (or boy) a pedicled preputial flap can be used to repair a stricture at any site and of any length in the urethra. Even in a circumcised and less well endowed patient it will usually be possible to get a patch to reach back to the bulbomembranous junction for more proximally sited strictures. If a pedicled penile skin technique proves impossible or impracticable then I would use pedicled scrotal skin as the next best option in an adult, working on the principle that pedicled and therefore vascularised tissue will have a predictable viability and 'take', without subsequent contracture. Because of the

excellent results with the 'pedicled patch' technique when compared with free graft techniques, I prefer to use it whenever possible, reserving the technique of urothelial patching for strictures in which a pedicled skin patch is impossible or impracticable, usually because of multiple previous operations (e.g. repeated surgery for hypospadias), particularly in children in whom scrotal skin is inherently much less satisfactory than in adults.

As with skin patching, the urethra is first prepared either by excision of the stricture, with restoration of urethral continuity where possible or by incision and laying open of the stricture. A urethral catheter is then passed and a template is made of the urethral defect.

During this first stage it is important to preserve as much as possible of whatever healthy spongy tissue of the corpus spongiosum there is, as this and the bulbospongiosus muscle will subsequently form the bed for the urothelial patch. This particularly applies to proximal bulbar strictures in the bulb of the corpus spongiosum. In such a case, rather than making a simple longitudinal incision through the spongiosum and into the urethra, a posteriorly based triangular flap of

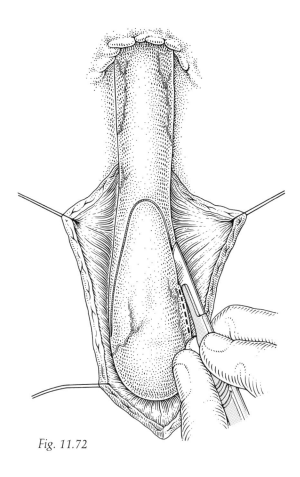

Fig. 11.72

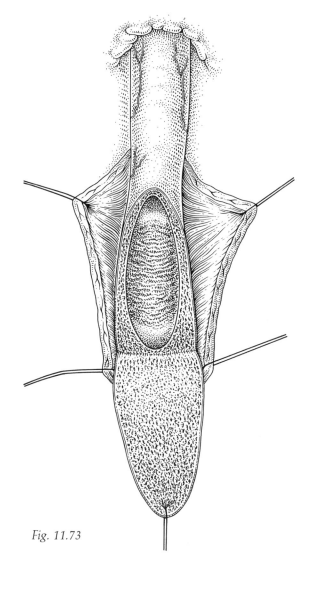

Fig. 11.73

healthy, unfibrosed spongy tissue is reflected (Fig. 11.72) before the strictured urethra is incised (Fig. 11.73), so that this can subsequently be used to cover the patch.

The urothelium is harvested from the bladder by a suprapubic incision exposing the bladder, which is distended by filling it with water. A vertical incision is made through the muscle of the dome of the bladder, taking care not to breach the urothelium, to allow the urothelium to bulge through the muscular incision. For this purpose a blunt-ended diathermy point is less likely to breach the urothelium than a scalpel. When urothelium bulges through, the incision is extended by gently teasing the muscle fibres apart to allow the required amount of urothelium to bulge through. When sufficient urothelium to form a patch (or tube) has been exposed, it is excised and the

bladder is closed around the customary suprapubic catheter. The patch is then trimmed to size and a few stab incisions are made so that blood oozing from the vascular bed of the graft during the early postoperative period can escape into the urethral lumen, so that haematoma formation will not prevent a 'take' (although whether or not this actually makes much difference I don't know). The patch is then sutured to the margins of the urethral defect with interrupted 4/0 Vicryl sutures (Fig. 11.74) and the previously reflected spongy tissue is then sewn over the patch to cover it (Fig. 11.75).

If a tube graft is required (usually only for penile urethral substitution in hypospadias 'cripples' — see below) the urothelium is formed into a tube and sewn into the urethral defect around a catheter as described above for a preputial skin tube graft.

Throughout a urothelial graft procedure, two points should be borne in mind. Firstly urothelium tends to dry out very quickly so it should be kept moist by irrigating it frequently with saline. Secondly it is important not to lose orientation of the graft. Once it is harvested it is difficult to tell which is

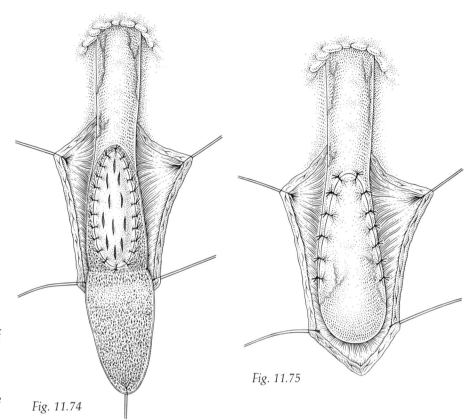

Fig. 11.74

Fig. 11.75

the epithelial surface and which is the subepithelial surface so some system of marking must be used to avoid this problem. Obviously a patch or tube graft will only take if the epithelial surface is inwards (into the lumen of the urethra) and the subepithelial (raw) surface is in close contact with the surrounding tissues which form the bed of the graft.

As with all one-stage bulbar urethroplasties, the bulbospongiosus muscle is carefully reconstituted around the completed repair and the wound is closed with deep interrupted mattress sutures. A catheter-gram is performed at 3 weeks, followed by a voiding cystogram. If these are satisfactory, the suprapubic catheter is removed 24 hours later after normal voiding has been re-established.

As always the flow rate and radiological assessment are repeated 6 months later to confirm a satisfactory result.

Buccal mucosal grafts
Buccal mucosa is a more recently introduced alternative to urothelium for free grafting. Like urothelium it can be used as either a patch graft or a tube graft and is particularly useful in hypospadias cripples (see below).

There are several advantages to buccal mucosa as compared with urothelium. It is easier to harvest (as it does not involve a laparotomy), it is tougher and it does not tend to develop the exuberance that urothelium shows on exposure to the atmosphere (see below). Like urothelium the donor defects can be closed primarily. The only precaution to be taken is to avoid damage to the parotid duct on the inside of the cheek. Small patches or tube grafts are taken from the inside of the cheek; longer tube grafts are taken from the inside of the lips.

Experience with buccal mucosa is limited at present but I would guess that before long it will replace urothelial grafting assuming that the initial satisfactory results are maintained.

Urothelial or buccal mucosa tube grafts and hypospadias cripples
A hypospadias cripple is a sorry sight. By the time most of them present as

such, all of the available skin for urethral reconstruction has been used and there seems no possibility of getting a satisfactory result. Sometimes the skin on the ventral aspect of the penis is fairly smooth (albeit scarred) or can be made so and it is possible to roll this into a neourethral tube in situ to anastomose to the bulbar urethra (as for the second stage of a two-stage urethroplasty — see below). The neourethra can then be covered by rotating a pedicled flap of scrotal skin up onto the ventral aspect of the penis. If this is not possible or, more commonly, unlikely to give a satisfactory result, a urothelial or buccal mucosa tube graft is a useful option.

The graft is harvested, prepared and rolled into a tube around a catheter as described above. The three important points when used in hypospadias cripples are that the external meatus should be skin lined, not urothelially lined; that the tube graft should be completely covered by intact skin; and that it should be under a bit of tension. If urothelium is exposed to the atmosphere it becomes thickened, polypoid and unsightly. If the graft is not covered by intact skin then fistulae develop from the graft suture line to the skin surface. If the tube graft is not sewn into place with a bit of tension to stretch it, it ends up like a concertina.

The operation begins with a glanuloplasty/meatoplasty to give a skin-lined meatus. A circumcision incision is made, including the meatus of the stenotic and otherwise unsatisfactory urethra (Fig. 11.76) and the penis is then degloved back to healthy urethra, stripping the skin and all the subcutaneous tissue including the dartos layer (such as it is) off the corpora cavernosa (Fig. 11.77). An alternative to circumcision degloving if the glans and meatus are satisfactory or if healthy urethra is proximal to the peno-scrotal junction, is to start with a midline

scrotal incision to split the scrotum in half and then to deglove the penis, working from the base distally, until the shaft of the penis can be evaginated. If the circumcision degloving is preferred but is not sufficient to reach back to expose healthy urethra then further exposure is gained through a perineal incision with subcutaneous tunnelling between the two to establish communication. The strictured urethral remnant is then excised and a graft of appropriate length prepared. After excising the urethral remnant and before sewing in the neourethral graft it is important to ensure that any chordee has been corrected by injecting the corpora with saline to produce an artificial erection.

A glans meatoplasty is usually performed by a MAGPI procedure as described by John Duckett. In a hypospadias cripple this is probably not possible. In such a case the glans is often small and a glansplasty as such is

not possible at all, so the meatus of the urethra can only be brought to the tip of the penis by tunnelling through the glans (see below). If the glans is a reasonable size, a glanular urethra can be created by defining a skin strip of appropriate width (Fig. 11.76), denuding the glans on either side of skin (Fig. 11.77) and then rolling the glans over, undermining when necessary, and closing it in two layers as shown in Figure 11.78.

The tube graft on its catheter is then positioned to bridge the gap and sutured to the proximal urethra with one end of the catheter passed up and into the bladder and the other end passed out through the meatus. This catheter serves as a urethral stent not as a sole means of urinary drainage. The graft is then 'put on the stretch' and the distal end is trimmed to the right length for anastomosis to the glandular urethra with the penis laid flat on the anterior abdominal wall to put it 'on the stretch'

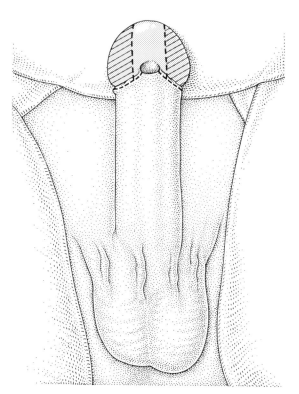

Fig. 11.76

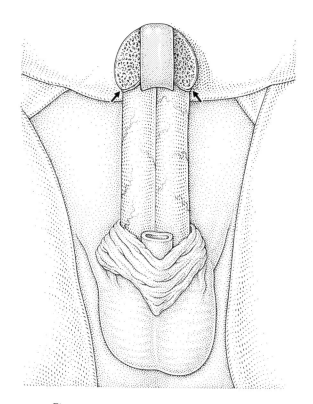

Fig. 11.77

(Fig. 11.79). Finally the degloved penile skin and subcutaneous tissue is rolled back over the neourethra and the circumcision incision is sutured. When the glans is not suitable for a glansplasty as described above, usually because it is too small, and when a urothelial tube graft has to be brought through to the tip of the penis, something has to be done to prevent the development of the exuberant urothelial reaction described above. The simplest technique is the one described by Philip Ransley. After a core of glans tissue has been removed to allow the tube graft to reach the tip of the penis and the graft itself has been trimmed to size, the distal 1 cm or so is removed and replaced by a slightly more generous free skin graft (to allow for contracture) so that the tip of graft at the glanular meatus will be skin rather than urothelium.

Postoperatively, the penis is held on the anterior abdominal wall with some adhesive tape for a week or so. A suprapubic catheter should be passed to complete the procedure. The postoperative management and catheter removal follow the usual pattern.

3. TWO-STAGE URETHROPLASTY

This is the technique of choice for long strictures complicated by infected false passages, fistulae or other gross periurethral complicating factors, or whenever the reconstruction is otherwise precarious. A two-stage procedure is also useful when there are multiple strictures or when there is a lack of suitable tissue for urethroplasty. None of these situations is very common these days so a two-stage urethroplasty is not commonly required.

Many of the principles have already been described in the last section. The main difference between a two-stage and a one-stage procedure is that there is an interval period after incision or excision of the stricture(s) and preparation of the urethra, and before final closure to allow time for any infection or other complicating factor to resolve. During this interval period the urethra is left open to view so that residual problems are more easily defined and treated.

The aims of the two-stage procedure are to incise or excise the stricture opening into healthy urethra at each end, to

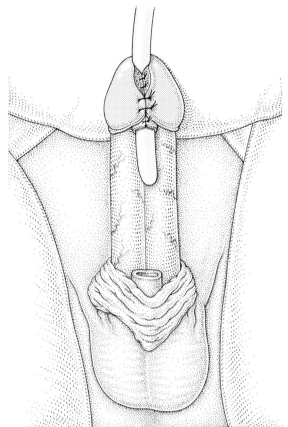

Fig. 11.78

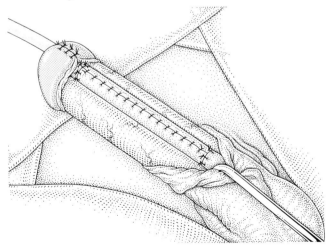

Fig. 11.79
The suture is best left on the deep aspect but is shown here superficially for clarity.

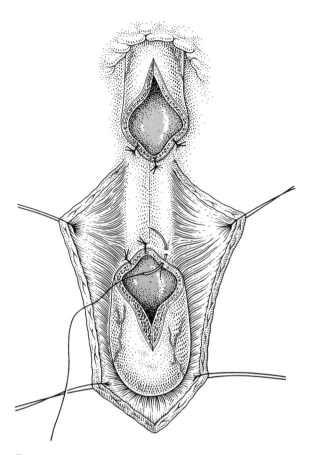

Fig. 11.80

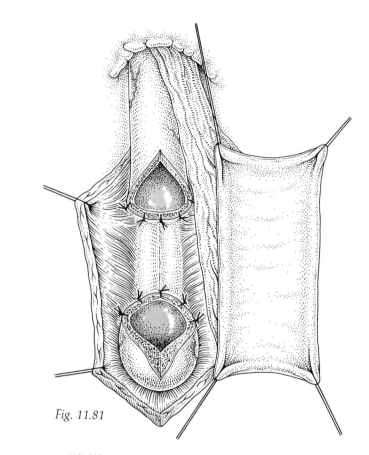

Fig. 11.81

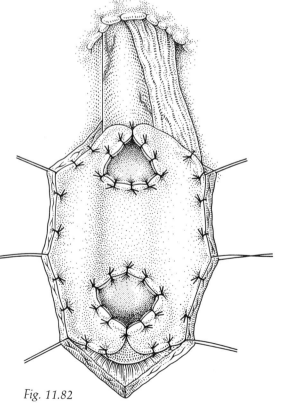

Fig. 11.82

bridge the gap when necessary with healthy skin, and to leave enough additional skin alongside so that this can be used for closure of the urethra at the second stage.

The counsel of perfection is to excise the stricture, spatulate the cut ends and fix the lateral aspects and cut ends flat to the underlying fascia of the corpora cavernosa (Fig. 11.80). More commonly the urethra is simply incised.

When the strictured segment of the urethra has been excised, a pedicled preputial/penile skin patch is prepared and brought through to the perineum (Fig. 11.81) to fill the gap between the two ends of the urethra. It is sutured at each end to the urethral margins and on each side it is tethered to the corpora cavernosa to fix it in place (Fig. 11.82).

The third objective, to bring in healthy epithelium for subsequent urethral closure, can be achieved in one of two ways. Firstly, if the strictured segment has been excised the patch used to 'fill the gap' can be made wide enough to allow it to be rolled in later to form a skin tube urethra, and this is obviously the most sensible thing to do. The alternative, in patients who have had their stricture incised (rather than excised), is to use scrotal skin. In practice, the first stage of the urethroplasty is completed by funnelling scrotal skin down to the margins of the repair so that this is always available in any case.

Scrotal funnelling

To form the scrotal funnel, all the subcutaneous tissue between the scrotal skin and the urethra must first be mobilised out of the way so that the scrotal skin can be retracted posteriorly to allow the original midline perineal skin incision to be closed horizontally. This is achieved by finger dissection, working superficially from the perineal aspect of the urethra. This finger dissection also makes it easier to get the scrotal skin down to the bulbar urethra in the depths of the perineal wound (Fig. 11.83), without tethering by the testes which would otherwise put tension on the skin and therefore on the subsequent suture line. The original midline perineal incision is then closed horizontally with interrupted 3/0 Vicryl mattress sutures. The scrotal skin in the depths of the funnel is then incised in the midline, along the raphe, over a length equal to that of the opened urethra so that the margins of the scrotal skin can be sutured to the margins of the urethra and the patch (when present) with interrupted 3/0 or 4/0 Vicryl sutures (Fig. 11.84).

At the end of the procedure a 16 F silicone-coated Foley urethral catheter is passed (in addition to the usual suprapubic catheter) and vaseline-gauze is placed between it and the underlying urethra. A further layer of vaseline gauze is placed over the catheter and the margins of the scroto-urethral suture line and this is then covered with a generous layer of gauze, which is in turn covered with cotton wool and held in place with a T-bandage or with a flexible adhesive tape such as Mefix. After 8–10 days, the bulk of the dressing and the urethral catheter are gently removed and the deep remaining part of the dressing is allowed to soak off in a bath. The suprapubic catheter is clamped off 7–10 days later (between the 15th and 20th postoperative day) and, if voiding is satisfactory, it is removed the next day.

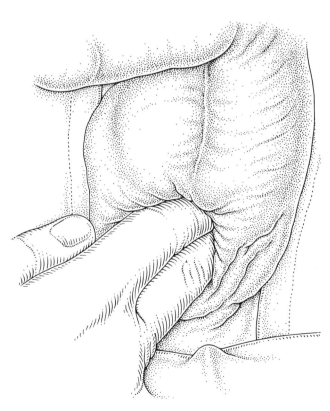

Fig. 11.83

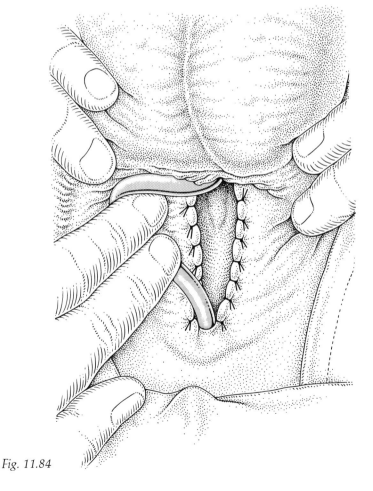

Fig. 11.84

Three months are then allowed for adequate healing of the ends of the urethra to the skin patch and the scroto-urethral inlay, at which time the appearances of the tissues and the calibres of the two ends of the urethra are assessed. If the assessment is satisfactory, the urethra is closed. If the appearances are not completely satisfactory, closure is deferred until they are. If there is stenosis of either of the ends of the urethra, this is corrected by incising through the stenosis (Fig. 11.85) and then rotating in a local flap (Figs 11.86–11.88). Urethral closure is deferred for a further 3-month period.

Urethral closure

If a pedicled preputial/penile skin inlay was performed at the first stage then at the time of urethral closure there should be a well 'taken' patch, at least 3 cm wide, clearly visible in the depths of the scroto-urethral inlay with a urethra of normal calibre at each end. The aims of urethral closure are to detach the scrotal inlay and to roll in the lateral aspects of the preputial/penile patch with the underlying bulbospongiosus to form a neourethra. In other words, the scrotal inlay plays no part in the urethral closure itself, it has simply served as a window during the interval between construction and closure to check the adequacy of the repair and to allow revision if necessary.

Urethral closure is begun by circumcising the patch and the open ends of the urethra to detach the scrotal inlay from them completely (Fig. 11.89) and expose the urethra at each end. The

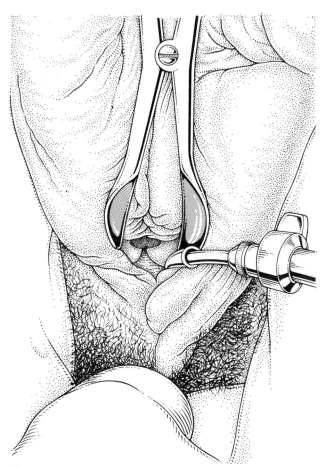

Fig. 11.85

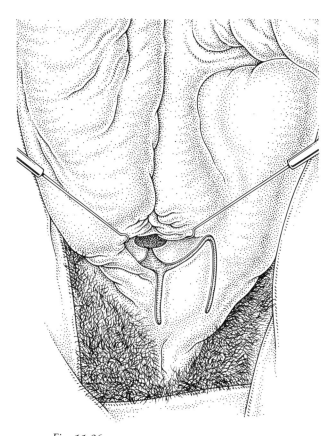

Fig. 11.86

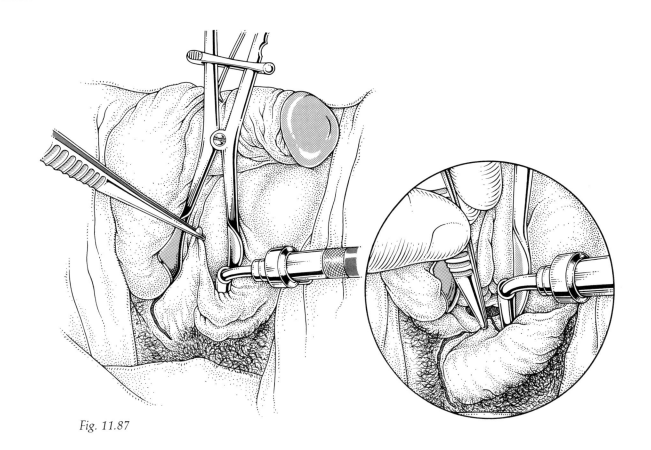

Fig. 11.87

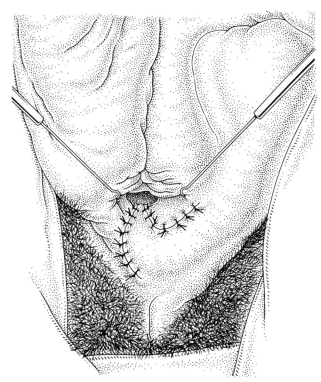

Fig. 11.88

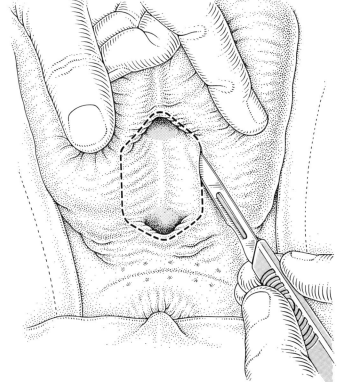

Fig. 11.89

patch with the underlying bulbospongiosus muscle is then undermined on each side for about 1 cm (Fig. 11.90), so that the sides can be rolled ventrally to form a tube around a 24 F Neoplex bougie within the urethra, trimming the margins where necessary to excise any redundant tissue. The urethra is closed with inverting 4/0 Vicryl interrupted sutures to approximate the epithelium followed by a second layer of 4/0 interrupted Vicryl sutures to close the bulbospongiosus over the top of the neourethra (Fig. 11.91). The repair is covered by a suprapubic catheter and a 16 F silicone Foley urethral catheter. The skin and subcutaneous tissue are closed in the usual way.

If the first stage of the urethroplasty consisted of 'stricturotomy' and scrotal skin funnelling without a pedicled preputial/penile skin inlay then obviously scrotal skin will have to be incorporated into the second stage of urethral closure. The principles of circumcision of the inlay and subsequent closure are however essentially the same and need not be detailed again.

Postoperative management and follow up are as for a primary anastomosis or a one-stage patch urethroplasty, as described in previous sections.

THE COMPLICATIONS OF PENILE AND BULBAR URETHROPLASTY

One-stage excision and end-to-end anastomotic reconstruction for short post-traumatic bulbar strictures is extremely successful with a success rate approaching 100%. This assumes that the case was properly selected (in other words it was truly short and post-traumatic), the stricture was stable and there were no complications, of which the commonest is that 'the catheter fell out' in the early postoperative period which tends to lead to extravasion and restricturing. Whatever the cause a recurrent stricture will require a patch technique to correct

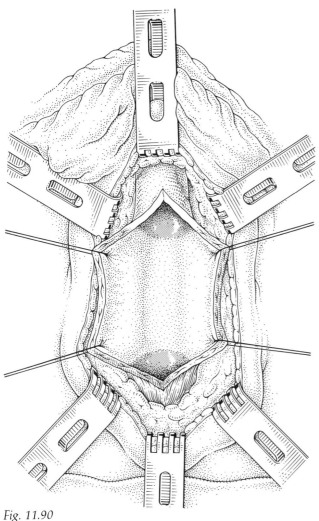

Fig. 11.90

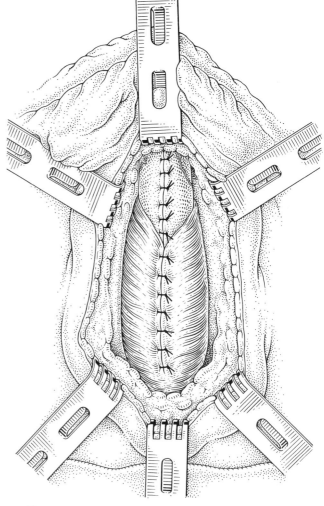

Fig. 11.91

it unless it is controllable by optical urethrotomy.

Whenever a patch is used problems may occur, although in 85% or thereabouts the results are satisfactory. Satisfactory results should not be equated with radiological perfection — postoperative urethrograms never look very pretty after a patch procedure; the best to be hoped for is relatively normal calibre. A normal flow rate is much more reassuring. The main problems (assuming that the catheters are not removed until the repair is radiologically satisfactory) are recurrent stricture or pouching/bagginess of the patch. Recurrent strictures tend to occur at either end of the patch, either because the stricture was insufficiently incised into healthy tissue or because the ends of the urethra were insufficiently spatulated or because of ischaemia at the apex of the patch. (The development of a stricture at a site remote from the urethroplasty is not considered to be a surgical complication but a further manifestation of a stricture-prone urethra.)

Bagginess and pouching seem to be inherent problems with any patch but certain factors make it worse. It is an inherent problem because the tissue of the patch is much thinner than the wall of the urethra itself and is therefore more likely to be 'blown out' on voiding. This is then compounded, at the distal end of the patch at its junction with normal urethra, by an 'anterior urethral valve effect' which accelerates the problem (Fig. 11.92 — here with a stone in the pouch below the 'valve' which has been arrowed).

The exacerbating factors are incorrect sizing of the patch, so that it is inherently baggy, failure to fix the urethral margins laterally at the site of the repair so that it tends to pouch ventrally, and lack of support from failure to overclose the bulbospongiosus.

If a major degree of ballooning of the patch occurs, particularly if complicated by stone formation (Fig. 11.93), the urethra should be reconstructed. If there

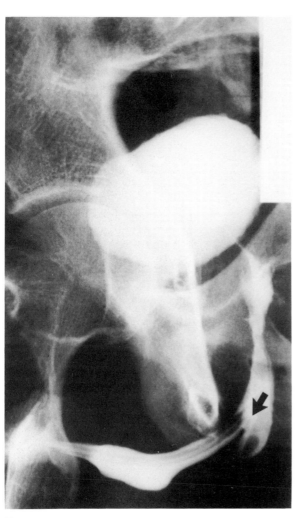

Fig. 11.92

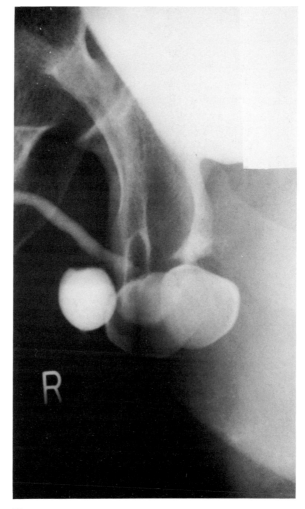

Fig. 11.93

is no associated stricture the redundant part of the patch is excised and the remainder is closed to give a urethra of even calibre. If there is an associated stricture (or strictures) the urethroplasty will usually have to be revised completely. Lesser degrees of bagginess can be left alone. Minor degrees of post-micturition dribbling as a result can usually be corrected by teaching the patient to empty the urethra by milking it manually. Loss of pulsatile ejaculation cannot be treated.

Impotence is not generally recognised as a complication of bulbar urethroplasty — it is certainly not talked about — but in my experience it does occur. It is less common after an anastomotic urethroplasty but occurs transiently in 30% of patch procedures. I am not sure what the explanation is but presumably it is related to interference with the blood supply of the corpus spongiosum. In most patients the impotence is only temporary but may last 12–18 months. Unfortunately in some patients the disability is permanent and will require specific treatment. The question of potency in relation to stricture surgery is one that has been sadly neglected to date.

MEMBRANOUS URETHRAL STRICTURES (Table 11.3)

There are three basic types of membranous urethral stricture:

1. strictures without urethral disruption — these are termed 'sphincter strictures' to differentiate them from the other two types;
2. strictures with urethral disruption, but without distraction or other complicating factors — 'simple strictures';
3. strictures with urethral distraction or other complicating factors — 'complex strictures'.

In general sphincter strictures are due to instrumentation, especially transurethral

Table 11.3　Membranous strictures

A. Sphincter strictures:
　— dilatation
　— if rapidly or repeatedly recurrent:
　　— optical urethrotomy + AUS
　　— transperineal bulbo-prostatic anastomosis + AUS + bladder neck reconstruction in post-prostatectomy patients
B. Simple strictures
　Short (<2 or 3 cm)
　　— optical urethrotomy or, if that fails,
　　— excision and transperineal (end-to-end) bulbo-prostatic anastomosis
C. Complex strictures
　Medium (3 or 4 cm)
　　— abdomino-perineal bulbo-prostatic anastomosis
　Long (4–8 cm)
　　— reroute urethra through the pubis

resection of the prostate, but may be due to pelvic fracture injuries. Strictures with urethral disruption or worse are almost always due to external injury — typically a pelvic fracture sustained in a road traffic accident.

SPHINCTER STRICTURES

The aim of treatment with sphincter strictures is to preserve sphincter function if at all possible, and urethral dilatation is therefore the treatment of choice. This is particularly so for strictures following transurethral resection of the prostate or bladder neck incision where the bladder neck continence mechanism has been destroyed and only the distal sphincter mechanism remains. Urethrotomy is contraindicated in such patients as this will destroy any remaining sphincter activity (if there is any remaining) if it extends more than 1–2 mm deep into the urethral wall.

If the bladder neck is competent, as might be expected if the stricture was due to external injury, and dilatation proves unsatisfactory, then a urethrotomy is a reasonable step to take. If that fails, an anastomotic urethroplasty (a transperineal bulboprostatic anastomosis) will be necessary, accepting

the loss of distal sphincter function and relying thereafter on bladder neck function for continence.

If the bladder neck is incompetent for whatever reason, urethrotomy or urethroplasty will leave the patient incontinent. Theoretically this might be controlled either by a bladder neck reconstruction or by implantation of an artificial sphincter (AUS). Unfortunately a bladder neck reconstruction (as described below) only gives satisfactory results in about 50% of patients; the rest remain incontinent to some degree, particularly in the much more common post-prostatectomy group. The alternative of an AUS is also unsatisfactory in this group because with a bladder neck cuff the fibrosis following a previous prostatectomy may prevent the device being effective, and with a bulbar urethral cuff the blood flow through the urethra may be critically impaired causing ischaemia and erosion because the urethral mobilisation that is required for a bulbo-prostatic anastomotic urethroplasty (if a urethroplasty was necessary) leaves that part of the urethra entirely dependent on retrograde blood flow which the cuff will then be compromising.

For these various reasons I try to avoid surgery in post-prostatectomy sphincter strictures if at all possible and persevere with urethral dilatation. If there are no local complicating factors in the urethra such as false passages, with or without stones or accumulations of debris, this will often work in controlling the stricture although an AUS may still be necessary to treat residual sphincter weakness incontinence. If urethral dilatation fails then the best approach appears to be a urethroplasty to deal with the stricture combined with bladder neck reconstruction (see below) to correct the incontinence. However as bladder neck reconstruction gives satisfactory control of incontinence in only 50% of patients I combine this with omental wrapping of the bladder neck reconstruction and placement of an AUS cuff around the omental wrap. The tubing of the AUS cuff is then left plugged off in the inguinal canal so that the rest of the components can be connected at a later date if necessary by a relatively simple procedure.

Bladder neck reconstruction is an important adjunct to AUS implantation in patients with post-prostatectomy sphincter strictures because even if it does not produce continence it does produce a more pliable and compressible prostatic urethra of more normal calibre, and one that will therefore be more easily occluded by an AUS cuff around it. In post-traumatic sphincter strictures the bladder neck and prostate are usually sufficiently pliable once they have been freed from the surrounding fibrous tissue during the course of the urethroplasty, so bladder neck reconstruction is not necessary before implantation of an AUS. Bladder neck reconstruction is therefore an alternative to AUS implantation in this type of patient rather than an adjunct as it is in the post-prostatectomy group and as an AUS gives better control of incontinence it is to be preferred in most patients.

UNCOMPLICATED TRAUMATIC STRICTURES

Strictures following partial urethral disruption, but without distraction or any other complicating factor, may be amenable to optical urethrotomy. In such instances the urethral sphincter mechanism has almost certainly been destroyed but bladder neck competence is usually unaffected and continence will therefore be maintained as long as detrusor function is normal. Even if there has been complete urethral disruption optical urethrotomy may still be effective because, after urethral disruption, the urethra distal to the site of injury tends to come to lie just in front of the proximal segment, rather than in direct continuity. As a result it is

often possible to cut back into the prostatic urethra with an optical urethrotome. With tight strictures it often helps to pass a suprapubic cystoscope simultaneously to visualise and illuminate the proximal end of the stricture. Indeed one sometimes finds that there is an obstructing inferior shelf or diaphagm rather than a true stricture at the site of injury, which can be incised downards to restore direct and unkinked urethral continuity.

If optical urethrotomy fails or the stricture recurs rapidly a transperineal anastomotic urethroplasty will be necessary as for short traumatic strictures of the bulbar urethra.

COMPLICATED TRAUMATIC STRICTURES

For strictures with distraction or other complications, neither dilatation nor urethrotomy is satisfactory, and a urethroplasty will usually be necessary. As with uncomplicated strictures the aim is to perform an anastomotic urethroplasty but because of the distraction, or other complication, a simple transperineal approach is sometimes inadequate because only the urethra distal to the stricture can be exposed and mobilised to any degree and the prostatic urethra above the stricture may be inaccessible. For this reason a combined abdomino-perineal approach is usually required for complicated strictures so that the urethra on both sides of the stricture can be exposed. This approach is sometimes called a transpubic approach but this is really a misnomer.

BULBO-PROSTATIC ANASTOMOTIC URETHROPLASTY

The principles underlying anastomotic urethroplasty for membranous urethral strictures are the same as those for

bulbar strictures as described earlier in this chapter.

In general it may be said that a bulbo-prostatic anastomosis per se is a relatively simple procedure, particularly with an uncomplicated stricture that can be repaired transperineally which is usually the case, but that the dissection and mobilisation necessary to achieve it and to deal with any associated problems in those few patients who require an abdomino-perineal approach may be expremely difficult and time consuming. Although it is usually possible to predict whether the stricture will require a simple transperineal bulbo-prostatic anastomosis or a complex abdomino-perineal reconstruction, this is not always the case, and the surgeon embarking on a transperineal repair of a pelvic fracture stricture must be prepared to proceed to an abdomino-perineal reconstruction if this proves necessary. Factors in favour of a simple repair are a short stricture segment, minimal distraction of the two ends of the urethra, a small amount of surrounding fibrosis and no complicating factors. Factors against a simple repair are a long stricture (due to distraction), dense fibrosis, incompetence of the bladder neck, fistulae, abscesses, stones, and false passages. Associated bulbar strictures pose additional problems that may preclude an anastomotic urethroplasty altogether and will be discussed separately.

A simple transperineal bulbo-prostatic anastomosis involves perineal exposure and mobilisation of the bulbar urethra, excision of the strictured segment and exposure of the apex of the prostate, spatulation of the prostatic urethra proximally and the bulbar urethra distally, anastomosis of the two ends, bulbar urethral fixation and overclosure of the bulbospongiosus. All of these stages are also part of an abdomino-perineal reconstruction, but this also involves retropubic exposure of the prostatic urethra to overcome the problem of distraction which makes the prostatic urethra inaccessible from the perineal approach.

A transperineal procedure takes about an hour. Blood loss is not usually significant but may be necessary, and it is a wise precaution to cross match 2 units just in case. The patient is admitted the day before operation.

A complex reconstruction may take 4–6 hours and blood loss may be considerable. Two days preoperative assessment are usually necessary to be sure that the patient is fit for surgery, to ensure that the urine is sterile and to ensure that 4 units of blood are available.

Once again Turner Warwick's work in this field must be acknowledged as it was he who was largely responsible for developing and refining the technique of bulbo-prostatic anastomotic reconstruction.

Technique

The patient is placed in the low lithotomy position and draped to allow full exposure of the abdomen and perineum. A preliminary urethroscopy is performed to ensure the normality of the bulbar urethra if this has not been performed beforehand.

1. Mobilisation of the bulbar urethra. The first step is to expose and mobilise the bulbar urethra. This is achieved through a midline perineal incision deepened down to the bulbospongiosus, which is divided in the midline and reflected laterally. The midline fibrous septum between the corpus spongiosum of the bulbar urethra and the fascia of the corpora cavernosa is then divided all the way up to the level of the stricture and the surrounding fibrosis (Fig. 11.94).

Posteriorly the bulb of the urethra is mobilised by ligating and dividing the two small superficial posterolateral arteries to the bulb and then mobilising it off the perineal body in the posterior midline up to the level of the stricture and then above that to the apex of the prostate (Fig. 11.95). The bulbar urethra is then divided through or immediately below the stricture and its surrounding fibrosis. The urethra is then trimmed until it is of normal calibre and with a healthy looking urothelium. The spongy tissue of the cut end of the bulbar urethra should look healthy and should bleed freely by virtue of its collateral blood supply from the glans and from the multiple small vessels that run between the corpora cavernosa and the penile part of the corpus spongiosum.

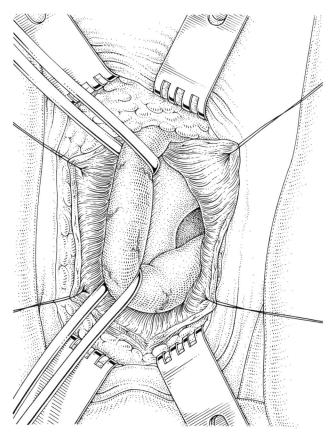

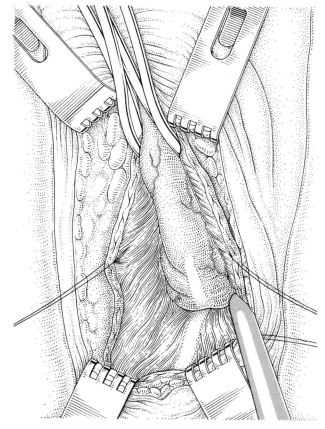

Fig. 11.94

Fig. 11.95

Any areas of unhealthy tissue should be excised. Then, until the anastomosis is performed, it is a good idea to cross clamp the end of the divided urethra with a bulldog clamp to prevent blood loss and to stop the otherwise irritating steady dripping of blood into the perineal wound.

Having mobilised the bulbar urethra, the next stop is to expose the apex of the prostate.

2. Transperineal exposure of the prostatic urethra. Many patients already have an indwelling suprapubic catheter; in those that do not a percutaneous suprapubic cystotomy is performed. For this purpose I use the needle, guidewire and dilators used to place an Amplatz tube for percutaneous renal access or alternatively the suprapubic catheter introducer designed by Will Lawrence. Either way, a large-calibre urethral sound can then be passed through the bladder neck and down the prostatic urethra until it is held up at the upper end of the stricture. Downward pressure with the sound pushes the apex of the prostate into the wound and shows, by palpation, where to incise through the stricture and surrounding fibrosis to reach and open up the prostatic urethra when the way through is not obvious (Fig. 11.96). The degree of downward mobility of the prostatic apex is often surprising.

It is at this stage that it will become clear, if it was not clear previously, whether or not a transperineal procedure will be possible. If the apex of the prostate, with the sound inside, is readily defined and accessible then a transperineal procedure is possible. If the apex of the prostate is difficult to palpate, usually because it is in the depths of a wound, then a combined abdomino-perineal ('transpubic') approach will be required (see below).

If the patient was not made impotent by the injury that gave him his stricture it

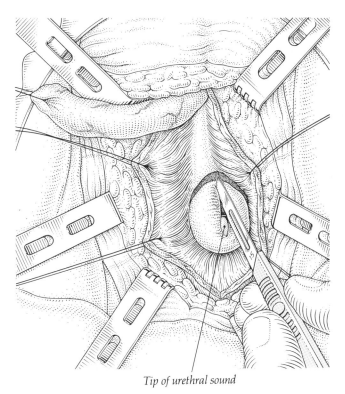

Tip of urethral sound

Fig. 11.96

is vitally important when incising down to the prostatic urethra and the bougie within it, to cut down on to the front of the prostatic apex and to avoid the posterior aspect of prostatic apex as far as possible. Any dissection posteriorly or posterolaterally risks damage to the nerves to the corpora cavernosa that are responsible for erection (see Ch. 3).

When a pathway through the stricture has been established the fibrous scar tissue that forms and surrounds the stricture is excised to expose healthy urothelium within the prostatic urethra and healthy tissue at the prostatic apex. During this excision the bulbar arteries (branches of the pudendal arteries) may be cut just below the apex of the prostate. These can bleed furiously if they have not been thrombosed by the original injury. Having cleared away the stricture and surrounding fibrosis the prostatic urethra (in an adult) should accept a 36 F bougie with ease.

It is important to identify the verumontanum within the prostatic urethra to be sure that it is indeed urethra and not a false passage. A longstanding false passage can look surprisingly like normal urethra.

This stage of the procedure is completed by tacking the urothelium of the prostatic urethra out to the 'capsule' of the prostatic apex to stop it retracting and to give a widely spatulated open end (Fig. 11.97). To achieve this some of the apical prostatic tissue will need to be excised on either side.

3. 'Transpubic' exposure of the prostatic urethra. If a transperineal approach fails to give adequate access to the apex of the prostate, a midline lower abdominal incision is made from the anterior aspect of the pubis to just below the umbilicus. The incision may need to be extended up to the xiphisternum later on in the operation to mobilise the omentum (see below), but such an extension is unnecessary at this stage.

The incision is deepened to expose the bladder extraperitoneally and a ring retractor is placed to hold the incision open. Fibrous tissue within the retropubic space that plasters the anterior and lateral aspects of the bladder and prostate to the front and side walls of the pelvis is then incised, or excised if it is particularly dense, to open the retropubic space widely. This fibrous tissue is usually particularly dense between the prostate and the pubis and may contain false passages or pockets of infection. During incision or excision of a fibrous plaque it is important not to damage the bladder neck, so it is helpful to open the dome of the bladder, well away from the bladder neck, to make it easier, by palpation from within, to avoid damage to the bladder and bladder neck and also to identify the upper end of any radiographically demonstrated false passages.

The main way of reducing the risk of damage to the bladder neck is to keep as close as possible to the pubic bone during the anterior dissection, literally carving the bladder and prostate off the bone if necessary.

It is during this early phase of the procedure that most of the blood loss will occur, particularly from veins in the depths of the anterolateral aspects of the retropubic space that become bound up in the 'concrete' of the haematoma–fibrosis and then get torn as the retropubic space is opened.

After the fibrous plaque has been incised or excised the apex of the prostate and the subprostatic strictured segment must be exposed by removing the posterior aspect of the pubis, the convexity of which obscures the view of this area. It is important to remember that it is the posterior aspect of the pubis that needs to be removed, not the superior aspect.

To expose the pubis, the rectus tendons must be separated right down onto the front of the pubis where they are inserted. To further clear the upper aspect of the pubis, the rectus tendons will then need to be reflected off their bony attachment for 1 cm or so laterally on each side (Fig. 11.98). The pubic periosteum is then incised horizontally down onto bone for about 2 cm on either side of the midline, as gouges and chisels tend to slip off periosteum. Using a hammer with either a gouge or a chisel, a trench is then cut, 5 cm wide or thereabouts, through the posterior aspect of the pubis (Fig. 11.99). When doing this for the first time one tends to worry about going through the lower end into the dorsal vein complex and causing torrential bleeding, but this never happens; firstly because the gouge/chisel is arrested by periosteum at the lower end, and secondly because much of the dorsal vein complex has been obliterated by thrombosis as a result of the original injury. After chiselling through the bone, the slivers usually need to be removed either with a cutting diathermy point, if they are still attached to the periosteum, or with bone nibblers. Chiselling proceeds until a trench of adequate width allows the apex of the prostate to be clearly seen. To help identify the upper end of the

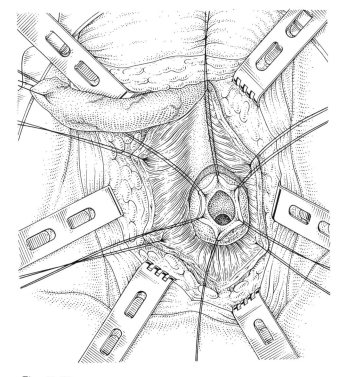

Fig. 11.97

stricture at the apex of the prostate, a large-calibre metal sound passed down through the prostatic urethra from above is helpful.

The next step is to open the prostatic urethra at the apex of the prostate by a vertical incision, cutting down onto the tip of the metal sound (Fig. 11.100). The prostatic urethra should be opened by a vertical incision about 2 cm long exposing the verumontanum on the posterior wall — assuming of course that the verumontanum is above the level of the stricture — to be sure that it is actually the urethra that has been exposed and not a false passage. The metal sound is then removed. The prostatic tissue around the edges of this incision is then trimmed away so that the urothelium can be tacked out (as with the transperineal approach) to the prostatic capsule to produce a widely spatulated, urothelially lined, opened end of the prostatic urethra that is about 1.5 cm in each axis (Fig. 11.101).

If there are no complicating problems to be dealt with, this stage of the procedure is complete and the surgeon goes on to the next stage of establishing a communication between the pelvis and the perineum. The two most common complicating factors are false passages bypassing the prostatic urethra and bladder neck incompetence.

False passages are usually anteriorly situated within the fibrous plaque that by now has been incised or excised. All

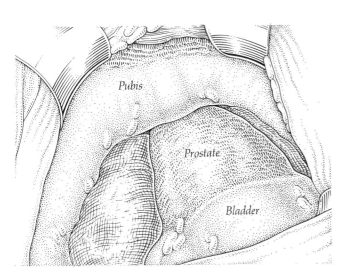

Fig. 11.98

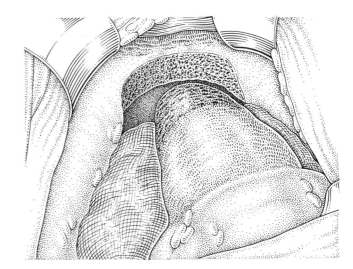

Fig. 11.99

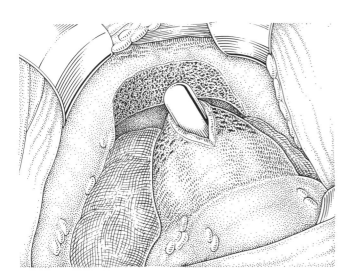

Fig. 11.100

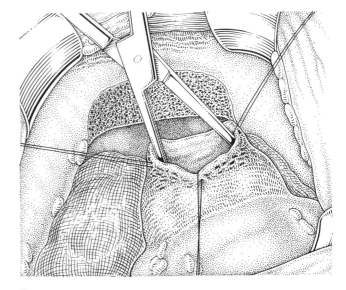

Fig. 11.101

that remains is to 'clean' the opening into the bladder in front of the bladder neck and close the opening with one or two sutures. Posterior false passages are best dealt with by gentle curettage and closure of the bladder opening, taking care to define the distal track of the false passage, so that it will not be incorporated into the subsequent bulbo-prostatic anastomosis. Large or infected posterior false passages are better dealt with by opening them up, if necessary formally opening up the plane between the prostate and rectum, as described in Chapter 3, so that a tongue of omentum can later be pulled through to obliterate the cavity.

Bladder neck incompetence is either due to:

— associated injury of the pelvic plexuses (more common in adults),
— injury at the time of the pelvic fracture (more common in children),
— encasement in fibrous tissue,
— iatrogenic bladder neck incision,
— traction injury from a balloon catheter.

Encasement in fibrous tissue will be corrected by the excision of the fibrous plaque. Direct injury or (iatrogenic) bladder neck incisions cause a radial defect in the circumference of the bladder neck, which can usually be reconstructed quite simply. Neurological damage or a traction injury produce a patulous bladder neck which can only be corrected either by a reduction procedure (see below) to narrow the bladder neck around a fine-calibre catheter or by accepting the problem, recognising that such a reduction procedure carries a fairly high failure rate, and implanting an artificial sphincter at a later date.

Having mobilised the bulbar urethra, prepared the apex of the prostate and dealt with any complicating factors, the layer of fibrous (scar) tissue between the pelvic and perineal dissections is incised

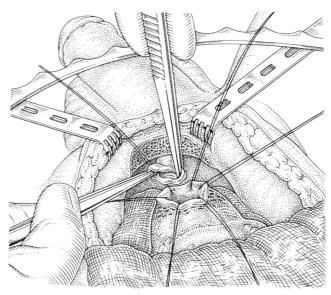

Fig. 11.102

to give a line of communication to the perineum. Then, having established a line of communication, fibrous tissue anterior to the apex of the prostate is incised or excised to produce a wide channel through which to pass the mobilised bulbar urethra to perform the bulbo-prostatic anastomosis (Fig. 11.102).

It is important to keep the dissection anterior. Dissection posteriorly risks damage to the nerves to the corpora cavernosa and consequent impotence if the patient was not made impotent by the original injury.

After severe pelvic fracture injuries the perineo-pelvic channel created in this way may be inadequate because of displacement of the pubic bones back onto the prostate and fibrous tethering between the two, or because of displaced bone as a result of the original pelvic fracture, or because of posterior fibrosis in relation to the apex of the prostate and the by-now excised stricture. Most patients with this type of injury will be impotent and if this is known to be the case beyond any doubt, then the posterior fibrosis can be incised as necessary to enlarge the channel with relative abandon. If the patient is potent but there is a severely

restrictive plaque of fibrous tissue posteriorly that will be sufficient to compromise the bulbo-prostatic anastomosis then the plaque will have to be incised despite the risk to the corporal innervation. To reduce this risk to a minimum the fibrous plaque (which I think in most instances is a grossly fibrosed perineal body) is incised strictly in the midline as judged by the position of the prostatic apex and the verumontanum. The full thickness of the plaque is carefully incised throughout its vertical extent back to the areolar layer between it and the anterior wall of the rectum to allow it to spring open, sometimes almost magically.

It is sometimes said that an alternative way of creating a sufficient channel to get the bulbar urethra up to the prostatic apex without tension is to chisel away the inferior pubic arch from below, if necessary separating the corpora for a centimetre or two at their point of fusion to allow more bone to be removed. My experience is that this does not give much space but does sometimes cause a lot of bleeding from the corpora which may be difficult and time-consuming to control and is no substitute for the posterior incision of a fibrotic perineal body.

4. *The bulbo-prostatic anastomosis.* Having ensured that the two ends reach each other without tension, the free end of the bulbar urethra is spatulated to prepare it for anastomosis to the spatulated prostatic urethra (Fig. 11.103). Because the natural arc of the bulbar urethra makes the dorsal wall shorter than the ventral wall and because the bulk of the spongy tissue of the proximal bulbar urethra lies ventrally and posteriorly, it is usually best to spatulate the bulbar end by incising it vertically for 1.5 cm in the ventral midline and then to rotate the mobilised bulbar urethra through 180° so that the bulk of the spongy tissue comes to lie anteriorly and the spatulated open end faces posteriorly. This has the twofold effect of gaining extra apparent length and of bringing the two spatulated ends into the most satisfactory position for the anastomosis between the two.

If there is any tension between the two ends when they are approximated (or when they quite obviously will not come together) a 4–5 cm full thickness wedge of the pubis should be removed (pubectomy — Fig. 11.104) and the bulbar urethra should be re-routed around one side of the shaft of the penis

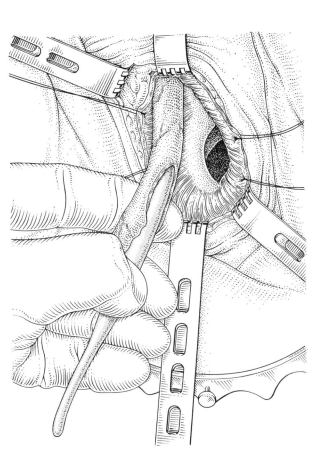

Fig. 11.103

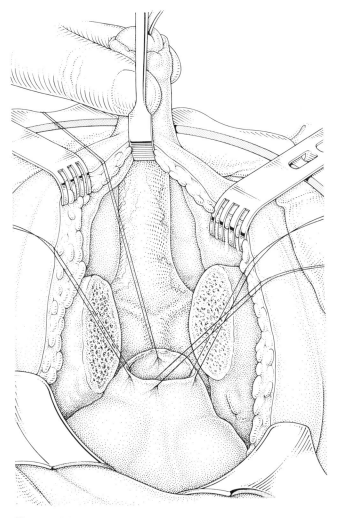

Fig. 11.104

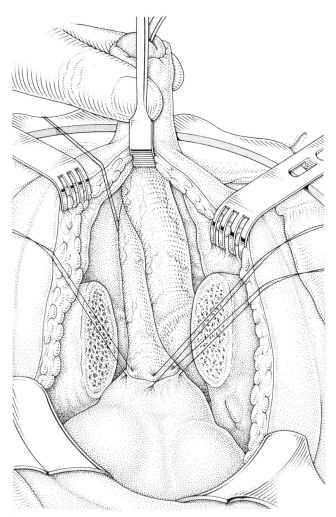

Fig. 11.105

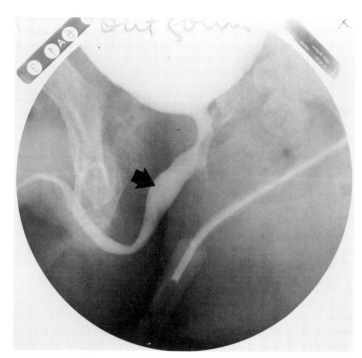

Fig. 11.106

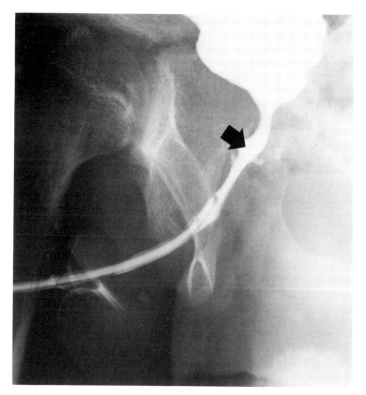

Fig. 11.107

and through the pubic gap (Fig. 11.105). This 're-routing', by eliminating the natural curve of the urethra down into the perineum and then up into the pelvis and allowing the urethra to run directly through the pubis to the front of the prostate, has the effect of giving another 2–3 cm beyond that which can be gained by the elastic lengthening achieved by mobilisation of the bulbar urethra. The effect of this can be seen by comparing Figure 11.106, which shows the appearance after a standard abdomino-perineal anastomosis, with Figure 11.107 which shows the appearance after a pubectomy and re-routing — the arrow in each case shows the site of anastomosis. The net result is that, with re-routing, a stricture 5–6 cm long or sometimes even longer can be corrected by bulbo-prostatic anastomosis.

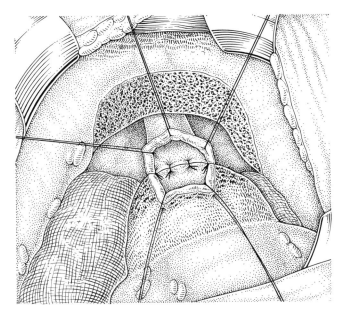

Fig. 11.108

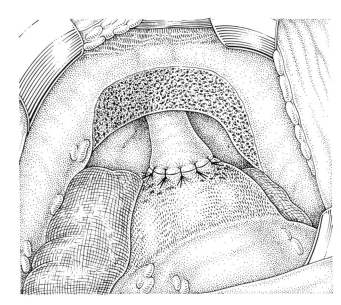

Fig. 11.109

With the abdomino-perineal procedure the bulbo-prostatic anastomosis is more easily performed from above than from below. About eight interrupted 4/0 Vicryl sutures will be placed in all. The first three are placed in the midline posteriorly and 0.5 cm on either side and then tied with the knots on the inside (Fig. 11.108). The next two are placed at the mid-lateral points and then tied with the knots on the inside. The final three sutures are placed in the anterior midline and between that and the mid-lateral sutures on each side and tied with the knots on the outside (Fig. 11.109). Each suture is about 0.5 cm from its neighbour, a little closer posteriorly where the weakest point of the anastomosis is, and each must achieve direct urothelial apposition between the two ends. Tying the knots on the inside achieves this more easily than tying them on the outside of the anastomosis. When the anastomosis is complete a 16 F silicone Foley urethral catheter is passed to act as a 'stent' for the anastomosis and urinary drainage is established by means of a 20 F Foley suprapubic catheter.

With a transperineal procedure the anastomosis is sometimes more difficult than with a pelvic approach because of the more restricted access. It is usually easiest to place the sutures first, taking care to pick up urothelium on each side with each stitch, and then push the bulbar urethra down along the sutures onto the prostatic apex and then tie them (Fig. 11.110).

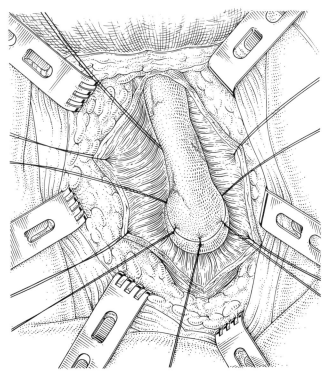

Fig. 11.110

As with all urethral reconstructions, the procedure is completed by a series of lateral tethering sutures on each side of the urethra, to fix the corpus spongiosum to the corpora cavernosa, and by overclosure of the bulbospongiosus. For transperineal repairs, the wound is then closed in the usual way.

For abdomino-perineal reconstructions the procedure is completed by omental wrapping of the anastomosis.

5. *The omental wrap.* Sometimes the omentum is sufficiently long for it to be brought down over the front of the bladder and prostate and wrapped around the anastomosis without mobilisation. More commonly some degree of mobilisation is necessary; sometimes the omentum must be mobilised completely. Tiresome as it is to have to mobilise the omentum after a long and tiring reconstruction, it is extremely important to do so to fill in the dead space: firstly to prevent adhesion of the anastomosis and of the

bladder neck to the raw bony surface of the partially excised pubis, secondly so that fibrosis does not recur and thirdly to provide a healthy supple support to the bladder neck and the anastomosis to maintain normal bladder neck function and to give the anastomosis its best chance of healing without restenosis.

Full omental mobilisation usually requires extension of the original midline incision up to the xiphisternum, so that the gastroepiploic vascular arcade is clearly demonstrated along the greater curvature of the stomach.

The first step is to lift the omentum up and dissect it off the transverse colon (Fig. 11.111) starting on the right-hand side on the right lateral border of the omentum and continuing across to the left side until the omentum is completely detached. The next step is to mobilise the omentum on the right gastroepiploic artery by dividing the gastric branches that run upwards from the arcade to the lower border of the stomach (Fig. 11.112). The vessels are

individually ligated and then divided between the ligatures, beginning at the most dependent part of the stomach where the vessels are longer, the gap between the vessels is larger and the thickness of the tissue between the arcade and the stomach is less than at the duodenal end. This is quicker with an LDS stapler (Autosuture) rather than with ligation–division. This separation of the omentum continues along towards the origin of the gastroepiploic artery from the gastroduodenal artery at the inferior border of the first part of the duodenum. Finally, the separation proceeds along the greater curvature of the stomach until either sufficient mobilisation has been achieved to allow the omentum to drop down into the pelvis comfortably, or until a gap is reached in the arcade indicating discontinuity between the right and the left gastroepiploic vessels, or until the omentum has been completely mobilised and the left gastroepiploic artery has been divided at its origin (Fig. 11.113).

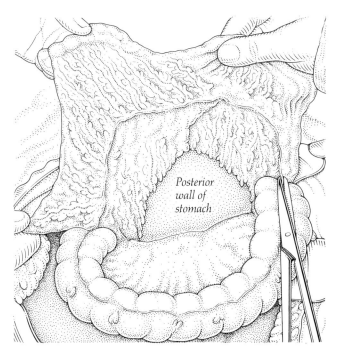

Fig. 11.111

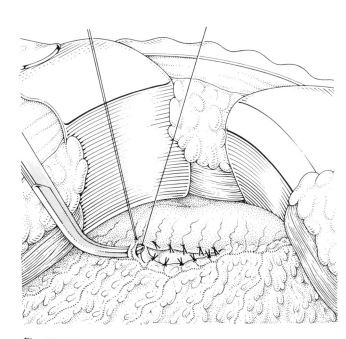

Fig. 11.112

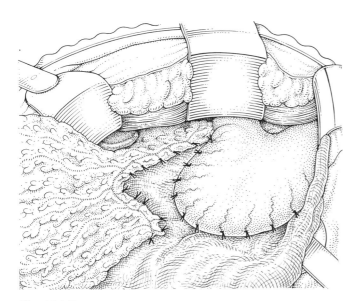

Fig. 11.113

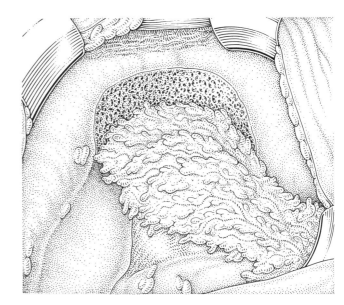

Fig. 11.114

The omentum is best brought down into the pelvis by passing it retroperitoneally deep to the right colon and its 'mesocolon', either by mobilising the right colon and hepatic flexure and then tacking it back to the posterior abdominal wall afterwards or by tunnelling behind the hepatic flexure and then between the right 'mesocolon' and Gerota's fascia and emerging at the pelvic brim, which requires a bit of practice.

The omentum is then tacked to the peritoneum of the side wall of the pelvis to obliterate any defects that may lead to postoperative intestinal obstruction and then brought through into the retropubic space (Fig. 11.114).

It is then tacked around the anastomosis, so that the latter is completely wrapped, and packed into the bony trench cut in the back of the pubis, leaving the most dependent part in the perineum where it is picked up when the bulbospongiosus is closed to hold it in place (Fig. 11.115). Further tacking sutures are placed as necessary to hold it in place around the bladder neck. A tube drain is then left in the retropubic space to drain any oozing.

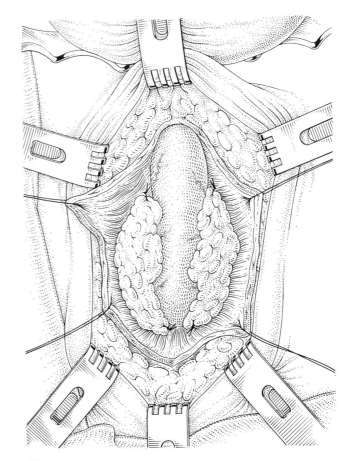

Fig. 11.115

Postoperative management

The postoperative management is the same as with other types of urethral reconstruction. The crucial factor as always is a catheter-gram at 3 weeks (2 weeks for healing, 1 week for surgical paranoia) before removing the catheters to be sure that the anastomosis has healed (Fig. 11.116). Figure 11.117 shows the same patient 6 months later. Note the dilatation at the site of the spatulated anastomosis.

If it is assumed that the patient has had a satisfactory radiological result at or about three weeks postoperatively then late complications are rare. If the X-rays at 3 weeks show extravasation then obviously the catheters should be left in until further radiological studies confirm that the anastomosis has healed satisfactorily.

Complications of bulbo-prostatic anastomotic urethroplasty

Restricture at the site of the anastomosis is rare assuming that there was no pre-existing bulbar urethral abnormality to reduce its vascularity, no tension at the anastomosis and no early postoperative extravasation. Of these, it is tension at the anastomosis in younger men and ischaemia in older men that are the main problems in most instances.

Unfortunately there are patients who develop late strictures both at the anastomosis and in the mobilised segment of the bulbar urethra for no apparent reason in whom, presumably, there is or was some obscure factor leading to a reduction in retrograde blood flow through the bulbar urethra or in whom the tension at the anastomosis was greater than realised at the time. Alternative culprits are a postoperative haematoma, urinary extravasation or local infection.

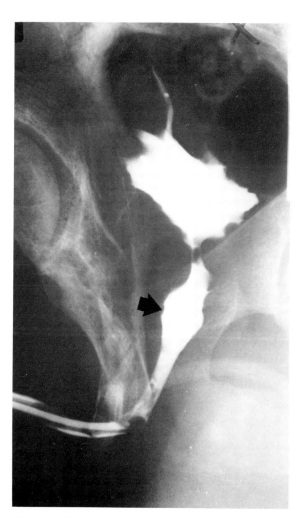

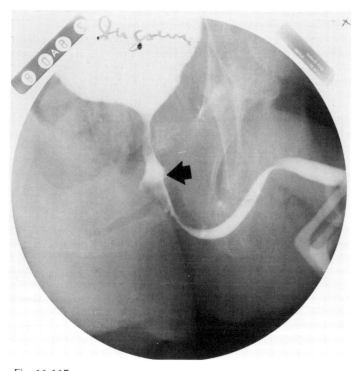

Fig. 11.117

Fig. 11.116

A short anastomotic stricture, particularly after transperineal bulbo-prostatic anastomosis, can often be treated by re-doing the operation—if necessary with transpubic rerouting of the urethra—if the remainder of the bulbar urethra is normal. Longer strictures cannot be treated in this way but may respond to optical urethrotomy. If that fails a pedicled patch procedure will be necessary.

Other complications include chordee, impotence and incontinence. Chordee is due to excessive mobilisation of the urethra and is sometimes inevitable if a tension-free anastomosis is to be achieved. Strictly speaking chordee occurs very commonly in the form of an erection that rises to only 90° (with respect to the anterior abdominal wall) rather than the usual acute angle. This does not usually cause any problem. Impotence, if it is truly due to the procedure itself and was not present beforehand, is usually the result of dissecting posterior to the prostate. Hence the reason for avoiding dissecting in this area except when it is necessary and then keeping strictly to the midline. Unfortunately, despite one's best attempts to avoid it in this way, postoperative impotence, both temporary and permanent, is distressingly common. As I mentioned earlier in this chapter the question of impotence in relation to stricture surgery is far from resolved. It is rarely discussed and it has never been adequately researched. Many people seem to think that this sort of surgery does not or should not cause impotence but I am quite sure that it does and always warn my patients that this might happen.

Postoperative continence is dependent on the function of the bladder neck as distal sphincter function will be almost completely destroyed by the original trauma and completely destroyed by the urethroplasty. If bladder neck function is normal then continence will be normal unless the patient has some associated urodynamic abnormality, the commonest of which is detrusor instability. Even without detrusor instability most men have urgency after a bulbo-prostatic anastomosis although not urge incontinence unless they try to hold beyond their normal bladder capacity.

If the patient is incontinent and this is due to bladder neck incompetence not to a detrusor abnormality, then an artificial urinary sphincter (AUS) should be considered. The problem with an AUS is that this will have to be placed around either the previously traumatised bladder neck or the recently mobilised segment of bulbar urethra in which blood flow is therefore retrograde. Theoretically at least, a bulbar urethral cuff may cause a critical degree of reduction of blood flow in the urethra between the cuff and the anastomosis leading to ischaemia and erosion of the device through the urethral wall. For this reason I prefer to implant the cuff of the device around the bladder neck rather than the bulbar urethra (despite the horrifying prospect of reopening the pelvis) as blood flow distally into the prostate is likely to be more secure than retrograde blood flow up the urethra through a bulbar urethra cuff. If a bulbar cuff site is chosen, a pressure-regulating balloon of the lowest range ($51-60 \, cmH_2O$) should be used to minimise the risk of secondary urethral ischaemia.

Occasionally one encounters voiding difficulty when the catheters are removed, presumably due to trauma to the pelvic plexuses at the time of the original surgery causing an acontractile bladder. Voiding is usually re-established eventually but the occasional patient (I have one) requires CISC thereafter.

Patients who have had a pubectomy are prone to two additional problems. Firstly there is a tendency to hernia development between the bone ends and in relation to the omental wrap.

Secondly there is a tendency for the base of the penis to drop back through the pubic gap giving apparent shortening of the penis. Some patients find this rather distressing—particularly those who were less well endowed in the first place.

THE PRIMARY TREATMENT OF A RUPTURED POSTERIOR URETHRA
(Table 11.4)

Urologists seem to be split (almost fanatically) into two groups on this issue — the 'temporisers' and the 'interferers'. The 'temporisers' stick in a suprapubic catheter and wait and see, the idea being that passing a urethral catheter might introduce infection or might turn a partial rupture into a complete rupture, thereby making matters worse. The interferers try passing a urethral catheter or get an emergency urethrogram and if either of these suggest a urethral rupture 'realign' the urethra immediately by one means or another, the idea being that urethral continuity should be maintained at all costs.

The first point to emphasise before taking the discussion any further is that these are rare injuries and that the majority are not due to severe external injury in a road traffic accident but due to a fall at work or something of that nature; the patient presents with little in the way of other injuries, is conscious and is able to cooperate. In such a patient all that is necessary is to wait and see if he can void spontaneously and, if not, to pass a suprapubic catheter. Such patients do not develop severe strictures unless made worse by surgical interference.

The problem patients are those admitted with severe multiple injuries, often life threatening. In these circumstances the question of trauma to the lower urinary tract is relatively unimportant. Here the risk of introducing infection by catheterisation is of trivial importance by comparison with the need to make a rapid diagnosis of the extent of injury and to monitor urine output as a means of assessing the response to resuscitation.

In such circumstances there would seem to be every reason to attempt (gentle)

Table 11.4

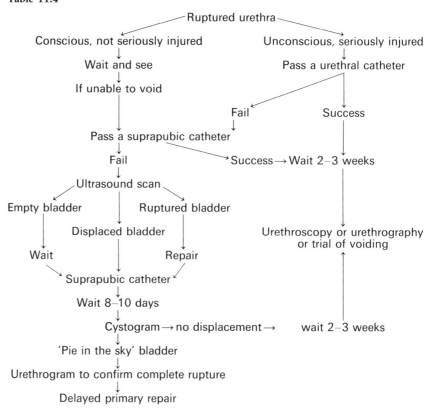

urethral catheterisation. If that succeeds then all well and good; if it fails a percutaneous suprapubic catheter is passed and left on free drainage until a cystogram is performed a week or so later (see below).

If the bladder cannot be found on attempted suprapubic catheterisation by someone competent in the technique there are three possible explanations: either the bladder is empty, or it has been ruptured, or there has been a severe distraction injury and it is no longer within the pelvis. An empty bladder is rare. A distracted bladder can usually be found if necessary by ultrasound or CT scan. If the bladder has been ruptured it should be explored and repaired. A suprapubic catheter is left in at the end and the urethra is then managed as described below.

The real question revolves around whether or not to operate on a ruptured urethra at the time of injury and in my opinion the answer is no — not immediately. Immediate surgical interference is more likely to make the ruptured urethra worse rather than better and opening the retropubic space is also likely to make bleeding worse if the pelvis is badly fractured. My philosophy is that there is little or nothing that one can do to prevent a stricture from developing. What one can and should do is to ensure that if a stricture develops then it should be one that is easily treated. Short strictures, those that are not associated with distraction, are easy to treat — by dilatation or optical urethrotomy at best or by a transperineal anastomotic repair at worst — and the results are good. Long strictures, usually due to distraction, are difficult to treat, always require an abdomino-perineal reconstruction and often end up with a less than satisfactory result. This is the situation to avoid if at all possible and so it is distraction that should be looked for in the early postoperative period and treated. If there is no distraction then I would advocate minimal interference so as to avoid making the effects of the original injury any worse.

My approach is to wait 8–10 days, firstly to see if the patient is going to survive his other injuries and secondly to get a cystogram through the suprapubic catheter to see where the bladder is. If it is more or less in the right place there may be a complete urethral rupture but there is no significant distraction and so at worst the patient will require a transperineal bulbo-prostatic anastomosis a few months later when he has recovered from the immediate injury.

If there is significant distraction on radiological assessment at 8–10 days (Fig. 11.118) then that is the best time to intervene but first of all the diagnosis of urethral rupture should be confirmed radiologically as considerable distraction can occur without rupture (Fig. 11.119). The rationale for waiting 8–10 days before exploring the rupture is that by that time the patient's general condition should be considerably improved and the pelvic haematoma can be evacuated without the bleeding starting all over again, but fibrosis has not yet set in and the urethral ends are still mobile. In my experience it is then a relatively simple matter to divide any residual ligamentous attachments of the prostate to mobile bone fragments, freshen up the proximal transected end of the prostatic urethra, push the distal end (bulbar urethra) back into the pelvis by pressure on the perineum and then tack the two together. Where necessary because of instability, external or internal fixation of the pelvic fracture is applied to prevent further displacement — when

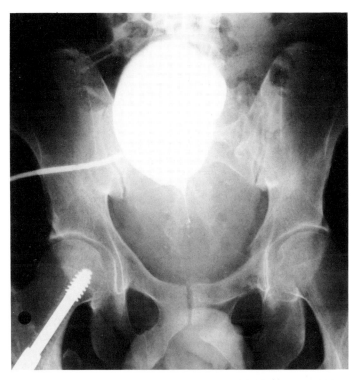

Fig. 11.118

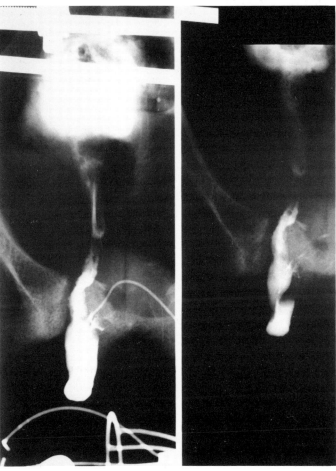

Fig. 11.119

the pelvis is unstable this is just as important as repairing the urethra, if not more so. If a stricture develops later on it will at worst need a simple transperineal repair to fix it. Left on its own a ruptured and distracted urethra will end up as a difficult stricture needing a complex and avoidable abdomino-perineal reconstruction.

If the patient presents much later than 10–12 days after his injury with an established distraction injury then the moment has been lost for the simple repair described above because the distracted tissues will have begun to lose their mobility. It is then best to wait for the haematoma–fibrosis to mature completely which generally takes 3 to 6 months. As it matures the fibrosis tends to pull the bladder and prostate back down to the pelvic floor thereby shortening the gap that will have to be bridged. In the meantime some surgeons find it impossible to resist the urge to attempt to re-establish urethral continuity endoscopically and allow urethral catheterisation until healing has occurred. This approach rarely, if ever, stops a stricture developing so there seems little point, particularly as most patients find a suprapubic catheter more comfortable.

One of the problems is that these are rare injuries and most urologists only see them occasionally at the time of injury (rather than later when the stricture has developed). Even then some patients are too ill to warrant urological attention in the face of more severe injuries; some survive only to die a few days or weeks later; and the rest are too small in number for any individual to conduct a trial to determine the best approach.

BLADDER NECK RECONSTRUCTION

I have mentioned bladder neck reconstruction in two circumstances: firstly with post-prostatectomy sphincter strictures when the bladder neck is iatrogenically incompetent and secondly in those instances of pelvic fracture injury when the bladder neck is incompetent, usually as a result of associated pelvic plexus injury.

In both instances the emphasis in treatment should be on the preservation of sphincter function and for this reason dilatation is the treatment of choice in the first instance. When this or urethrotomy fails to control the stricture a urethroplasty will be required but this will leave the patient incontinent so something else must be done to restore continence. In most patients with a pelvic fracture injury the best option is implantation of an artificial sphincter around the bladder neck. Here the bladder neck, although incompetent, is

reasonably supple and of reasonably normal calibre. After prostatectomy the bladder neck may be neither of these and a cuff at this site may not therefore work efficiently. On the other hand a cuff around the bulbar urethra is prone to problems after the urethra has been mobilised for a bulbo-prostatic urethroplasty as discussed above. For this reason the best option for post-prostatectomy sphincter strictures, and occasionally in other situations, is to reconstruct the bladder neck and prostatic urethra to make it more normal in calibre and more supple. Then, to be on the safe side, an AUS cuff can be wrapped around the reconstruction leaving the tubing plugged off in the groin so that it is readily available to connect to the rest of the components at a later date if the bladder neck reconstruction is not sufficient on its own to give continence.

Figure 11.120 shows the typical radiological appearance of a patient with a post-prostatectomy sphincter stricture.

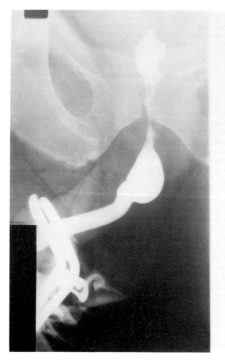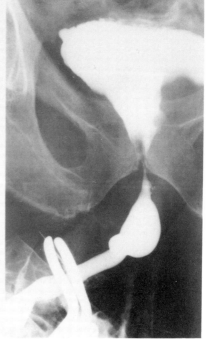

Fig. 11.120

The stricture is first explored transperineally and the bulbar urethra is mobilised in the usual way for a bulbo-prostatic anastomosis. The prostate is then mobilised retropubically and opened in the anterior midline by an incision running along the anterior bladder wall through the bladder neck and prostate to the upper end of the stricture where the prostate is transected (Fig. 11.121 — the ureters have been catheterised for orientation).

The posterior half of the bulbo-prostatic anastomosis is then performed (Fig. 11.122). Next the prostatic urothelium is narrowed to about 12 mm in width so that it will be about 12 F in calibre when rolled into a tube, by stripping urothelium off the prostate on either side of the midline (Fig. 11.123). The prostatic urethra is then reconstituted in two or three layers (Fig. 11.124) and wrapped with omentum.

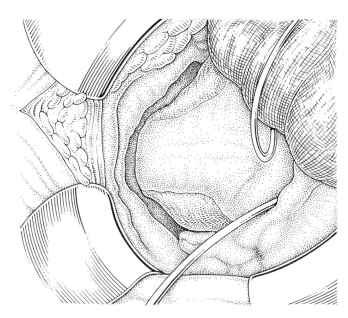

Fig. 11.121

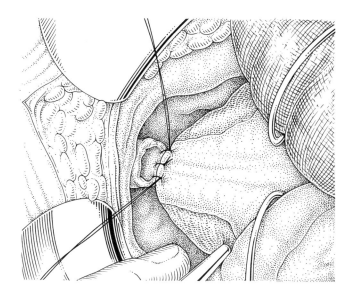

Fig. 11.122

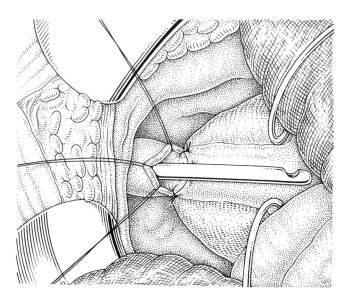

Fig. 11.123

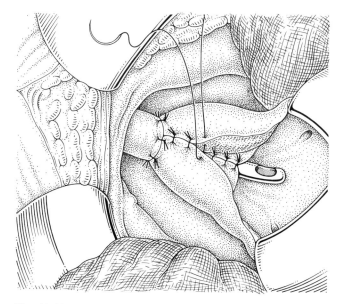

Fig. 11.124

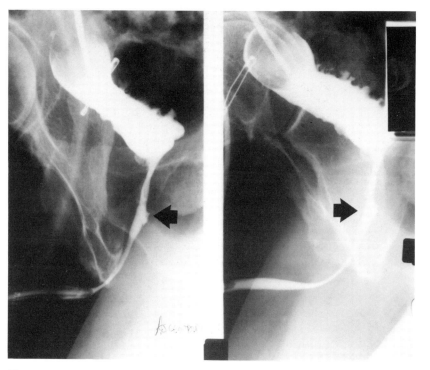

Fig. 11.125

amenable to optical urethrotomy). Bladder patch urethroplasty is also useful for recurrent strictures after a previous bulbo-prostatic anastomosis when a simple revision is not possible.

Unfortunately these patch procedures are only helpful when the lumen of the urethra is still reasonably patent. If the membranous urethra has been obliterated a patch procedure may be impossible. Then the only options are: either to mobilise the bulbar urethra, if its condition looks good enough (e.g. a mild bulbar stricture in a young man), accepting the risk, and to perform a bulbo-prostatic anastomosis; or to form a pedicled preputial/penile skin tube to bridge the gap; or to use a bladder tube to bridge the gap as described in Chapter 14; or to perform a two-stage scroto-urethral inlay procedure, similar to that described for bulbar strictures, but extending more proximally up to the verumontanum which is often the safest option.

Figure 11.125 shows the radiological appearance at 3 weeks with a more normal prostatic urethral calibre above the spatulation of the bulbo-prostatic anastomosis (arrowed).

BULBOMEMBRANOUS STRICTURES

The success of bulbo-prostatic anastomosis for membranous urethral strictures is dependent on having a normal bulbar urethra that can safely be mobilised throughout its length without prejudice to its viability because of its good retrograde collateral blood supply. This retrograde blood flow may be critically impaired by spongiofibrosis associated with a coexisting bulbar stricture. If the bulbar urethra is mobilised in such a situation, ischaemia between the area of stricture/spongiofibrosis and transected end of the bulbar urethra will usually lead to further stricturing between the site of the previous stricture and the bulbo-prostatic anastomosis which may be sufficient in degree to cause total obliteration of this segment of the urethra.

Thus when strictures at both sites coexist each must be treated separately and using a technique or techniques that do not require the bulbar urethral mobilisation that is necessary for an anastomotic urethroplasty. As always, optical urethrotomy should be tried first. If that fails it is usually possible to rotate in a pedicled preputial or penile skin patch to perform a patch urethroplasty of both strictures, certainly in an uncircumcised man, but not always in a circumcised patient. One alternative is to use a pedicled scrotal skin patch as described above; the other is to treat the membranous stricture by a bladder patch urethroplasty and then to treat the bulbar stricture by a pedicled preputial/penile skin patch urethroplasty (assuming of course, that it is not

BLADDER PATCH URETHROPLASTY

The incision and preliminary exposure for this procedure are as for the pelvic part of a combined abdomino-perineal bulbo-prostatic anastomosis. The subprostatic urethra is exposed with chiselling of the posterior aspect of the pubis as necessary and incision or excision of any fibrous retropubic plaque. The membranous urethra is then incised vertically along its axis from healthy prostatic urethra above, down to healthy proximal bulbar urethra below (Fig. 11.126). This usually requires excision of more of the pubis than is necessary for a bulbo-prostatic anastomosis and it is important that this should be sufficiently extensive to allow a good margin of healthy urethra to be exposed and incised distal to the stricture. It will be appreciated that there is a limit to the inferior extent of this exposure beyond which this approach is

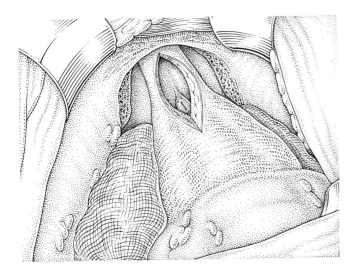

Fig. 11.126

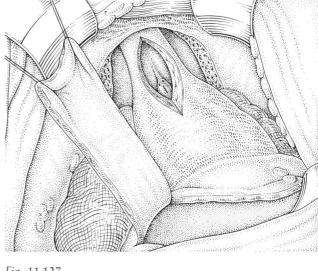

Fig. 11.127

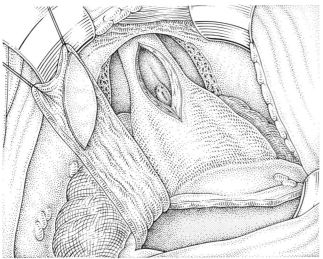

Fig. 11.128

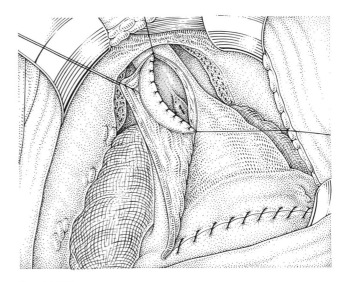

Fig. 11.129

impossible, in which case a two-stage scroto-urethral inlay procedure will be necessary.

Having opened the stricture, a wedge of prostate is excised on each side of the upper end of the stricturotomy to splay out the urothelium.

A flap of bladder wall is then raised with a width equal to the length of the stricture and running from one side of the bladder to the other with the base

of the flap arising in the region of the lateral vascular pedicle (Fig. 11.127).

The urothelium of this full thickness bladder flap is then removed from the full length of the flap with the exception of the part at the end that will serve as a patch to close the urethra. This must be trimmed carefully to size (Fig. 11.128). The bladder is then closed carefully and the usual suprapubic and urethral catheters are passed.

The bladder patch is then anastomosed carefully with interrupted 4/0 Vicryl sutures to the margins of the opened urethra ensuring good urothelial apposition all the way round (Fig. 11.129). The omentum is then mobilised and tacked down into the pelvis to cover the anastomosis and fill in the bony defect in the pubis.

The usual postoperative management plan is followed.

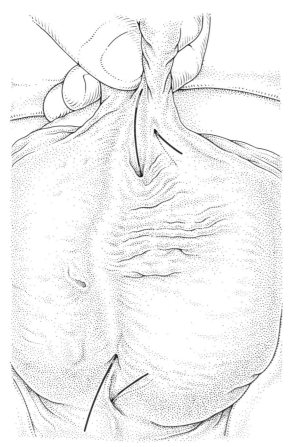

Fig. 11.130

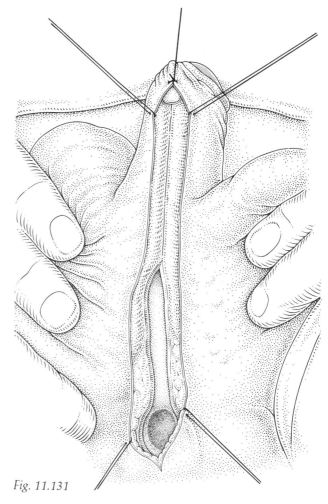

Fig. 11.131

OTHER STRICTURE PROBLEMS

Most of the strictures that will be
encountered can be treated by one or
other of the procedures described above
but each stricture must be treated in its
own right and the surgeon must be
prepared to adapt and modify his
technique according to the operative
findings. For the vast majority of
strictures a one-stage technique will
almost always be possible using the
anastomotic technique for short strictures
and the pedicled patch technique for
longer ones. Other techniques are only
rarely required. Two-stage techniques
can however be very useful on
occasions, particularly with complicated
strictures or otherwise unusual problems.
If there is any doubt about the likely

integrity of a patch urethroplasty a
scroto-urethral inlay should be
performed to leave the reconstruction
open to view during the early phase of
healing, opening the full length of the
urethra if necessary, and closing it at a
second stage.

Figure 11.130 shows an example of such
a patient with a congenital problem, the
exact nature of which is lost in the mists
of time. He was left with an obliterated
urethra and multiple fistulae illustrated
with bits of nylon thread). The whole
thing was opened up from the prostatic
urethra to the fossa navicularis (Fig.

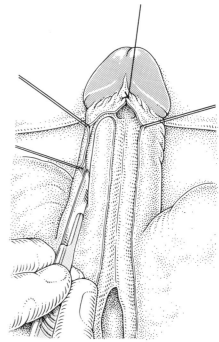

Fig. 11.132

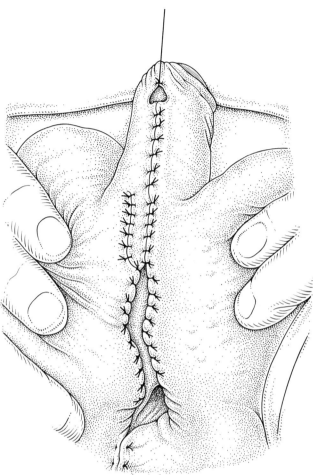

Fig. 11.133

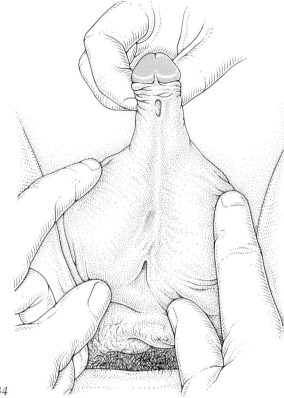

Fig. 11.134

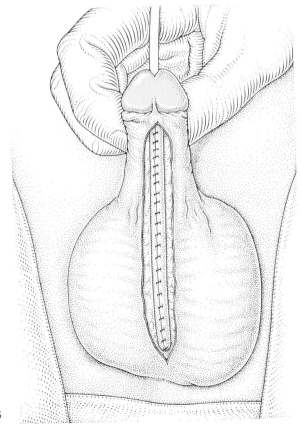

Fig. 11.135

11.131) revealing a sequestered strip of
ventral bulbar urethral wall that was
worth preserving. A flap of penile skin
(Fig. 11.132) was rotated down to the
peno-scrotal region (Fig. 11.133) so that
the eventual closure would have the
best quality skin and the skin was closed
around the urethral remnants. Six
months was allowed for healing and
then, when the whole length of the
proposed urethra looked smooth, regular
and stable (Fig. 11.134) it was rolled
into a tube (Fig. 11.135) in the usual
way.

THE FUTURE OF URETHROPLASTY

At the time of writing this chapter there is considerable interest in a new form of treatment for urethral strictures — implantation of an endoprosthesis (or stent) to hold the urethra open after the stricture has been incised by optical urethrotomy. The short-term results with this technique have been very satisfactory and it will undoubtedly prove to have an important place in the management of strictures. What that role will turn out to be is not yet clear.

Basically strictures can be divided into three types: short post-traumatic strictures in an otherwise normal urethra suitable for an anastomotic urethroplasty, usually in young men; longer strictures in an otherwise normal urethra, suitable for a one-stage patch urethroplasty, usually in young and middle-aged men; and long strictures complicated by some other factor, particularly by a generally stricture-prone urethra, in elderly men. It is in the latter group that I would imagine that endoprosthetic surgery will find its main role. I can also see a role for endoprosthetic surgery for long strictures in young men with an otherwise normal urethra but I would be a little unhappy about its general use in such circumstances, basically because I feel a little unhappy about the use of any prosthesis in someone with decades of life yet to live.

As for short strictures, I think that the results of anastomotic urethroplasty are so good that it is unlikely that endoprosthetic surgery will replace it except in unusual circumstances.

REFERENCES

Probably the most complete and readable overview of strictures is by Blandy, and this review also describes his techniques for one-stage and two-stage scrotal skin urethroplasty. It is unfortunately a little dated.

More than anyone else Turner Warwick has made strictures his own personal subject. Numerous references to his work could be cited — the one given below is the most up to date and covers most aspects of urethroplasty.

This chapter has been expanded beyond, perhaps, what the subject deserves because there are many important principles of reconstructive surgery described here for the first time in this book. Principles such as wide access, adequate mobilisation, tension-free anastomosis, epithelial apposition, urothelial preservation and the like will be reiterated throughout the remainder of the book. One particular principle — the mobilisation of pedicled preputial skin patches — owes much to the work of Duckett although it was in fact described earlier by Yaxley. Again, many references to Duckett's work could be cited and the one given here is (or was) simply the latest.

The most detailed description of the use of urothelial grafts is that of Li et al (1981), who also have the greatest published experience of the technique.

The reference to Euan Milroy's experience with the endoprosthetic stent and to Orandi's publication are added for completeness.

Blandy J P 1980 Urethral stricture. Postgraduate Medical Journal 56: 383–418

Duckett J N, Snow B W 1988 Hypospadias repair. In: Mundy A R (ed) Current operative surgery — Urology. Bailliere Tindall, Eastbourne, pp 119–139

Li Z-C, Zheng Y-H, Sheh Y-Z, Cao Y-F 1981 One-stage urethroplasty for hypospadias using a tube constructed with bladder mucosa — a new procedure. Urologic Clinics of North America 8: 463–470

Milroy E J G, Chapple C R, Elden A, Wallsten H 1989 A new stent for the treatment of urethral strictures — preliminary report. British Journal of Urology 63: 392–396

Orandi, A 1972 One-stage urethroplasty: Four year follow up. Journal of Urology 107: 977–980

Turner Warwick R T 1988 Urethral stricture surgery. In: Mundy A R (ed) Current operative surgery — Urology. Bailliere Tindall, Eastbourne, pp 160–218

Yaxley R P 1968 Another one-stage hypospadias operation. Australian and New Zealand Journal of Surgery 38: 63–65

Chapter 12

Vesico-vaginal and other fistulae

VESICO-VAGINAL FISTULAE

There are few disasters, short of death, greater than the sudden onset of more or less total incontinence in an individual who previously had normal continence. Vesico-vaginal fistula is such a disaster.

It is not usually difficult to make the diagnosis. The onset of more or less total incontinence by day a week or so after a hysterectomy (or, where such problems are still common, a complicated childbirth) will raise the suspicion in even the most obtuse gynaecologist. However, if the fistula is small there may be normal voiding with insensible incontinence between times. Indeed, apparent continence at rest, at least for short periods, with incontinence only on activity stimulating stress incontinence is sometimes seen with a moderate-sized fistula if the pelvic floor musculature is capable of retaining urine within the vagina. Symptoms alone are not therefore always reliable. However, the presence of a pool of urine in the vaginal vault, however small, should always suggest the presence of a fistula even if the fistula itself cannot be seen.

The diagnosis is usually substantiated by a 'three pad test' and then confirmed by cystoscopy and EUA. With tiny fistulae, the fistula itself may not be visible but early on its site will sometimes be indicated by a patch of oedema or inflammation, usually just above the interureteric bar which is the usual site for fistulae. If no fistula is seen but there is a strong suspicion that a fistula nonetheless exists, the other two tricks to try are vaginal air insufflation—looking for bubbles in the bladder endoscopically—or intravesical instillation of dilute methylene blue—looking for leakage vaginally.

When the patient has previously been treated for carcinoma of the cervix, or any other malignancy, the edge of the fistula should be liberally biopsied to look for residual or recurrent disease.

Any other suspicious areas on EUA should also be biopsied. A CT scan is another important investigation in such patients to look for residual or recurrent disease.

If no fistula is seen, an IVU is arranged to look for a uretero-vaginal or, more rarely, a uretero-uterine fistula. With an endoscopic diagnosis a micturating cystogram is not really necessary for simple fistulae but in complex fistulae after previous pelvic radiotherapy may show accessory tracks or cavities. An IVU is a sensible precaution in all fistulae because of the close proximity of many fistulae to the intramural segments of the ureters and because a procedure that has damaged the bladder may damage the ureter coincidentally.

Most fistulae these days, in the developed world, occur after a simple hysterectomy. They are small; they are situated close to the interureteric bar; they are due to a combination of devascularisation of that area of the bladder during its dissection off the front of the cervix and anterior vaginal wall and overdistension of the bladder in the early postoperative period because the patient was not catheterised; they usually present when the patient is still in hospital recovering from the procedure, and they are usually otherwise uncomplicated. These fistulae and others like them may be termed simple fistulae.

Factors which make a fistula a complex fistula include:

1. very large size;
2. involvement of the bladder neck or urethra or both;
3. extensive fibrosis;
4. underlying disease (especially cancer and previous radiotherapy);
5. associated rectal or other fistula;

—anything in fact that alters things such that a simple repair, as described below, would not be possible.

In practice the common denominator making a fistula complex in the vast majority of instances is a history of a Wertheim's hysterectomy and radiotherapy for carcinoma of the cervix. It is rare to find an unusually large fistula, extensive fibrosis and associated rectal or other fistulae in any other situation. Previous surgery is often cited as a complicating factor but in my opinion this simply makes a simple fistula into a more difficult simple fistula rather than a complex fistula.

Post-irradiation fistulae, as will be discussed later in this chapter, are so different from simple fistulae that they deserve to be regarded in a class of their own, principally because the effects of irradiation on the bladder and urethra are such that closure of the fistula alone rarely returns the urinary tract to normal.

With a simple fistula there is rarely any reason to do other than treat it directly. It used to be said that 3 months or so should be allowed to elapse to allow the local tissues to 'settle down' but this is unnecessary and simply leaves the patient wetter for longer. All things being equal, if a fistula does not dry up within a few days of catheterisation and treatment of any associated urinary infection there seems to be no reason not to proceed to surgical repair unless there is some complication, such as a coexisting deep vein thrombosis for example, making it safer to wait.

With complex fistulae the question is whether to repair the fistula or go for a simpler option such as urinary diversion. My practice is to explain both procedures and their possible complications to the patient and let the individual make up her own mind. The only proviso, in patients recently treated for carcinoma of the cervix, is that the operative findings may dictate an ileal conduit.

REPAIR OF A SIMPLE FISTULA

For decades the argument has raged as to the relative merits of vaginal and retropubic repair of simple fistulae. To a large extent this is as much an argument between gynaecologists with extensive experience of vaginal surgery and less of retropubic surgery, and urologists with a predominantly or exclusively retropubic experience. Another factor is that vaginal repair is a lesser procedure than a retropubic repair but this argument is largely offset in fistulae to the vaginal vault (as is the case with post-hysterectomy fistulae) by the higher success rate of retropubic surgery.

My feeling is that the most important factor is the accessibility of the fistula as this determines whether or not a fistula can be *easily* repaired by a vaginal approach. If not, I feel it is safer to repair it *easily* by a retropubic procedure than with difficulty by a vaginal procedure. The main consideration must be to guarantee to close the fistula at the first attempt.

These days the majority of fistulae in the Northern Hemisphere are post-hysterectomy and are therefore high in the vaginal vault. Thus, unless the fistula is attacked within a few days of its appearance before fibrosis has developed, the surgeon's ability to define the necessary tissue planes adequately is restricted in a vaginal approach by the limited access when compared with a retropubic approach. It is my view therefore that the retropubic route is better because it is more reliable, except in the (these days) rare instance of an obstetric fistula on the anterior vaginal wall.

Obstetric fistulae can be closed by the retropubic approach but, being on the anterior vaginal wall, are just as easily closed transvaginally with lower operative morbidity. The principles are the same as in the retropubic approach but the procedure more closely resembles repair of a urethro-vaginal fistula (see below).

Massive obstetric fistulae destroying the bladder neck and most of the urethra more closely resemble the urovaginal continence type of urogenital sinus described in Chapter 14 and treated by one of the neourethroplasty techniques described in that chapter. The technique described on pages 309–313 is generally the most appropriate.

Preoperative preparation
There is no special preparation other than to ensure that the urine is sterile. The patient's blood group should be known and her serum saved but blood loss seldom warrants transfusion.

Position
The patient should be supine and draped for a lower abdominal incision.

Technique
The general principle is excision of the fistula and a two-layer closure of both the vagina and the bladder with interposition of the omentum between the two to keep the two suture lines apart and thereby prevent recurrence. The requirement for omental interposition means that a midline lower abdominal incision should theoretically be used in preference to a transverse incision; with a transverse incision, although it is nicer for the patient, the omentum may not be sufficiently accessible. In practice the omentum is often found to be stuck onto the region of the fistula and in addition it is kinder to the patient to reopen the incision that she has already had. If necessary a second incision (upper midline) can be made to mobilise the omentum if the original incision was a Pfannenstiel.

The bladder is opened through an incision in its dome and a ring retractor is placed within the bladder to hold it and the incision open (Fig. 12.1). If the ureteric orifices are close to the fistula they are catheterised. The fistula is then circumcised, the aim being to incise through the full thickness of the bladder wall, then to enter and open up the

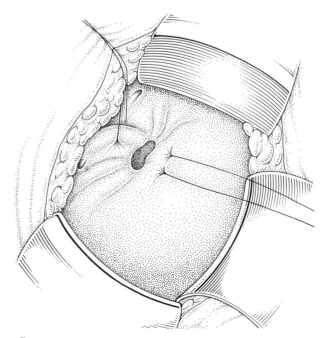

Fig. 12.1

plane between healthy bladder and healthy vagina, then to continue this all the way round the edge of the fistula. As the bladder and vagina are only usually in contact below the fistula (because the fistula is usually in the vaginal vault following a hysterectomy) the plane will only be found inferiorly. Above the fistula an incision through the bladder wall will usually expose adherent loops of bowel and omentum in relation to the vaginal vault closure and the fistula. When the correct plane has been found it is opened up superiorly (Fig. 12.2) and inferiorly (Fig. 12.3). These incisions are then joined on either side of the fistula, taking care not to damage the terminal/intramural ureter during the lateral mobilisation where the ureter is often close. As the tissue plane between bladder and vagina is opened up the fistula is progressively circumcised.

When the fistula has been fully circumcised in this way the edges are undermined in the correct plane so that there is no fibrosis tethering the vaginal vault to the bladder base and there is a 2 cm margin of mobilised bladder wall all the way round. Indeed the elasticity of the bladder wall causes the margins of the bladder to retract and this makes the hole look much bigger than the original fistula. However, with no fibrosis to tether the bladder it is usually easy to approximate the edges of the bladder transversely without tension. If the fistula is larger than usual this may not be possible without further undermining in the plane between the bladder and vagina. Another problem is when the bladder is collapsed and unpliable, usually because of prolonged catheterisation, making it difficult to retract or mobilise. The solution here is to bivalve the bladder in the coronal

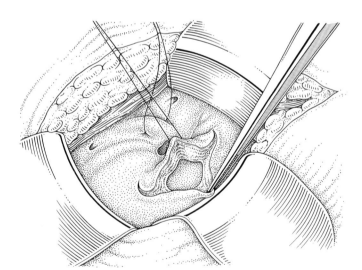

Fig. 12.2

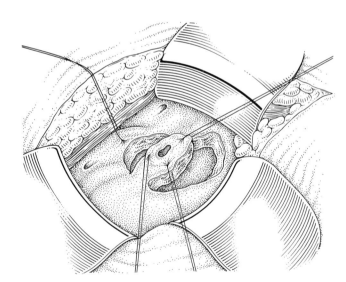

Fig. 12.3

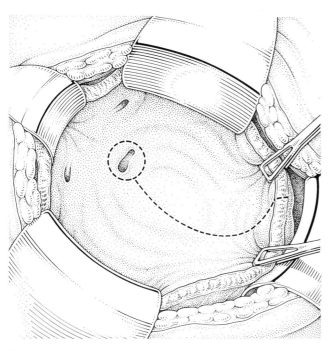

Fig. 12.4

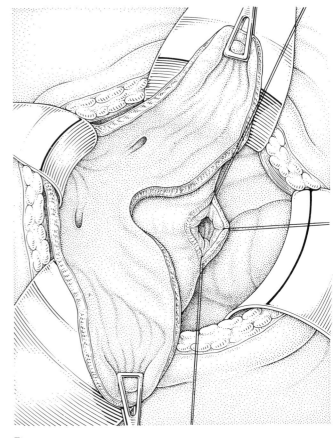

Fig. 12.5

plane (Figs 12.4, 12.5) which effectively mobilises the bladder in two halves on each lateral vascular pedicle.

Whether or not bivalving of the bladder is necessary (and it rarely is), it is usually easier to find the correct plane and to mobilise the bladder with the fistula and vagina intact. When the bladder has been mobilised the fistula is excised (Fig. 12.6) from the vagina leaving healthy vaginal margins in the depths of the bladder incision. The vagina is then closed in two layers with interrupted inverting 3/0 Vicryl sutures (Fig. 12.7). If all the tethering between the vagina and bladder has been divided, this should be easily accomplished.

The omentum is then interposed between the vagina and bladder and sewn there to cover the vaginal suture line and keep it separated from the bladder closure (Fig. 12.8). The omentum is often stuck down onto the vaginal vault and is therefore easily interposed but occasionally it needs to be mobilised for this purpose as described in Chapter 11. The bladder is then closed in two

layers, again with 3/0 Vicryl (Fig. 12.9). A suprapubic catheter is left in the bladder at the end of the procedure and for 10 days thereafter.

Postoperative care
The suprapubic catheter is clamped on the tenth postoperative day for a trial of voiding. Assuming there is no problem it is removed the next day.

If the repair has been close to the ureters or if the intramural ureter was involved, making a ureteric reimplantation necessary, an IVU is arranged 6 weeks or so later. If this is satisfactory, no further follow up is required.

COMPLEX FISTULAE

Complex fistulae are most commonly vesico-vaginal or vesico-urethro-vaginal fistulae following combined radiotherapy and hysterectomy for carcinoma of the cervix. Several factors distinguish a complex vesico-vaginal fistula of this type from a simple fistula of the same size and site:

1.   The potential for residual or recurrent malignant disease.
2.   Impaired tissue healing as a result of irradiation. This includes not just a failure of healing of any suture line, which is a well recognised complication of radiotherapy, but also a failure of healing around a reconstruction within the pelvis, resulting sometimes in loss of the usual obliteration of potential spaces by the fibrosis that normally occurs with healing. This is important because if a

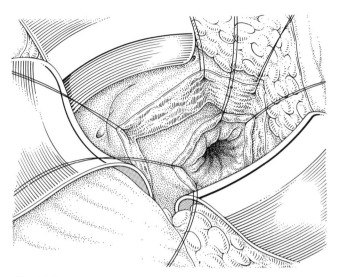

Fig. 12.6

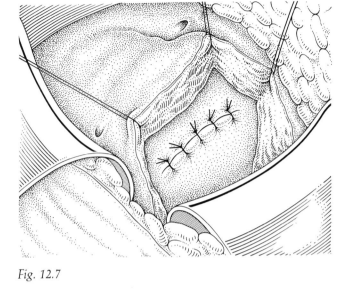

Fig. 12.7

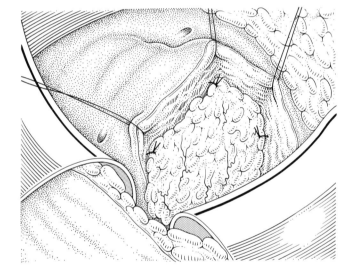

Fig. 12.8

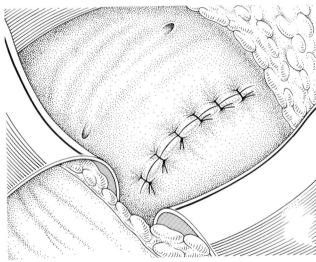

Fig. 12.9

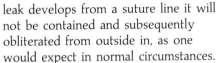

leak develops from a suture line it will not be contained and subsequently obliterated from outside in, as one would expect in normal circumstances.

3. Retropubic fibrosis beyond the area of the fistula itself reducing the mobility of the tissues of the pelvis and increasing their stiffness thereby disturbing most of the factors on which a simple repair, as described above, depends.

4. The possibility of pelvic plexus injury as a result of the hysterectomy causing a poorly compliant acontractile bladder, bladder neck incompetence and a distal sphincter mechanism of fixed resistance allowing both sphincter weakness incontinence and sphincteric obstruction.

5. Sphincter weakness incontinence and, commonly, detrusor instability as a result of radiotherapy.

In addition to these five basic points:

6. These fistulae are often large.
7. They are often close to or involve the bladder neck.
8. They often directly involve other structures, particularly the rectum, or indirectly involve them by adhesions or through abscess cavities.
9. They are often made worse by inadequate attempts to treat them surgically when they first develop.

Complex fistulae always look less of a problem than they really are. The first step in dealing with these patients is a thorough assessment. This should include:

Cystoscopy and EUA including biopsy of the edges of the fistula and any other suspicious areas. The state of the bladder and urethral urothelium should be noted and the capacity of the bladder should be assessed as far as it is possible to gauge. (A Foley catheter through the fistula from the vagina, with its balloon inflated, may provide sufficient occlusion to allow this to be reasonably assessed.) The thickness of the bladder wall and the urethral seal — is it like a 'drainpipe' or does it look fairly normal? — should also be noted.

Proctoscopy, colonoscopy. In patients who have had radiotherapy proctoscopy allows inspection and biopsy of the rectal mucosa, looking for gross evidence of radiation proctitis and microscopic evidence of radionecrosis. This gives a further assessment of the radiotherapy reaction in the pelvis although, in fact, one can get a fairly good idea as to how bad the radiotherapy reaction is from the state of the skin over the pubis and sacrum. In patients with rectal fistulae, colonoscopy supplemented by a barium enema assesses the normality or otherwise of the colon proximal to the fistula. The particular point to look for is irradiation stricture of the sigmoid colon.

IVU to look for secondary upper tract changes.

CT scan of the pelvis (and abdomen) to look for secondary spread of a tumour and assess the density of the fibrotic reaction in the pelvis.

Armed with this information and bearing in mind that the inside of the pelvis is probably worse than it appears to be, patients can be roughly allocated to one of three groups:

1. Vesico-vaginal fistula with a relatively normal bladder: in other words what appears to be an otherwise 'simple' fistula in a patient who happens to have had radiotherapy. It is likely in such cases that the hysterectomy rather than the radiotherapy was the cause of the fistula. The treatment of such patients is relatively straightforward. This is unfortunately unusual.

2. Vesico-vaginal fistula with an overtly abnormal bladder (and vagina) either because of severe urothelial changes, a small bladder capacity, poor bladder compliance or the sheer size of the fistula. Simply closing the fistula in such patients is not worthwhile in this type of situation even if it is possible because the patient is likely to suffer just as much with the irradiation cystitis. Curative surgery for such patients would therefore require a subtotal cystectomy and substitution cystoplasty but even so they are likely to have problems from incompetence of their sphincter mechanisms whether or not they are involved by the fistula itself. In such patients the radiotherapy appears to be a more important aetiological factor than the hysterectomy. If the urethra is involved in the fistula or is compromised by excision of the fistula-related mass then a substitution urethroplasty may also be required.

3. Vesico-vagino-rectal fistula, usually associated with an overtly abnormal, indeed useless bladder and vagina, representing a more severe type of radiotherapy reaction or surgical trauma.

In theory the broad principles of treatment, whichever group the patient falls into, are the same as for a simple fistula: mobilisation of the tissues around the fistula by opening out the tissue plane between; tension-free inverting closure of healthy edges; and interposition of healthy viable tissue to keep the two suture lines apart.

In patients in Group 1 it will be relatively easy to apply all of these general principles and, unless the fistula is close to or involving the sphincter mechanisms, the result should be satisfactory using a technique like that described above for a simple fistula.

Patients in Group 2 (the largest group) cannot be treated in this way because the effect of radiotherapy on the bladder causes the bladder wall to be plastered to the wall of the pelvis with dense fibrosis all around the bladder and around the fistula in particular making it very difficult to open up the plane between the vagina and bladder base at the lower edge of the fistula without damaging either or both in the process. Even if the planes were opened and the edges of the fistula mobilised satisfactorily, the fibrosis will almost certainly prevent a tension-free closure of the two viscera. And even if the fistula were to be dealt with satisfactorily, and with no symptoms due to irradiation cystitis, it would be impossible to predict whether the patient would be continent because the competence of the sphincters could only be guessed at preoperatively and if the patient turned out to be incontinent it would be a nigh impossible task to go back into the pelvis and perform anti-incontinence surgery.

Thus patients in this group cannot be treated like those with simple fistulae or like those in Group 1. They require a subtotal cystectomy to remove the fistula and the surrounding unhealthy bladder, followed by substitution cystoplasty to replace the diseased bladder with a healthy, low-pressure substitute of good capacity. To ensure low pressures, particularly in the presence of sphincter weakness, a pouch type or 'detubularised' substitution cystoplasty should be performed. The vagina is treated in the same way if it is affected — by excision and substitution. The two viscera are then wrapped with omentum to keep the suture lines apart and to help with healing.

For a young, fit, healthy and highly motivated woman this may be an entirely reasonable proposition but unless all of these criteria are satisfied a continent or conduit urinary diversion might be a better option and should be discussed with all patients. This question and the procedures used for continent diversion were described and discussed in Chapter 8 when we were considering irradiation cystitis and its treatment.

The same considerations apply to patients in Group 3 but because of the rectal problems there are two further conflicting factors. On the one hand simultaneous rectal reconstruction increases the scale of surgery, increases the risk of complications, reduces the range of tissues available for each individual reconstruction (there are only a certain number of options available which then have to be divided up between the three areas requiring reconstruction — bladder, vagina and rectum) and would therefore tend to deter both the surgeon and the patient. On the other hand the prospect of having both an ileal conduit and a colostomy would tend to push all but the most phlegmatic patient towards reconstructive surgery.

Another option of course is to reconstruct one system and divert the other; for example cystoplasty and colostomy, or colo-anal reconstruction and an ileal conduit or continent urinary diversion. Superficially, this alternative has considerable attractions, particularly colo-rectal reconstruction and a continent diversion (if it works) because it seems a smaller undertaking and leaves the patient looking nearly normal. It has the additional advantage that a failed continent diversion is often more easily and satisfactorily managed than an incontinent cystoplasty. In practice however it is probably no less a procedure than a total reconstruction because the advantage with a continent diversion of not having to excise the bladder remnant and deal with the vesico-vaginal fistula is probably offset by the greater difficulty with the colo-rectal/anal reconstruction when the bladder and surrounding fibrosis are still in place. Certainly, once the fistula-related mass and the surrounding fibrosis have been cleared out of the pelvis and the bladder, vaginal vault and rectum have been trimmed back to

healthy tissue ready for reconstruction, the subsequent stages are fairly straightforward. Furthermore, excision of the fistula-related mass has two other advantages — it rids the patient of a chronically infected, discharging and often painful abscess cavity and it allows a much more accurate histopathological assessment of the patient's disease status.

All these factors must be discussed with the patient because the patient's motivation is all important. The surest way to lose her confidence is by failing to ensure that she is fully informed; if, subsequently, there is a finding or complication requiring a further procedure or a different outcome, it should not be a shocking revelation. Above all the likelihood of a long slow postoperative recovery and the probable need for secondary revision procedures should be stressed. Again a continent or conduit diversion may be in the patient's best interests.

PELVIC RECONSTRUCTION

Preoperative preparation
This is the same in principle as for substitution cystoplasty or implantation of an artificial sphincter. As it is a very extensive surgical procedure which will usually take several hours and blood loss will be considerable, 6 units of blood should be cross matched. In view of the likely scale and duration of surgery it is wise to take steps to ensure adequate nursing care for the first 24 hours postoperatively in an intensive care or equivalent unit.

Position
The patient is placed supine on the operating table with the legs in the low lithotomy position and is draped for a full length midline abdominal incision. The inside of the legs should also be exposed in case there is the rare need for a gracilis muscle graft or for a substitution vaginoplasty using myocutaneous gracilis flaps.

This position gives access to all tissues that might be needed.

Procedure
As stated earlier there are three procedures or groups of procedures.

1. Excision of the fistula and closure leaving the bladder and vagina otherwise intact.
2. Excision of the bladder and vaginal remnants around and above the fistula followed by reconstruction by means of a substitution cystoplasty using an ileocolonic pouch type of cystoplasty, with or without a substitution urethroplasty depending on whether or not the urethra is involved, and either closure of the vaginal vault or substitution vaginoplasty.
3. Excision of the bladder, vaginal and rectal remnants around the fistula (pelvic clearance) followed by reconstruction by means of a subsitution cystoplasty using an ileocolonic pouch type of cystoplasty, with or without a substitution urethroplasty; substitution vaginoplasty; and reconstruction of the rectum.

Substitution cystoplasty using an ileocolonic pouch was described in Chapter 10. This pouch type of 'detubularised' cystoplasty should always be used in patients such as this to ensure the lowest possible intravesical pressures because of the high incidence of associated sphincter weakness incontinence.

The procedures that need to be described here are:

— differences in the technique of 'simple' fistula closure,
— pelvic clearance for reconstruction,
— ano-rectal reconstruction,
— total substitution cystourethroplasty,
— combined substitution cystoplasty and vaginoplasty using colon,
— and the alternative technique of substitution vaginoplasty using myocutaneous gracilis flaps.

They will be described in this order as this is the order in which they would be performed (excluding the technique of closure of an apparently 'simple' fistula in a patient with a vesico-vagino-rectal fistula requiring a complete pelvic visceral reconstruction).

CLOSURE OF AN APPARENTLY SIMPLE FISTULA

In theory, if the patient has been properly selected, this should be no different from closure of a simple fistula as described earlier on in this chapter. In practice, even if the bladder appears normal it has nonetheless been irradiated, is less pliable and is more prone to healing problems. Dissection must therefore be more meticulous, the technique of bisecting the bladder is more often necessary, and omental deployment is more important. Even if the fistula is small enough and low enough to be approachable vaginally, this approach (in my opinion) is contraindicated because of the risk of making matters worse and possibly irretrievably worse.

It may also be extremely difficult from the retropubic approach, because of intense fibrosis, to get adequate separation between the bladder and vagina at and below the lower edge of the fistula both for excision and closure of the fistula itself and for creation of sufficient space for the omental interposition. Rather than persist with a retropubic approach with the risks of an inadequate repair or of further damage to the bladder or vagina I recommend separating the urethra from the anterior vaginal wall from below, as for the opening stages of a Stamey-type procedure (Ch. 6), in order to open up the correct plane below the fistula. Then, when the fistula has been closed (or after substitution cystoplasty) the omentum can be pulled through this channel and incorporated in the introital wound closure to hold it in place.

Occasionally, the omentum is inadequate or absent, particularly after gastric surgery or after multiple intra-abdominal procedures of any type. In these circumstances one or both labial fat pads might be adequate. Failing that a gracilis muscle flap can be mobilised and pulled through a subcutaneous tunnel to the introitus, then passed up the tunnel between the bladder/urethra and the vagina and sutured in place from above. This procedure is described later on in this chapter.

PELVIC CLEARANCE PRIOR TO RECONSTRUCTION

This involves subtotal cystectomy, a correspondingly wide excision of the vaginal vault around the fistula and a similar excision of the rectum back to relatively healthy tissue. This is then built on by subsitution cystoplasty and colo-rectal reconstruction with either closure of the vaginal stump or substitution vaginoplasty, depending on the patient's age and inclination. As the distal colon is going to be used for the rectal reconstruction and the proximal colon/terminal ileum will be used for substitution cystoplasty and vaginoplasty the normality or otherwise of the colon is crucial. If the colon is deficient (for example after a previous sigmoid colectomy) or diseased (e.g. extensive irradiation damage to the sigmoid colon) then there may simply be 'not enough to go round'. The myocutaneous gracilis flap technique may be used for the vaginoplasty but in an older or obese patient this may not be feasible making vaginal closure mandatory irrespective of the patient's wishes, unless they would prefer that any available colon be used for vaginoplasty rather than cystoplasty. These factors must obviously be discussed with the patient preoperatively. Hence also the importance of preoperative barium enema.

Pelvic clearance starts with the subtotal cystectomy, aiming to preserve the bladder neck and the subureteric part of the trigone assuming these are not involved by the fistula. This can be extremely difficult, not only because of the fibrosis around the fistula but also because of the plastering of the bladder to the front and side walls of the pelvis. The general principles however are the same for subtotal cystectomy for interstitial cystitis (Ch. 8), namely wide opening of the retropubic space all the way round both sides, division of the superior vesical pedicles, ureters and the upper part of the inferior pedicles, bisection of the bladder in the coronal plane from the bladder neck anteriorly to the upper margin of the fistula posteriorly, and then excision of the bladder using a diathermy point to incise along the margins of the trigone laterally and below the fistula posteriorly to thereby excise the bladder.

Stay-sutures are then placed to hold the bladder remnant forwards while it is separated from the anterior vaginal wall. The vagina is then widely opened from the front to the back below the level of the fistula and then around the vagina to separate the vagina from the rectum or, if there is a fistula posteriorly, to circumcise the fistula from the rectum. Some patients will previously have had an end colostomy in the left iliac fossa with closure of the rectum just above the fistula (Hartmann's procedure) making this relatively easy. If necessary the circumcision of the fistula from the rectum is facilitated by a finger in the rectum to guide the dissection.

The posterior vaginal wall must always be carefully mobilised from the anterior rectal wall so that each can subsequently be sutured easily and then separated, the one from the other, by omental interposition. To achieve this, free margins of at least 1 cm will need to be created and the margins of the bladder, vaginal and rectal remnants should all preferably be staggered so that the

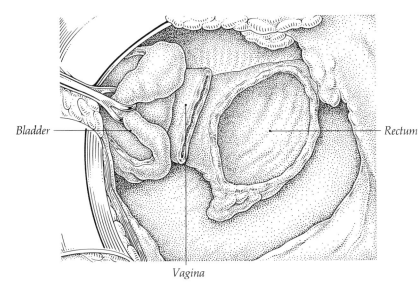

Bladder —

— Rectum

Vagina

Fig. 12.10

subsequent suture lines will not be juxtaposed (Fig. 12.10 — here the posterior wall of the bladder is being pulled forward with a pair of Babcock's forceps to show the transected vagina behind).

The posterior wall of the rectum should be disturbed as little as possible other than to ensure an adequate edge for subsequent closure, as this will provide sensation.

It is important to remember the rationale for leaving these 'bits' behind. The urethra and anal canal will provide sphincteric control for their respective viscera and the trigone and posterior rectal wall provide sensation. These must therefore be preserved if at all possible with as much of their normal blood supply as possible (but reckoning that they can survive on the pudendal and other collateral supply if necessary). On the other hand, there is no advantage to preserving the vagina unless there is enough of it to be functionally useful. A few centimetres of hypersensitive, constricted, irradiated vagina is no use to the patient or the surgeon. It is better to excise it down to the introitus and substitute it, as described below, with an introital suture

line where the blood supply is better and the anastomosis is easier. An introital anastomosis also gives the greatest degree of dissociation (or 'stagger') between the bladder, vaginal and rectal suture lines, minimising the risk of recurrent fistula.

It is easy to describe this mobilisation process; it is not so easy to do. If there is a 'Richter' scale of fibrosis then the pelvic 'clag' one finds in such patients must register at least 8 and usually nearer 10. All too often in practice, despite the most detailed preoperative assessment, one is left with several equivocal biopsy results, some radiological contrast studies which simply confirm the presence of a fistula and a CT scan report a yard (0.9 metres) long but adding little or nothing to the solutions of the two questions that really need answering:

— is there residual or recurrent cancer?
— is this operable?

Given that the tissue planes which largely determine operability are apparently destroyed by radiotherapy and that CT scanning is more or less useless at distinguishing between fibrosis and tumour this unsatisfactory situation

is not entirely surprising, albeit disappointing. The surgeon is therefore usually left to decide the answers to these two questions himself. My guiding principles are:

— the question of malignancy within the pelvis is often only decided after careful serial sectioning of the resected exenteration specimen and the best one can therefore often achieve preoperatively is the exclusion of disease outside the pelvis and particularly in the paraortic nodes, the liver and the lungs. If these areas seem clear then the fistula (and the rest of the pelvis) is treated on its own merits.
— If the patient would be happy with a urinary or faecal diversion or both and this would relieve her symptoms or if her general health is against resection and reconstruction, then diversion it is. If the patient is young, wants a reconstruction rather than a diversion, suffers from pain or chronic infection in the pelvic mass and understands the scale of the surgery proposed then resection and reconstruction is her best option.
— No mass is inoperable until you have tried and failed and if you are likely to fail you shouldn't be trying.

The crux of operability is the development of the fascial planes of the pelvis which, although they may seem obliterated by radiotherapy, can usually be developed with patience. Development of the relevant fascial planes in turn allows development of the vascular pedicles so that these can be controlled. The best way of doing this is first to develop fully the retropubic space taking care not to go through the obturator fascia and cause bleeding from the obturator vessels; then to open the plane on either side of the recto-sigmoid junction down to Waldeyer's fascia and then work anteriorly on each side onto the posterior aspect of the lateral pedicles. Having defined the pedicles it may then be possible to divide the relevant part down to and including the ureter, but preserving the inferior vesical and middle rectal vessels. If the whole pelvis is set in concrete, as it often is, then a precise dissection and mobilisation will not be possible. In such cases the best way of dealing with the problem is to divide the whole of the lateral pedicle which is, in effect, the whole of the anterior division of the internal iliac artery. Once this is divided the pelvic mass will become sufficiently mobile to allow resection of the mass without endangering the parts of the viscera to be left behind.

To achieve this the next step after clearly defining the anterior and posterior aspects of the lateral pedicles is to open the endopelvic fascia in the retropubic space in front of the lateral pedicle and then to go under the pedicle on each side putting a sling round the pedicle to define it. With the lateral pedicle clearly defined on each side it is often easiest just to cut through quickly and then oversew the margin afterwards to control any bleeding points as the tissue does not take clamps or ligatures well. The amount of bleeding is often only slight as the vessels are more or less set in concrete.

In this way and having divided the ureters and ovarian vessels at the pelvic brim, the apparently fixed solid pelvic mass is liberated from all but its inferior attachments to the urethra, vagina and anal canal. The dome of the bladder is first excised from the trigone below the level of the fistula through an incision in the anterior bladder wall. The vagina is then divided transversely below the fistula from before backwards and the rectum is then opened anteriorly below the fistula. The whole mass can then be circumcised from the anterior rectal wall or, if the patient has had a Hartmann's procedure, circumcised with the rectal stump from the posterior rectal wall. Division of Waldeyer's fascia will give additional posterior mobility if necessary to allow resection of the specimen.

Obviously, if it is at all possible to preserve the terminal branches of the anterior division of the internal iliac artery (the remainder of which will be divided by the manoeuvre described above) it is best to do so to maintain the best possible blood supply to the vesicourethral and anorectal remnants from the pudendal and other perineal vessels.

It is important, having got through the fascial layers of the pelvic floor (the endopelvic fascia and Waldeyer's fascia), to take care not to damage the puborectalis and the other muscles of the pelvic floor. They are often surprisingly healthy looking, considering the state of the other pelvic tissues; they have an important function, particularly for anal continence; they provide a landmark for the lowest possible limit for resection without compromising postoperative function; and they protect the pudendal vessels which lie deep to them and on which depends the vascularity of the urethral/vesical, vaginal and to a lesser extent the anorectal remnants.

Having thus cleared out the pelvis from front to back, the reconstruction proceeds initially from back to front.

RECTAL RECONSTRUCTION

If the patient has not previously had an end colostomy excision of the fistula will have left a large hole in the front of an otherwise intact rectum. This defect is closed with two obliquely orientated layers of inverting sutures, assuming that the colon is otherwise normal. Preoperative biopsies of the rectum and the findings of the barium studies and endoscopy and biopsy of the colon above are crucial in determining 'normality' in this respect. If the rectum was previously closed off with an end colostomy above, or if there is obvious radiation damage to the sigmoid colon with gross narrowing of the lumen and

thickening of the colonic wall then the colon is divided at a point where it is relatively healthy and then mobilised to reach down to the rectal stump. This may mean mobilising the whole of the left colon from the splenic flexure downwards. The proximal cut end of the colon is then spatulated on its antimesenteric aspect and then carefully sutured to the rectal stump with 12 inverting interrupted 3/0 Vicryl mattress sutures. This repair should be protected by a proximal, transverse defunctioning colostomy, no matter how good the repair looks.

Sometimes the closure of the rectum is so low that it is easier to do it transvaginally assuming, as is usually the case, that the vaginal length after the pelvic clearance is almost non-existent. Figure 12.11 shows such a case. On vaginal examination all that remains of the vagina is a transverse band with the bladder prolapsing through the fistula anteriorly and the rectum prolapsing through posteriorly. After pelvic clearance vaginal access for the anorectal reconstruction is excellent, especially anteriorly (Fig. 12.12).

It should be remembered that after the pelvic reconstruction has been completed the rectal repair, particularly the posterior part of the anastomosis, will be the least accessible part of that reconstruction. The greatest care should therefore be taken with this anastomosis because it will be extremely difficult to go back and revise the posterior suture line transabdominally if there are any postoperative problems with the anastomosis. Problems of the anterior suture line may be correctable transvaginally if there is any failure of healing but the transvaginal route will not give access posteriorly. For the same reasons the rectal reconstruction also takes priority with the omental wrap.

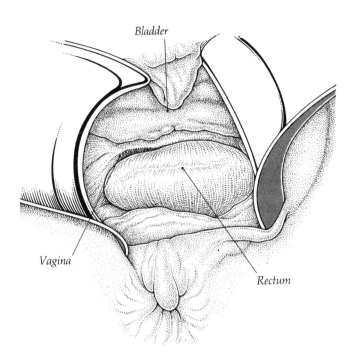

Fig. 12.11

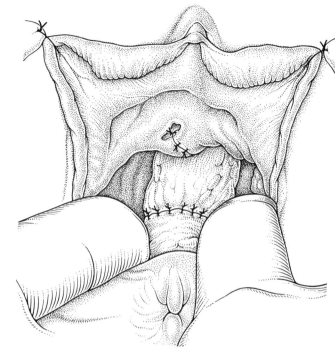

Fig. 12.12

TOTAL SUBSTITUTION CYSTOURETHROPLASTY

The best result after the exenteration procedure to remove the fistula-related mass will be to leave the bladder neck and the subureteric part of the trigone onto which a pouch type of substitution cystoplasty can be anastomosed.

Sometimes, however, either the fistula involves the bladder neck and urethra, or the urethra is damaged peroperatively or it is functionally useless from the combined effects of the hysterectomy and radiotherapy, particularly if the patient had pre-existing simple stress incontinence.

When the trigone, bladder neck and urethra are present but not functional, it may be possible theoretically to implant an artificial sphincter and get it to work but the risks are high, with infection, erosion and failure of adequate urethral compression by the cuff because of intramural and periurethral fibrosis at the top of the list of reasons. As a result the overall success rate of an AUS in such a situation in my experience is only 25% and so I only use it when there is no alternative.

If an artificial sphincter is implanted it should be with an omental wrap around the urethra within the cuff and another wrap around the cuff, to reduce the risks to a minimum. An artificial sphincter should only be implanted if the urethra and bladder neck look healthy and the trigonal margins bleed freely at the time of the subtotal cystectomy; and if the vagina is to be preserved (another sign of relatively healthy tissues) so that there is no vaginoplasty suture line close to the AUS cuff through which the cuff might erode. If a vaginoplasty is necessary or if any of the other conditions are not satisfied then an AUS should not be implanted as infection or erosion will be almost inevitable.

It is important to remember in patients like this, irrespective of the fistula, that if there is both a bladder abnormality and a urethral sphincteric abnormality causing incontinence then unless the urethral abnormality is particularly severe it is more important to correct the bladder problem. Thus even a quite severely compromised urethral sphincter mechanism may be able to give a reasonable degree of continence if the small capacity, poorly compliant bladder above it is replaced by a low-pressure pouch-type substitution cystoplasty of good capacity.

Another theoretically attractive alternative to give a competent 'sphincter mechanism' whether or not a bladder outflow tract is still present is to put an AUS cuff around the distal end of a colonic cystoplasty. Unfortunately, although I have two patients with a satisfactory system of that type, the procedure usually fails because the AUS cuff is not designed to compress a tube with the configuration of the urethra (thick wall, narrow lumen) not a structure with the configuration that gut has (thin wall, large lumen). Another alternative is to form an ileal urethra and then to intussuscept it into a substitution cystoplasty with the intussusception acting as a continence mechanism through which the patient self catheterises to void (see Ch. 15). Again that is not entirely satisfactory in this situation because the ileum may have been irradiated, because of mucus discharge from the neourethra, because the intussusception is not always reliable as a continence mechanism, because it is not always easy to catheterise through, and because it is not always possible to get an ileal segment down that far for anastomosis to the meatus.

The best alternative, particularly when the urethra has had to be removed because it is involved in the fistula, is to perform a complete substitution cystourethroplasty. The best way of achieving this is using the colonic cystourethroplasty technique described in Chapter 8 for irradiation cystitis for either substitution cystourethroplasty or continent diversion. With this technique all the tissue for reconstruction comes from outside the irradiated area. Unfortunately this technique may be undesirable if there has been extensive loss of the sigmoid colon due to irradiation colitis with stricture formation as it uses about one third of the total length of the colon. If the length of available colon is restricted the amount of colon used for the substitution cystoplasty can be reduced by incorporating more ileum than usual, assuming it is not too heavily irradiated. A reasonable length of colon can therefore be left for water reabsorption from the faeces to reduce the risk of severe postoperative diarrhoea. The other alternative for substitution urethroplasty is to form a neourethra from a pedicled strip of labial skin and then to anastomose it to a substitution cystoplasty by means of a submucosal tunnel technique which will act as a continence mechanism through which the patient self catheterises to void.

Technique
The strip of labial skin will need to be as long as possible to give the maximum neourethral length which in turn will give the maximum possible length for the tunnelled implantation

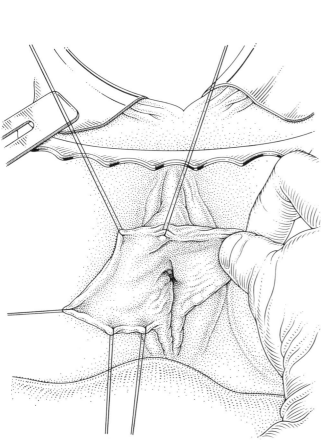

Fig. 12.13

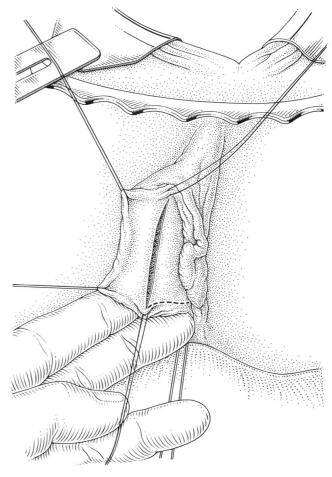

Fig. 12.14

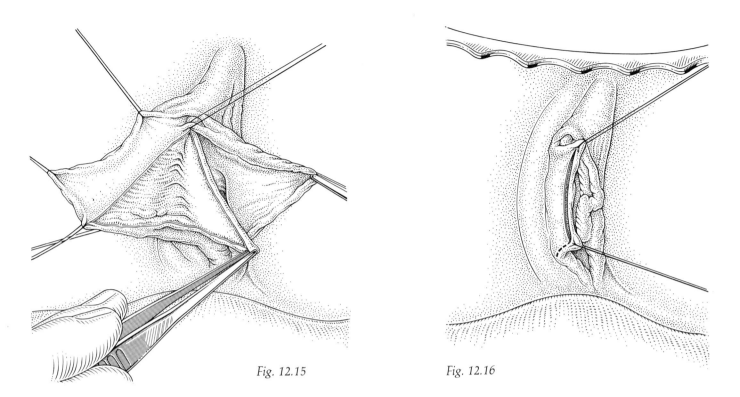

Fig. 12.15

Fig. 12.16

into the cystoplasty on which continence depends. The base of the strip will be alongside or just below the clitoris and the neomeatus will be situated at this site making it more accessible than a normal meatus for self catheterisation. The width of the strip will be a little less than 1.5 cm — sufficient when the strip is tubularised to hold a 12 F catheter within it comfortably.

Such a strip of inner labial skin is outlined on the inner aspect of the labium minus (Figs 12.13, 12.14). The skin alone is incised taking care not to damage the underlying subcutaneous tissue which will form the vascular pedicle. If the labium minus is too small to give an adequate skin tube then the skin of the inner aspect of the labium majus is used.

Having incised through skin alone, the skin on either side of the strip is reflected off the subcutaneous tissue (Figs 12.15, 12.16) so that the strip is isolated on its pedicle (Fig. 12.17). The

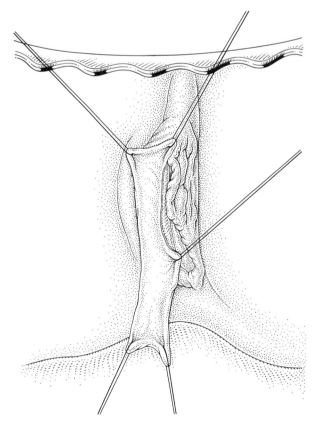

Fig. 12.17

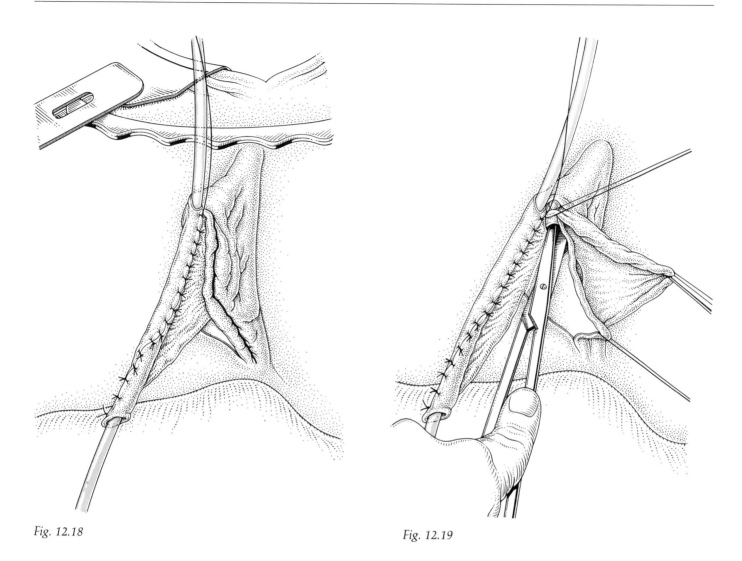

Fig. 12.18

Fig. 12.19

strip is then carefully closed around a 12 F catheter to form a neourethral tube (Fig. 12.18).

A tunnel is then made beneath the inferior pubic arch between the pedicle and the inner labial skin (Fig. 12.19) so that the lower end of the neourethra can be pushed through into the pelvis for anastomosis to the cystoplasty (Figs 12.20, 12.21).

Essentially this technique is a modification of the pedicled preputial patch technique described in Chapter 11 for the treatment of urethral strictures in men.

With the neourethra in this definitive position the labium is reconstructed. If labium minus skin has been used then the fat pad from the ipsilateral labium majus is used to support the neourethra and separate it from the labial skin closure.

The pelvic end of the neourethra (Fig. 12.22) is then anastomosed to the lower end of the substitution cystoplasty by

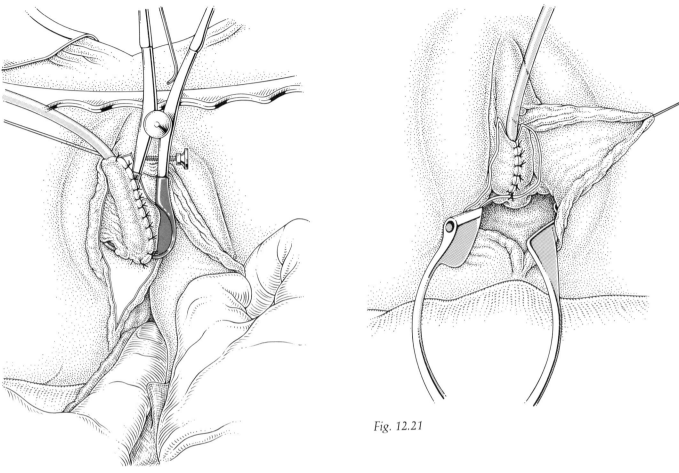

Fig. 12.20

Fig. 12.21

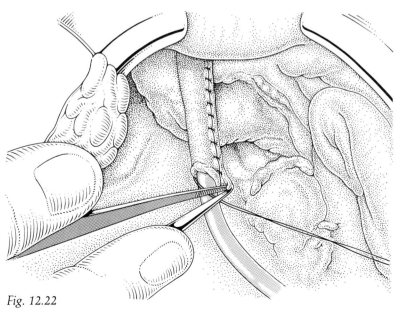

Fig. 12.22
Looking into the retropubic space.

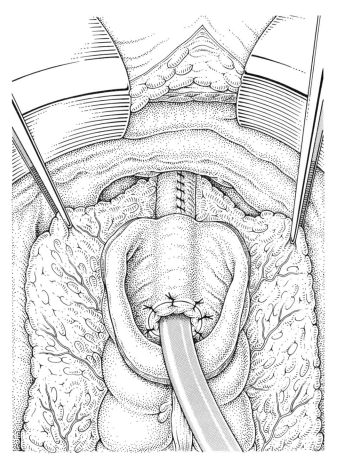

Fig. 12.23

COMBINED CYSTOPLASTY AND VAGINOPLASTY USING COLON

The simplest and best technique for vaginal reconstruction after exenteration is to use part of the colon that has been raised on its ileocolic and marginal vascular pedicle for the substitution cystoplasty. This technique is basically the same as for substitution cystourethroplasty with a colonic neourethra.

Technique
Carefully preserving the pedicle itself, the distal one quarter or thereabouts of the right colon is divided between the vascular arcades (Fig. 12.24). The proximal three quarters then becomes the cystoplasty and the distal quarter the vaginoplasty (Fig. 12.25). The easiest way of proceeding from then on is to close the distal end of the colon that will then become the vaginal vault; then to proceed with anastomosis of the cystoplasty segment to the bladder/urethral remnant or to the neourethra; then to wrap that anastomosis with omentum and wrap the colo-rectal anastomosis similarly; then to anastomose the vaginoplasty segment of colon to the vaginal remnant or introitus transperineally, with interrupted Vicryl mattress sutures spaced about 0.5 cm apart. Before starting the anastomosis it is important to be sure that the omental wraps are well in place and that suture lines will not be juxtaposed.

SUBSTITUTION VAGINOPLASTY WITH MYOCUTANEOUS GRACILIS FLAPS

Irrespective of sexual function, a neovagina of healthy tissue from outside the irradiated area is useful to separate and support the cystoplasty and the colo-rectal reconstruction, particularly as there is a limit to the amount of omentum available. The neovagina therefore acts in part as an omental

means of a submucosal tunnel — the longer the better (Fig. 12.23). It is often difficult to make such a tunnel under colonic mucosa in which case either the mucosa should be incised and reflected and the neourethra sewn into the gap so that re-epithelialisation will occur over the neourethral skin tube thereby creating the desired effect, or alternatively a taenia coli is incised down to the mucosa from outside the distal end of the cystoplasty and the neourethra is sewn into the trench thereby created. The latter is more difficult because of the limitations of access.

Postoperatively suprapubic and urethral catheters are left in for about three weeks until there is radiologically conclusive evidence of anastomotic

healing. As always the urethral catheter is removed first under radiological control, instilling contrast as it is withdrawn to ensure that there is no anastomotic leak. If this is satisfactory contrast is then instilled through the suprapubic catheter to fill the bladder to confirm that all is well. If this is also satisfactory the suprapubic catheter is clamped and the patient begins self catheterisation. When she has been self catheterising for 24 hours without difficulty the suprapubic catheter is removed.

If either the urethrogram or the cystogram show a leak then both catheters are retained for another two weeks and the X-ray studies are then repeated.

substitute. Myocutaneous gracilis (MCG) flaps are used when, and only when, gut cannot be used because it is deficient or has already been used extensively in other areas of the reconstruction. Even if the entire MCG flap is unnecessary or there is an adequate 'native' vagina the vascularised gracilis muscle alone might be useful in this role of supplementing the omentum (see below — prostato-rectal fistulae).

Thus MCG flap vaginoplasty is used as a source of non-irradiated healthy tissue to support and separate the reconstructed lower urinary and lower intestinal tracts and to fill out the pelvis as well as to provide a neovagina.

The factors that make the compound gracilis myocutaneous flap suitable are that:

1. It has a well and easily defined single neurovascular pedicle in most subjects.
2. Vessels from the muscle run through to supply the overlying skin to a predictable degree.
3. Having mobilised the flap, the wound can be closed primarily.
4. The muscle is expendable.
5. The flap has an axis of rotation, about its vascular pedicle, that allows it to reach the perineum and vagina.
6. The size of the flap is suitable for perineal and vaginal reconstruction.

The relevant anatomical features are shown in Figure 12.26. The common, superificial and deep femoral vessels are shown in black and the anterior branch of the obturator nerve in white, lying on adductor longus and supplying the gracilis by means of a discrete and well

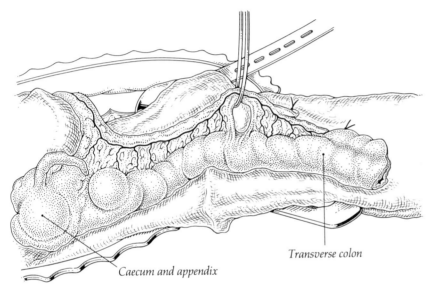

Transverse colon

Caecum and appendix

Fig. 12.24

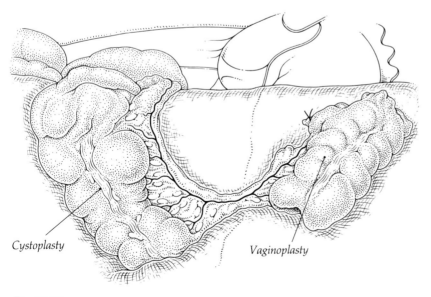

Cystoplasty

Vaginoplasty

Fig. 12.25

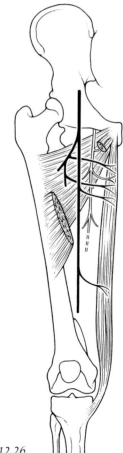

Fig. 12.26

defined and proximal neurovascular bundle. The aim of the procedure is to mobilise the skin over the middle third of the gracilis with the subcutaneous tissue and gracilis itself, including its fascial sheath, and bring it through a subcutaneous tunnel to the introitus where, with its partner from the other side, it will be formed into a pouch which will be pushed into the pelvis and sutured to the margins of the introitus. This procedure is possible because the blood supply to the skin is derived from the underlying muscle. The muscle is in effect the vascular pedicle of the skin.

The problems with the MCG flap technique are threefold.

1. The flap is bulky, although this rarely causes any trouble.
2. There is occasionally a distal vascular supply to gracilis and this impairs the viability of a flap based on the proximal neurovascular bundle just described. In such circumstances the procedure has to be abandoned.
3. The procedure is easy in a slim patient but in a woman with flabby thighs it is difficult to be sure which part of the skin of the inner aspect of the thigh is meant to be anatomically related to the gracilis. Hence there are problems with skin viability. The procedure is best avoided in such patients. Indeed it is only used as a last resort in all patients — colon, as described above, is much better.

For these reasons the technique is only used in carefully selected patients when a colonic substitution vaginoplasty is not possible.

Technique
First of all the landmarks are marked on the skin of the inside of the thigh (Fig. 12.27). The anterior margin of the flap is marked by a line along adductor longus and the posterior margin along the semimembranosus. The proximal limit of the flap is one handsbreadth below the origin of gracilis from the ischiopubic

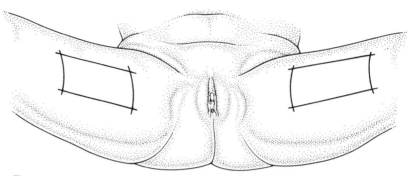

Fig. 12.27

ramus and the distal limit is where sartorius (and the saphenous vein and nerve) cross the anterior border of the muscle, about a handsbreadth above the knee. The patch will be an oval within the confines of this rectangle.

The anterior or superior margin of the oval is incised first and deepened down to and through the fascia of adductor longus, except at the two ends where it goes down to but not through the fascia of gracilis itself. During this dissection care should be taken not to damage the saphenous vein and nerve, particularly at the lower end of the incision. Within the sheath of adductor longus, finger dissection will open up the full length of the incision to expose the neurovascular bundle emerging at the upper end of the incision between addutor longus and adductor brevis. (Fig. 12.28 — the left MCG flap is being raised.)

The posterior margin is then incised and deepened down to and through the fascia of semimembranosus. Finger dissection within the semimembranosus sheath will show where to break through to join up with the anterior incision (Fig. 12.29).

The upper and lower limits of the flap should by now have deepened down to but not through the gracilis fascia. At the lower end gracilis is transfixed with one or two stitches within the sheath, to prevent it retracting, and is then transected.

Having mobilised the flap, a subcutaneous tunnel is made through to the introitus. This is an easy dissection other than at the fascial attachment that tethers the skin to the ischiopubic ramus which will need to be cut through sharply. It is obviously important that the tunnel is sufficient to transmit the flap. The flap is then brought through to the introitus and the procedure is repeated on the other side (Fig. 12.30).

It is a good idea to test the viability of the flaps before going any further, but before doing so it seems sensible to let them lie in their present position for a few minutes for the vessels of the neurovascular bundle to settle in their new position and for any 'spasm' to resolve. During this time the donor sites can be checked for haemostasis. The viability of the flaps is tested by giving intravenous fluorescein. After a few minutes the flaps will fluoresce under ultraviolet light (with the other lights in the operating theatre switched off). Any non-fluorescing areas are presumed to be devascularised and non-viable and are excised.

Additional trimming of the edge of each flap that will be sutured to the introitus may be necessary to allow it to sit comfortably. Whether or not this will be necessary will be obvious when the flap is being pulled through the subcutaneous tunnel. Any skin left in the tunnel when the flap is otherwise fully through will need to be excised.

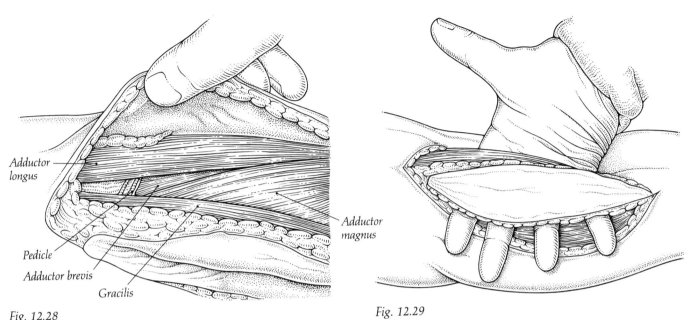

Adductor
longus

Pedicle

Adductor brevis

Gracilis

Adductor
magnus

Fig. 12.28
The upper medial aspect of the left thigh.

Fig. 12.29

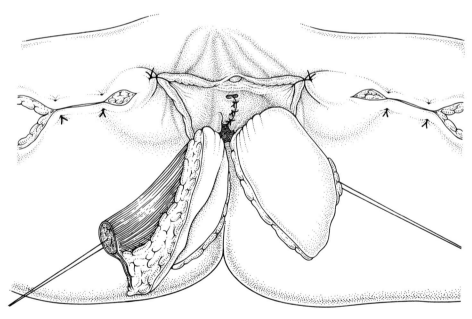

Fig. 12.30

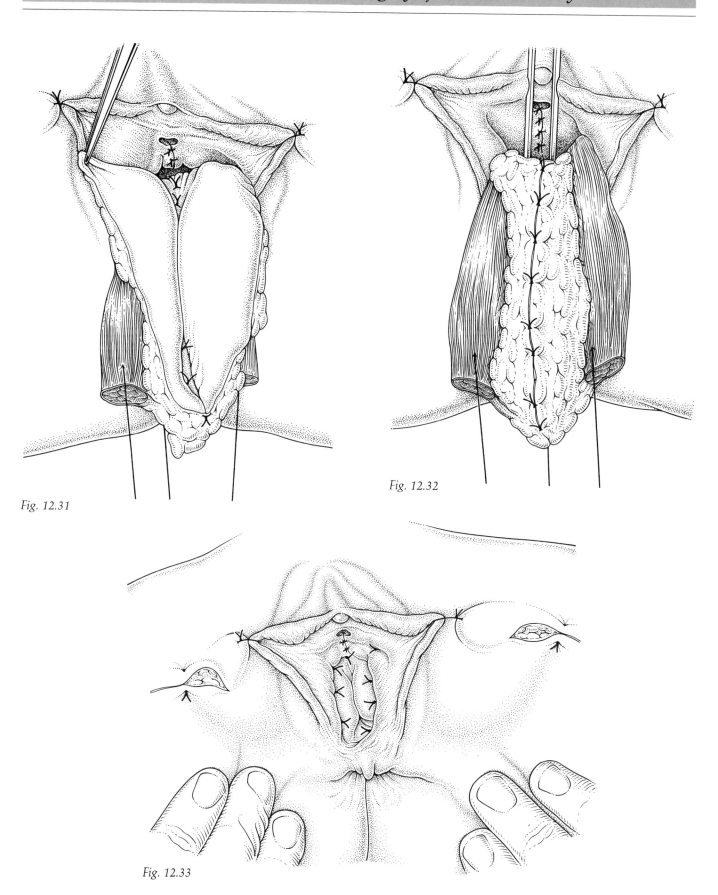

Fig. 12.31

Fig. 12.32

Fig. 12.33

The flaps are then sewn together to form a pouch (Figs 12.31, 12.32) with a subcutaneous 3/0 Vicryl stitch to hold the subcutaneous fat together and interrupted mattress sutures of Vicryl to hold the skin edges together on each side. The muscles on either side of the pouch are approximated over the dome of the pouch by loosely tying the stay-stitches together.

The pouch is then invaginated through the introitus (Fig. 12.33) and sewn in place with interrupted mattress sutures. Before invagination the colo-rectal reconstruction, cystoplasty and omental wraps should have been completed. Access to these suture lines will be difficult once the neovaginal pouch is in place. The pouch will easily allow two fingers (Fig. 12.34) and is therefore large enough for sexual intercourse.

The donor defects are then closed (Fig. 12.35).

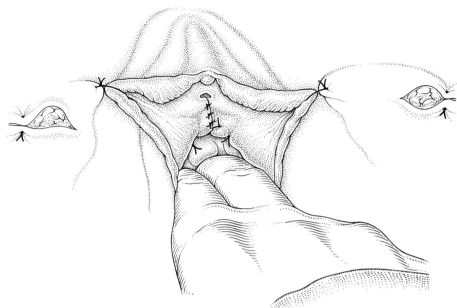

Fig. 12.34

POST-OPERATIVE MANAGEMENT AFTER PELVIC RECONSTRUCTION

There is no specific aspect that differs from the routine care of patients with a cystoplasty or colo-rectal anastomosis. The urinary catheters are removed after about 2–3 weeks when a urethrogram and cystogram have shown that all suture lines and anastomoses have healed and the covering colostomy is closed at about 3 months after a barium contrast study has shown that the anastomosis has healed.

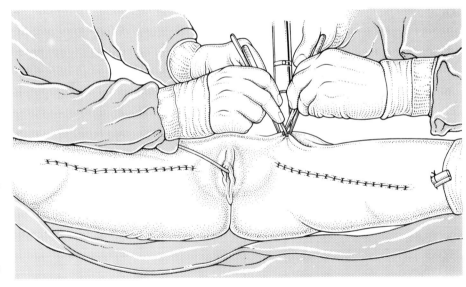

Fig. 12.35

The two problem areas are the vesico-urethral anastomosis, if a pedicled labial skin tube–substitution cystoplasty anastomosis was performed, and the colo-rectal anastomosis. With the former a fistula may develop between the vesico-urethral junction and the suture line of the labial skin closure. The labial fat pad that should have been interposed between the two should prevent this but if a fistula does develop it should be easy to close with mobilisation of the other labial fat pad to cover the repair.

If the colo-rectal reconstruction fails to heal on its posterior aspect causing a leak into the presacral space it will be almost impossible to revise with a substitution cystoplasty and vaginoplasty in front and such a deeply situated anastomosis. In such cases it is best to regard the defunctioning colostomy as permanent. If it fails to heal anteriorly, close to the vaginoplasty, a recto-vaginal fistula usually develops between the adjacent suture lines. The fistula is usually short, direct and easy to close transvaginally with interposition of whatever tissue is available.

The neovaginoplasty should cause no problems if colon has been used as long as the marginal artery and vein that supply it have not been damaged by previous irradiation, in which case the neovagina may be devascularised and ischaemic and will slough. I have seen this once. If MGC flaps were used there should be no problem if the viability of the flaps was checked peroperatively, but there is sometimes some marginal necrosis of the flaps which causes a discharge and then heals spontaneously. Occasionally fat or muscle necrosis in the pelvis may lead to pelvic sepsis and an abscess—we have seen this on one occasion.

Sexual intercourse should be avoided until the neovagina has been examined under an anaesthetic (Figs 12.36, 12.37)

and complete healing has been ensured. A lubricant is unnecessary with a colonic neovagina but will be required with MCG flaps as there is no natural lubrication of the skin.

It is important to emphasise to the patient before her reconstruction and to re-emphasise afterwards during the early days when everything seems to be going well that recovery is slow after such surgery and following previous radiotherapy. It is often weeks and sometimes months before the X-rays are satisfactory, the catheters come out and the covering colostomy can be closed. During this time patients often get extremely depressed after all they have been through and when recovery appears so painfully slow. It is absolutely vital however that catheters

and stomas are not done away with until it is absolutely and unequivocally certain that the need for them is past. In other words all anastomoses must be radiologically sound beyond any doubt. The penalty of succumbing to the entreaties of a miserable patient anxious to be rid of it and prematurely removing a catheter or closing a stoma can be a catastrophic anastomotic breakdown with dire consequences.

If there has been no major irradiation damage to the right side of the colon and the sigmoid colon, and if preoperative investigation and histopathological assessment of the resected fistula-related mass shows no evidence of residual or recurrent cancer, then the incidence of postoperative complications should be low apart from

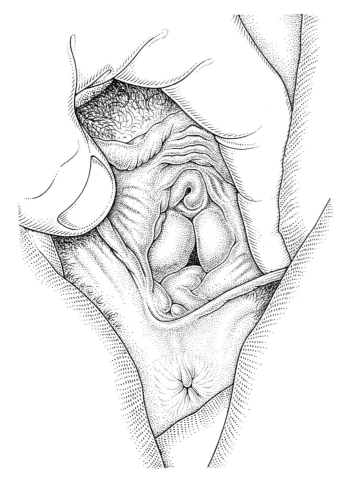

Fig. 12.36

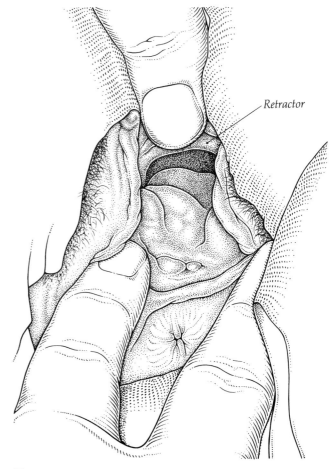

Retractor

Fig. 12.37

the two 'minor' anastomotic problems mentioned above. If there is residual or recurrent malignancy it usually involves the vault of the neovagina or the colo-rectal reconstruction causing either a bloody vaginal discharge, or large bowel obstruction, or a recto-neovaginal fistula or a combination. In such circumstances the best palliative measure is a Hartmann's procedure to direct the faecal stream through an end colostomy with closure of the rectum to exclude the fistula.

One of my patients developed a recurrent fistula between the colo-rectal suture line and the neovaginal vault because of chronic, irradiation-induced osteomyelitis of the left ischium with sequestrum formation. This resolved with removal of the sequestrum and packing of the bony cavity with muscle combined with excision of the fistula and revision of the neovagina and colo-rectal suture line, after a temporary Hartmann's procedure. In this lady recurrent malignancy was excluded preoperatively by CT scanning and biopsy.

Urinary continence after this type of reconstruction should be expected to be adequate rather than good in most patients. Those who have had a cystourethrectomy and substitution cystourethroplasty usually fare better but with a higher incidence of niggling postoperative complications. Those in whom the urethra and part of the trigone were preserved with substitution cystoplasty alone have a smoother postoperative course but usually have a degree of stress incontinence, unless the state of the pelvis was good enough to allow implantation of an AUS, which is rare. Persistent stress incontinence is best left untreated because of the high risk of complications unless the degree of incontinence is sufficiently debilitating to warrant conversion of the cystoplasty to a conduit or continent urinary diversion.

VESICO-COLIC FISTULA

These are almost always due to diverticular disease of the colon and the treatment is sigmoid colectomy and closure of the bladder defect. The bladder will then heal if the colo-rectal anastomosis is kept away by omental interposition.

URETERO-VAGINAL AND URETHRO-VAGINAL FISTULA

Uretero-vaginal fistulae and uretero-uterine fistulae are not really reconstructive problems (except to the patient, who has got one). They are treated either by ureteric reimplantation, either directly into the bladder or into a psoas hitch or by nephroureterectomy, depending on the state of the kidney.

Urethro-vaginal fistulae are usually secondary (in the UK) to an anterior repair or excision of a urethral diverticulum. If the bladder neck is competent they are usually asymptomatic and do not require treatment. If the bladder neck is incompetent, as is often the case, or they are otherwise symptomatic then the urethral defect is closed in two layers around a urethral catheter, a labial fat pad is pulled across to cover the repair and the vagina is then closed. If the distal sphincter mechanism is involved or if the fistula is larger than usual then a formal urethral reconstruction will be necessary, as described in Chapter 6.

PROSTATO-RECTAL AND URETHRO-RECTAL FISTULAE

Apart from congenital fistulae associated with anorectal atresia the majority of these are secondary to surgical trauma, usually a difficult prostatectomy or a difficult anterior resection of the rectum. They are rare.

Low fistulae involving the bulbar urethra are more commonly associated with urethral disease, usually a stricture, than rectal disease and are relatively easy to deal with by excision of the fistula, urethroplasty (when indicated), closure of the rectal defect and interposition of healthy local tissue.

With high fistulae the problem is access. Having got at the fistula it is usually relatively easy to close it. There are theoretically two approaches — transperineally and transabdominally — in practice both may be necessary. Ideally the aim is to expose the fistula, freshen the edges, close either side and interpose healthy tissue, leaving the patient with indwelling, suprapubic or urethral catheters and a covering colostomy until the repair has been shown radiologically to have healed. If adequate access can be gained transperineally then all of these aims should be achievable. The perineal incision should extend sufficiently far posteriorly, curving to one side of the anus, to allow separation of urethra enclosed within the bulbospongiosus from the anal canal posterior to or through the perineal body. This is usually deepened with relative ease up to the level of the prostate and the lower margin of the fistula.

At this stage the lower end of the fistula is opened so that the circumference of the fistula can be defined and incised to allow separation of the rectum from the prostate. The rectum is usually more mobile than the prostate and the rectal defect is therefore more easy to close, particularly when the fistula follows a prostatectomy. Furthermore with a finger in the rectum it is more easy to mobilise the rectum and palpate the fistula and also to check the adequacy of the closure. The rectum also holds stitches well assuming it is not intrinsically diseased.

The prostate, by contrast, is less mobile, less easy to see, does not allow palpation from within and does not hold stitches so well.

The key to closure is getting through the upper margin of the fistula and into the plane between the upper prostate or bladder neck and the rectum. If you can do this and get good separation of the structures then as long as the hole in the back of the prostate is not too large it should be possible to close it.

If it is not possible to separate the prostate from the rectum at the upper end of the fistula, if the rectum is diseased, if the margins of the prostate have been shredded or if the hole in the back of the prostate is too large then a synchronous abdominal approach will be necessary, firstly to define more clearly the plane between the rectum and the prostate and bladder neck, and secondly to make the rectal mobilisation easier. There is a third advantage in this approach and that is that if it still proves impossible to close the prostate adequately then it will be possible to pull the omentum through the tunnel between the prostate and rectum — which is desirable in any case — to keep the two apart, allowing the prostate to heal by second intention.

It might seem attractive theoretically to expose the fistula from above through an incision in the front of the bladder neck and prostate but the access and view are poor, the fistula cannot be mobilised by this route so the perineal approach will be necessary anyway, and if the prostate can be closed from above it can probably be closed from below more easily.

To improve the view you need good assistance and good light. Deaver-type retractors with fibre-light attachments are very helpful.

(Throughout this section I have assumed that the patient already has a defunctioning colostomy. If not one will be needed for 3 months or so to cover the repair while it is healing.)

REFERENCES

Simple fistulae are dealt with in almost any urological or gynaecological text
book. Complex fistulae are not really dealt with adequately anywhere.

Chapter 13

Bladder cancer and related problems

Until recently cancer was not a subject which sprung immediately to most urologists' minds as a field of reconstructive endeavour. To those of us brought up on 'wrench-out' cystectomies and similar heroic gestures this is perhaps not surprising but reconstruction has gone hand in hand with cancer surgery in other specialities for many years, notably in the head and neck and recently this approach has spread to urology with the widespread enthusiasm for continent diversion after cystectomy and Patrick Walsh's radical prostatectomy technique.

Two aspects distinguish the reconstructive approach to bladder cancer (and other pelvic cancers): the way the cystectomy is performed, to minimise the damage to the structures that are going to be left behind, specifically the membranous urethra and its innervation, and the way the bladder is replaced, by substitution cystoplasty rather than by an ileal conduit urinary diversion. Both seem to be laudable aims but there are several objections that are consistently raised against them.

The first objection is that the reconstructive approach may not be an adequate 'cancer operation'. (This sounds to me as though it may not be sufficiently mutilating.) The answer of course is that if the operative findings dictate a field of excision that precludes a subsequent reconstruction then so be it — but that is not usually the case if the patient has been properly selected.

The second objection is that it is much quicker to do a standard 'wrench-out' with an ileal conduit than a more careful cystectomy with substitution cystoplasty. My answer is that it takes me 3–4 hours to do a radical cystectomy and substitution cystoplasty and I have seen some surgeons take that long just to do the ileal conduit, let alone the cystectomy. In any case speed does not make a procedure a good one by that criterion alone. The third

objection is that after previous radiotherapy (which is usual in some countries including the UK) the cystoplasty–urethra anastomosis may not heal well. This may be true, although it has never been that much of a problem in my experience, but the same applies to the use of irradiated ileum for a conduit.

Overall, a 'reconstructive' approach to cystoprostatectomy is generally associated with less blood loss, less general operative trauma to the patient and hence a smoother postoperative course. These factors justify the 'reconstructive' approach even if an ileal conduit is preferred to a substitution cystoplasty. Even then there is little difference to the surgeon — in both there is a gut segment; in both the ureters are plumbed into one end; and only the fate of the other end is different: with one onto skin, and the other onto the urethra — but there is a major difference to the patient, all the difference between incontinent abdominal wall urinary drainage and continent urethral urinary drainage.

The question arises with pelvic tumours in general as to what are the least requirements that allow reconstruction of the pelvis after an adequate 'cancer operation'. To some extent this question was considered in the last chapter when discussing complex fistulae in women. There is as yet no adequate substitute for the anal sphincter so this must be retained. For rectal sensation part of the rectal wall must be retained. Thus the anal canal, part of the posterior (preferably) rectal wall and the puborectal sling with their innervation must be retained. The entire vagina can be satisfactorily replaced with colon if necessary and the entire lower urinary tract in women can be replaced by the cystourethroplasty technique described in the last chapter. In men an equivalent technique for cystourethroplasty is less satisfactory because full length skin tube urethral substitutions are difficult,

although not impossible, so one should normally aim to retain the membranous (sphincter-active) urethra and its innervation when disease considerations permit. This is not much to leave behind and leaves the surgeon more than sufficient scope for an adequate 'cancer operation' in most patients.

In the remainder of this chapter we will consider applying these principles first to bladder cancer and then to other pelvic tumours that do not allow a simple excision and restorative procedure.

CARCINOMA OF THE BLADDER

The role of cystoprostatectomy in the treatment of bladder cancer is controversial. Two factors that influence the continuing debate about the relative merits of surgery and radiotherapy in locally advanced disease are the problems of impotence as a result of the cystoprostatectomy and the psychological problems of urinary diversion. Most men who are potent before their operation would prefer to remain so and most patients would prefer to void urethrally rather than through a stoma. Indeed, given the choice, many men would rather be incontinent through the urethra into a condom drainage device rather than incontinent through the abdominal wall into a stoma bag. Thus, when a cystoprostatectomy is deemed necessary, a potency-preserving cystoprostatectomy would seem preferable to a standard 'wrench out' and if the nature of the bladder tumour allows preservation of the urethra a substitution cystoplasty would seem to be a better option than an ileal conduit. If the bladder tumour is multifocal or if the bladder neck or prostatic urethra are involved or if for any other reason a urethrectomy is necessary then although an attempt to preserve potency is desirable, reconstruction of the urinary tract is much more difficult although not impossible. The only other alternative to ileal conduit diversion, and much more practicable than an attempt at cystourethroplasty, is a continent diversion using the technique described in Chapter 8 for either cystourethroplasty or continent diversion in women.

The technique of potency-preserving cystoprostatectomy is described in Chapter 2. It owes much to Walsh's description of his technique for radical prostatectomy and the anatomical work that led up to it. Needless to say it is not possible to guarantee the potency of male patients undergoing this procedure, firstly because the operative findings may dictate a wider than usual excision, secondly because the relevant nerves are still liable to a traction injury during the course of the resection, thirdly because diathermy damage may occur if there is difficulty in controlling haemostasis and, fourthly, in patients who have had previous radiotherapy, because the anatomical landmarks may be obscured or the procedure made otherwise more difficult by fibrosis. In my experience, 60–70% of patients in whom both of the neurovascular bundles to the corpora appear to be undamaged at the end of the procedure are potent postoperatively. If one or both of the bundles are damaged then impotence seems to be the rule. In the same series neurovascular bundle damage occurred in nearly 75% of salvage cystoprostatectomies, usually by accident, but only in about 20% of elective procedures, usually because the operative findings dictated a wide excision.

Continence is more of a problem because the acceptability of the procedure really hangs on this question. In my series, 60% are continent both subjectively and objectively both by day and by night, 10% more are continent by day but incontinent at night and a further 15% have a degree of sphincter weakness on urodynamic testing but have no symptoms. For all practical

purposes, 85% are dry. The remaining 15% have subjective and objective sphincter weakness giving them the symptoms of stress incontinence of whom one third also have an element of overactivity of the cystoplasty. Sphincteric competence or loss of it is obviously related primarily to the ability to preserve all or part of the sphincter-active urethra and its innervation. This however is only one part of the problem of continence after a cystoprostatectomy and substitution cystoplasty although it is certainly the most important part. Another part of the problem, although less important for daytime continence, is the inevitable loss of bladder sensation after a total cystectomy. Despite this, most patients develop some sensation of 'bladder' filling, but nevertheless, voiding is usually 'by the clock'. This is usually sufficient almost to guarantee daytime continence but unless an alarm clock is used during the night to wake the patient at appropriate intervals, bedwetting will occur, unless the capacity of the cystoplasty is sufficient to contain the volume produced. This may not be the case if the patient likes to have an uninterrupted sleep of 8 hours or so. It is often therefore a choice between complete continence or a full night's sleep. Night-time continence is more affected by loss of bladder afferent activity after cystectomy because these afferents, in the normal situation, are responsible for the reflex rise in urethral sphincter activity as the bladder fills. When there is no bladder afferent activity, urethral sphincter activity is low and does not increase as the bladder fills. During the daytime the patient can compensate for this by voluntary contraction of the pelvic floor muscles in general and of the pubourethral sling in particular but at night this is impossible and so incontinence is much more likely.

Neither of these considerations is much of a problem in male patients because stress incontinence is easily controlled by implantation of an artificial sphincter

around the bulbar urethra, which may also help bedwetting in patients in whom sphincter weakness is present if not troublesome by day, and because a sheath-type collecting device can be used at night if the patient chooses to have an undisturbed night's sleep.

In female patients these problems are more significant because there is no easy way of containing sphincter weakness incontinence in women to compare with the sheath. An artificial sphincter would therefore have to be implanted and, given that cystectomy causes a partial devascularisation of the urethra and that the AUS cuff would be very close to the cystoplasty—urethral suture line, the incidence of complications is likely to be high. In any case disease considerations make a cystourethrectomy desirable in most patients.

Thus in women a substitution cystourethroplasty would usually be more appropriate, in which case a continent diversion might be preferable in those who have previously been treated with radiotherapy to keep out of the irradiated field, and the risk of complications with either of these approaches makes the alternative of a conduit diversion more appealing for many, particularly for older patients.

The third part of the problem of continence after cystectomy and substitution cystoplasty is the contractility of the gut segment used for the cystoplasty. To a large extent the question of contractility is related to the questions of capacity and emptying ability. The obvious aim is to produce a large capacity, low-pressure substitute bladder that will empty completely. The two most widely used methods by which a large capacity neobladder can be achieved are by using a long length of right colon, which by its very nature gives a large capacity, or by detubularising a length of ileum or an equivalent length of terminal ileum and adjacent right colon to compensate

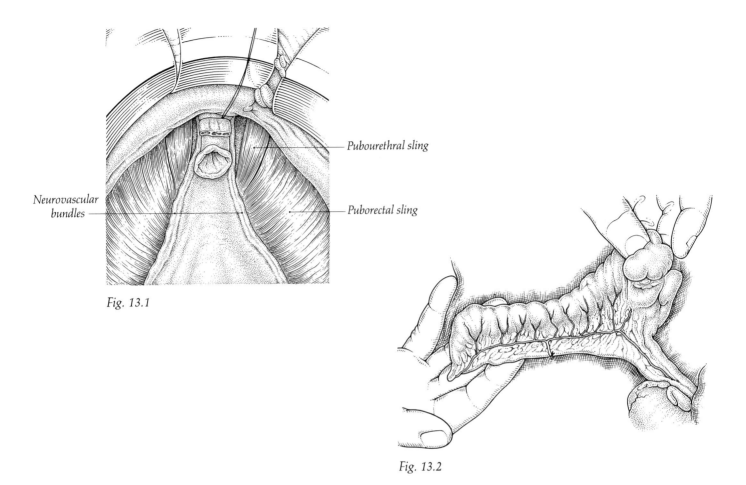

Neurovascular bundles

Pubourethral sling

Puborectal sling

Fig. 13.1

Fig. 13.2

geometrically for the smaller calibre (and therefore capacity) of this segment of bowel. A similar capacity can be achieved by either means and if the total capacity *is* similar then at any lesser capacity the contractility of either will be much the same. The difference between the two lies in their emptying ability. In my experience, a 'straight' right colon segment will be more likely to empty spontaneously without the need for self catheterisation and a detubularised cystoplasty will be less likely to empty spontaneously with an increased likelihood of needing self catheterisation.

My experience is that if the distal sphincter mechanism of the membranous urethra and its innervation are preserved then the patient will be continent by day if not by night with a 'straight' right colon cystoplasty of adequate

capacity and will not need to self catheterise to empty. If the sphincter or its innervation is damaged or in any other way deficient then incontinence is more likely and a few patients may subsequently need to have their cystoplasty 'detubularised'. In practice problems of cystoplasty contractility only occur in about one third of those men with more severe degrees of sphincter weakness who have previously had radiotherapy and even then do not occur sufficiently often to make detubularisation worthwhile as a matter of routine.

Preparation, technique and follow up
The technique of cystoprostatectomy and of 'straight' substitution cystoplasty have already been described in Chapter 3 and Chapter 8 respectively. The technique of detubularised (or pouch) substitution cystoplasty for use when the right colon is short or when the patient has had radiotherapy has been described in Chapter 10. Only the colo-urethral anastomosis needs to be described here. The technique of cystourethroplasty and its use for continent diversion has been described in Chapter 8.

At the end of the cystoprostatectomy the pelvic floor will look like Figure 13.1 with the membranous urethra visible within the sling of the pubourethralis, lying on the anterior wall of the rectum. A 'straight' cystoplasty is prepared in the usual way (Ch. 8, Fig. 13.2) and

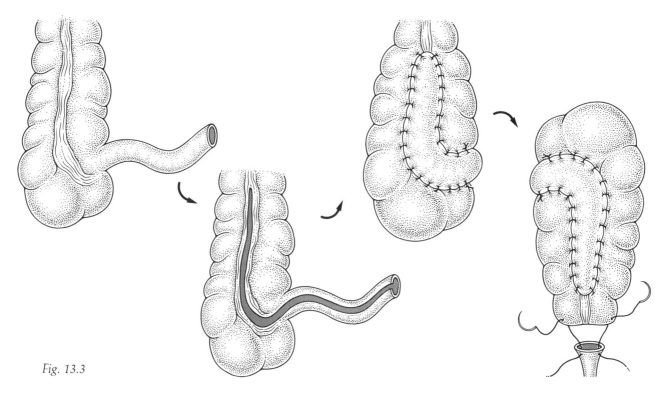

Fig. 13.3

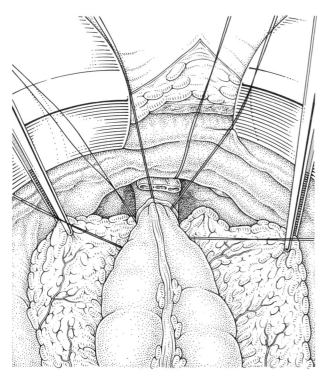

Fig. 13.4

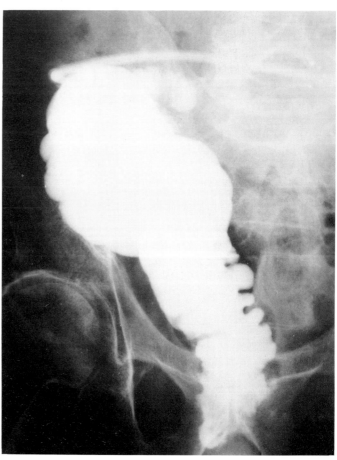

Fig. 13.5

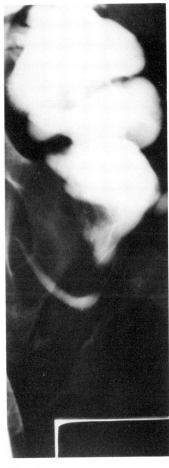

Fig. 13.6

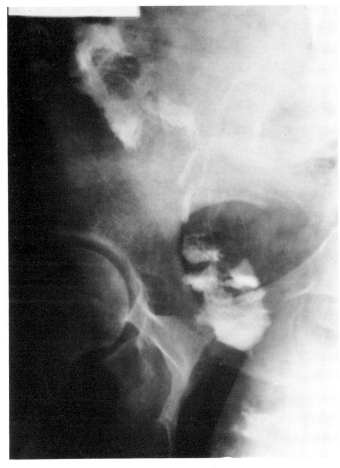

Fig. 13.7

detubularised if necessary (Ch. 10, Fig. 13.3).

Following the colo-urethral anastomosis an omental wrap is necessary to help healing, to restrict extravasation, to keep the area supple and to stop the anastomosis becoming stuck to the pubic symphysis. It is easiest to mobilise the omentum first and lay it down and suture it in place behind the urethra with sufficient length to wrap it round the front.

Next the colonic end of the cystoplasty segment is narrowed by putting one or two inverting mattress sutures at each end so that the lumen is reduced to about the size of a fingertip. This narrowed end of the colon is then anastomosed to the urethra with 6

interrupted 3/0 Vicryl sutures (Fig. 13.4) taking care to pick up the full thickness of both the colonic and the urethral walls and taking care also not to tie the sutures too tightly. It is important to take all possible steps to ensure the preservation of sphincter function.

The sutures are placed first; the colon is then slid down the sutures into place; the knots are then tied. The procedure is completed by finishing the omental wrap and a drain is left in the retropubic space. A 16 F Foley urethral catheter (to prevent cross adhesions) and a 20 F suprapubic catheter are left in for two weeks postoperatively.

Two weeks postoperatively a filling cystogram is obtained (Fig. 13.5). If there is no leak from the anastomosis

the urethral catheter is removed and a voiding study follows immediately (Figs 13.6, 13.7). If the X-ray studies are satisfactory the suprapubic catheter is clamped for a trial of voiding and removed the next day if voiding is satisfactory. If there is a leak the catheter is left on free drainage until the leak has healed.

Immediately after removal of the catheters most patients will void half-hourly for the first 24 hours and be incontinent by night. They should therefore be given a condom drainage device to use at night. Over the next 48 hours their daytime frequency improves to a voiding pattern of once every hour or so. This then gradually improves over the next 6–8 weeks to 3–4-hourly voiding or better. As daytime frequency and continence improve, so night-time continence develops.

Three months postoperatively the patient is evaluated subjectively and objectively. By this time the long-term urodynamic pattern of the cystoplasty and the distal sphincter mechanism should have declared itself — any further substantial improvement in frequency daytime continence and bedwetting is unlikely. Regardless of symptoms a video-urodynamic study is performed in all patients to act as a baseline for the future and any symptomatic patients are offered further treatment at that stage (e.g. (usually) implantation of an AUS for sphincter weakness).

OTHER PELVIC TUMOURS

This book is not the place for a description of radical prostatectomy, radical hysterectomy or anterior (or other) resection for carcinoma of the rectum. These are standard procedures that are well described elsewhere.

There are, in general, three types of pelvic tumours that have presented to me as 'reconstructive' problems:

— There are those tumours with multisystem (lower urinary tract, genital tract and lower gastrointestinal tract) involvement but with no evidence of distant spread, where an excision and multisystem reconstruction is the preferred option.
— There are those tumours that are so large that they are seemingly inoperable unless the reconstructive surgeon can find a way.
— There are those tumours that are so rare that nobody else really knows what to do with them. Many of these, in my experience, also fall into the 'size' category.

Tumours with multisystem involvement. These are mainly carcinoma of the cervix and other gynaecological

tumours, carcinoma of the sigmoid colon in women, carcinoma of the rectum in men and rare sarcomas of the pelvic viscera or supporting tissues in descending order of incidence. Most present with external bleeding, a fistula or voiding/bowel dysfunction.

Bulky, rare tumours. These tend to present as voiding difficulty, subacute large bowel obstruction or as a palpable mass. These are tumours such as haemangiopericytoma, leiomyosarcoma and rhabdomyosarcoma that usually cause symptoms by virtue of their mass effect rather than the visceral involvement.

Assessment
Three main questions arise:

1. Is it worth trying to get it out? In other words, is this tumour localised with no evidence of metastases or is it causing such symptoms that it is worth trying to get it out regardless?
2. Is it possible to get it out?
3. Is there anything that can be done to improve the chances of getting it out or reducing the morbidity of getting it out?

Metastases are best excluded by CT and bone scanning, supplemented by appropriate specific investigations where indicated. CT scanning should also tell you whether it is possible to excise the tumour but my experience is that CT is not particularly helpful in this respect.

The main limiting factor for excision is fixation to the side wall of the pelvis. Even then some sarcomas may still be resectable if they are fixed anteriorly to the pubis or the pubic rami as these areas of bone are relatively easy to remove 'en bloc' with the tumour. On the other hand fixation to the region of the hip joint or to the ischium makes the tumour relatively unresectable unless the loss of lower limb function (or indeed the limb itself) is acceptable.

The other limiting factor is size. The sheer bulk of the tumour may prevent adequate mobilisation. Size, like mobility, is probably as well assessed by examination under anaesthesia as by any other modality.

There are essentially three ways of shrinking a tumour to make it easier to resect. In most instances none of them help. Some radiosensitive tumours may respond to preoperative radiotherapy but if they are radiosensitive then this will usually be the preferred definitive treatment. Some tumours, notably the embryonal rhabdomyosarcomas, are chemosensitive but such chemosensitivity is otherwise rare. Finally very vascular tumours may be shrunk or at least devascularised (thus reducing the morbidity of surgery) by finding the feeder vessels arteriographically and embolising them. For this reason arteriography by an experienced vascular radiologist, with a view to embolisation, is always worthwhile if the tumour looks as though it is going to be a real surgical challenge. Some particularly large tumours can only be removed piecemeal if they fill the pelvis to such a degree as to make it impossible to gain control of the vascular pedicles. Debulking of the tumour by taking a chunk out of it, although strictly speaking 'bad form', may be the only way of creating space within the pelvis to get at the major vessels. If this is to be done without the patient exsanguinating then it helps to have the tumour as devascularised as possible.

Thus in the absence of a preoperative histological diagnosis of the tumour type, the principal methods of assessment are an EUA, appropriate endoscopy, a CT scan of the chest, abdomen and pelvis, and a bone scan, with supplementary arteriography for very bulky tumours. If the tumour has been biopsied then more specific investigations may be necessary. Indeed it may be a type of tumour that is better treated by another surgeon!

Surgical technique
Plenty of blood must be cross matched and available. All possible options must have been discussed with the patient including the potential need for a temporary or permanent urinary diversion or colostomy or both. The anaesthetist should be encouraged to spend as much time as he/she likes in getting in all the necessary lines (although they don't usually need much encouraging). In other words, catastrophic blood loss and equal difficulties in other respects should be expected and anticipated.

Unless extrapelvic (or transpelvic) extension dictates otherwise, the only sensible incision is a long midline incision from the front of the pubis up as high as necessary. After the incision has been made and a suitable retractor placed, a proper 'EUA' can be performed.

Before a complete excision starts the tumour must be mobilised by mobilising the respective viscera and gaining control of the vascular pedicles. There are certain danger areas. The aorta, vena cava, common and external iliac vessels are obviously potential problems but are easily visible and should not cause difficulty. The danger areas from which there may be bleeding which may be difficult to see and control are: posterolaterally along the course of the anterior divisions of the internal iliac vessels, laterally in the obturator fossae and later on, with more extensive tumours, from the branches of the posterior divisions of the internal iliac vessels posteriorly, from the pudendal vessels and their branches laterally and from the dorsal vein complex (in males) anteriorly. It is easy to get carried away by the tumour itself when mobilising it and to lose anatomical orientation so these danger areas should regularly be brought to mind.

Sometimes, as indicated above, a tumour is so bulky that it fills the pelvis completely and prevents access to the vascular pedicles. The only way to deal with this is to take a chunk out of it to allow the retraction that will give this access. Obviously once you have done this you are committed to excising it (and doing so pretty damn quickly sometimes!) so it is important to know whether you can finish what you have started. In general, if the tumour is mobile in the vertical axis of the pelvis (i.e. if it can be moved up and down) then it is resectable and a piecemeal removal can be attempted in the reasonable expectation of eventual complete excision. This may be 'untidy' surgery but sometimes it is the only surgery possible.

If the lateral pedicle of the anterior division of the internal iliac vessels needs to be controlled quickly then the quickest and easiest way of doing this is by the manoeuvre (described in Ch. 3) of opening the endopelvic fascia in the retropubic space and then passing a right-angled forceps backwards, under the pedicle, to emerge posteriorly on the lateral aspect of the rectum. A sling can then be passed round the pedicle or it can be cross clamped. A simple vascular clamp across the internal iliac artery is obviously helpful if all else fails but this alone is not as effective as getting around the lateral pedicle as it does not control the venous or collateral circulation. With patience it is often possible to get a sling around the lateral pedicles even with very bulky tumours. It is certainly always worthwhile trying.

Bleeding from the obturator fossa is only usually a problem when the bulk or site of the tumour restricts access. On the other hand it is relatively easily controlled, until there is access, by a swab or pack held firmly in place with a deep, wide-bladed retractor. Arterial bleeding is usually easy to control because the artery can be seen, clipped and ligated. Venous bleeding is more

difficult because the exact site can be difficult to see. Stitching is usually more successful than reducing the whole area to charcoal with diathermy.

Bleeding from greater sciatic notch is worrying because of the risk of damage to the sciatic nerve and its roots and because it is an area with which most surgeons are not familiar. As with the obturator fossa it is best to pack the area and leave definitive haemostasis until the access is better and the exact bleeding point(s) can be identified accurately.

Bleeding from the dorsal vein complex should never be a problem because it should always be possible to ligate it before transecting it. If the ligature slips or if it is so chunky or fibrosed that there is bleeding despite the ligature then a transfixion stitch will usually regain control. It is pointless to try and cross clamp the whole chunk of tissue and diathermy usually makes the bleeding worse.

Bleeding from the pudendal vessels only occurs when the dissection has gone through the pelvic floor musculature. The pudendal vessels are vulnerable (in either sex) on the lateral side wall of the pelvis in Alcock's canal. More importantly, the bulbar arteries in the male are vulnerable more medially as they run to the upper limits of the bulb of the corpus spongiosum.

If the pelvis is to be reconstructed after the tumour has been excised then there are certain basic requirements. Obviously it is best if the excision of the tumour leaves the majority of the pelvic viscera intact, as when excision of a sigmoid colonic tumour mass involving the uterus and the dome of the bladder (or similar tumour mass arising from the uterus or ovary) leaves the majority of the bladder wall, vagina and the rectum intact. In such circumstances reconstruction is a simple matter.

Tumour masses arising from the cervix, prostate, bladder base or rectum are much more of a problem because the excision is more likely to compromise urethral and anal sphincter function, or to damage their innervation, particularly urethral innervation. Nonetheless an adequate 'cancer operation' is usually still compatible with reconstruction.

The soft-tissue sarcomata of the pelvis are not untreatable by virtue of size alone. In the absence of metastases these tumours usually kill by their local effects and if they can be excised then every effort should be made to do so if excision is likely to give a better quality of life than palliation. I have on several occasions excised a hugh pelvic tumour mass when the alternative would have been to leave the mass and simply divert the urinary and faecal streams. Some might regard this as heroic surgery and nothing more but I have never had occasion to regret it because of the better quality of life it produces and because, in the absence of overt metastases at the time of the surgery, the behaviour of these unusual tumours is so unpredictable. Adequate guidance on how to deal with these tumours is lacking in the literature because of their rarity and the surgeon therefore has to rely on the 'Journal of Clinical Impression'.

Even if the patient is unreconstructible after excision of the mass, excision with (continent or conduit) urinary and faecal diversion may still be worthwhile if it relieves the patient of the presence of an obvious abdominal mass or of troublesome symptoms caused by the tumour. If the minimum requirements for reconstruction can be met, so much the better. These, as mentioned above, are: a urethra with an innervated sphincter mechanism to which a substitution cystoplasty can be anastomosed (although a total substitution cystourethroplasty is possible in women as described in Ch. 12); an intact innervated pelvic floor musculature; and an intact anal canal with a normally innervated sphincter mechanism and enough of a rectal cuff to provide sensation to which the colon can be anastomosed.

As with all major pelvic reconstructive operations, anastomoses should be wrapped with omentum and proximal vents — ureteric, suprapubic and urethral catheters and a proximal colostomy — should be freely used and not removed until there is objective evidence of satisfactory healing.

Chapter 14

Congenital problems

Congenital problems include hypospadias, exstrophy, epispadias, and the urogenital sinus and cloacal abnormalities. With the exception of hypospadias these are rare conditions, even for someone who specialises in dealing with this type of problem, but they warrant discussion because there are several interesting points of treatment that are relevant to other situations. With most of these abnormalities, unlike many of the conditions discussed in this book so far, the main problem is with the bladder outflow rather than the bladder itself. With epispadias, urogenital sinus and cloacal abnormalities the bladder is often of normal structure and capacity, although its innervation may be abnormal. The urethra is deficient or even absent and, in urogenital sinus and cloacal abnormalities, the urethra and vagina are joined at some varying point and reach the perineum through a common channel.

Hypospadias, exstrophy in either sex and epispadias in males are more properly dealt with in early life by paediatric urologists and will not be discussed here. It could obviously be argued that female epispadias, urogenital sinus and cloaca are also more properly dealt with by paediatric urologists but because, in girls, the anatomical deformity of epispadias is not as obvious as it is in boys and because incontinence may be the only symptom of female epispadias and some urogenital sinus problems, they often go unnoticed and untreated in early childhood. It is common also, at the other end of the symptomatic spectrum to find some patients with more severe malformations treated by urinary diversion alone leaving the primary problem untreated until the patient presents as a teenager for undiversion and reconstruction. These problems will be discussed first, followed by a discussion of the problems faced when dealing with exstrophy patients who have had less than satisfactory results from primary

treatment in the neonatal period. Finally, as most other aspects of vaginoplasty will already have been discussed, substitution vaginoplasty in the Mayer–Rokitansky syndrome will be described.

FEMALE EPISPADIAS

The condition is rare but easily recognised. The external meatus is obviously abnormal and patulous and the clitoris is bifid (Fig. 14.1). A plain X-ray of the pelvis shows separation of the pubic symphysis (Fig. 14.2) and an IVU shows a small capacity bladder with an incompetent bladder neck (Fig. 14.3). Urodynamically the distal sphincter mechanism is also incompetent and endoscopically the urethra is patulous and short.

The traditional treatment is by a Young–Dees–Leadbetter (YDL) type of

procedure to reconstruct the bladder neck leaving the natural urethra, the meatus and the clitoris untouched. Whilst this is of little importance to very young girls, the appearance is somewhat more distressing to older girls so I prefer to add the Hendren touch and deal with these simultaneously, coincidentally giving a longer urethra and a more even urethral calibre, rather than the inverted trumpet shape which the YDL procedure produces. These may or may not be of additional benefit for continence.

Preoperative preparation
No special preparation is needed other than to ensure that the urine is sterile and that blood has been crossmatched.

Position
The patient is placed in a low lithotomy position to give perineal access and also allow a Pfannenstiel approach to the retropubic space.

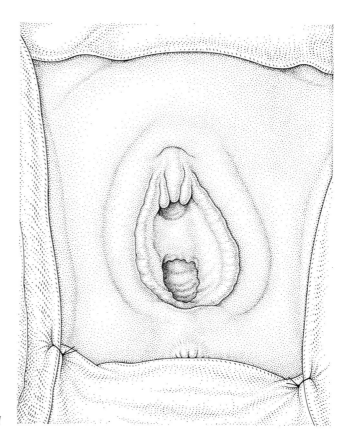

Fig. 14.1

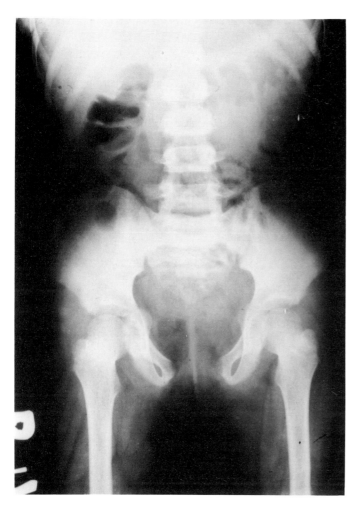

Fig. 14.2

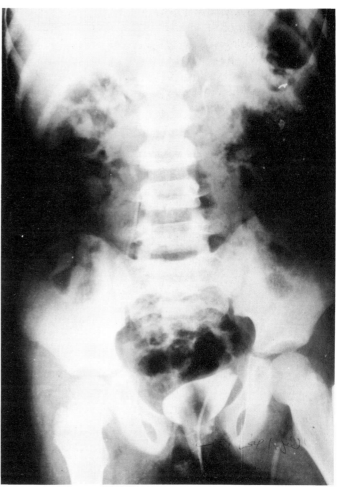

Fig. 14.3

Procedure

The bladder, bladder neck and urethra are exposed from above through a Pfannenstiel incision in the usual way and the pubourethral ligaments and the fascia between them are carefully incised to expose as much as possible of the distal urethra.

Attention is then turned to the perineum. A vertical incision is made along the medial aspect of each half of the clitoris and this is then extended upwards and inwards on each side so that the two incisions meet over the lower mons (Fig. 14.4). These incisions are extended downwards to the meatus and up the urethra towards the bladder neck, excising the redundant part of the anterior urethral wall.

These incisions up the urethra continue upwards until they are clearly seen from within the pelvis. The mobilised segment of the urethral wall with the attached skin is then pulled through into the pelvis and the excision of the redundant anterior urethral wall, up to the bladder neck, continues from above (Fig. 14.5). The strip is then transected at this point and the bladder neck and bladder are then incised longitudinally and opened up as a continuation of the urethral incision/excision. The perineal incision and the distal urethra can then be closed with two layers of interrupted 4/0 Vicryl sutures. As part of this closure, the two halves of the clitoris are united.

The next step is to convert that part of the bladder (the trigone) below the level of the ureteric orifices into a tube that will become a proximal extension of the urethra. Before doing so the ureters may need to be (and usually are) mobilised and reimplanted at a higher level using the Cohen advancement technique.

To get the right calibre of the 'urethra' is not easy because the bladder tends to become oedematous and thickened peroperatively. Furthermore the worry, whilst preparing the trigone to form a neourethra, is always that it will be too small so for both of these reasons it often ends up being too large. The aim is to get a neourethral tube of about 12 F calibre. If the excision of the anterior wall of the epispadiac urethra has been carried out properly then the calibre of this part of the urethra, after it has been closed with interrupted sutures, will be about this size. To convert the trigone into a neourethral tube of about 12 F means stripping the urothelium of the bladder neck and trigone leaving a midline strip a little less than 1.5 cm wide posteriorly between the ureteric orifices as an upward extension of the urethra and of equal width, and removing the rest of the urothelium from the bladder below the level of the ureters (Fig. 14.6). The full thickness of the bladder wall on the left-hand side of this strip is then mobilised carefully from the underlying vagina and the lateral half of this flap is excised. On the right-hand side of the preserved urothelial strip, the part of the bladder from which the urothelium was stripped is also carefully mobilised from the underlying vagina as a flap but in this instance the flap is preserved (Fig. 14.7).

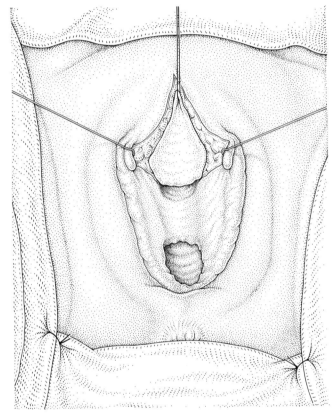

Fig. 14.4

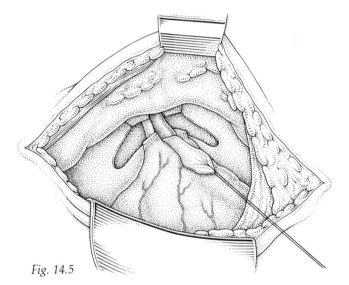

Fig. 14.5

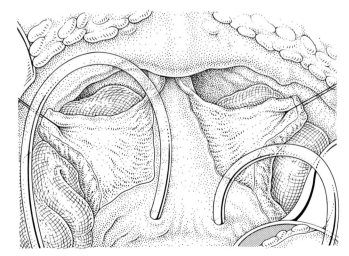

Fig. 14.6

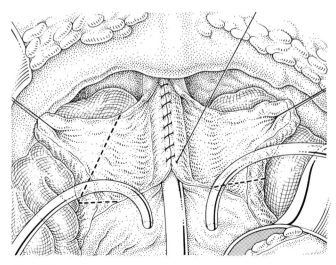

Fig. 14.7

This is a procedure that is easier to describe than perform because the urothelial stripping is often difficult and the bladder wall is easy to damage.

The trimmed left side is then sutured to the right urothelial margin suturing urothelium to urothelium (Fig. 14.7) and then muscle to muscle around a 10 or 12 F catheter depnding on the size of the child (Fig. 14.8). It is important to get urothelial apposition with the first layer and a secure stitching of the second layer to maintain that apposition.

The preserved bladder flap on the right-hand side is then wrapped over this neourethral tube and sutured in place (Figs 14.9, 14.10). The urethral catheter is then removed and replaced to check that it is easily catheterisable before the closure of the wound begins. The bladder is closed in the usual way with a suprapubic catheter, to drain the urine for the first 10 days, and a retropubic wound drain. As always the omentum is brought down to cover the reconstruction and separate it from the back of the symphysis.

In this, as in other neourethroplasties in females, the aim in theory is to produce a competent urethra. In practice the aim is to produce a tube with sufficient intrinsic resistance to hold urine in, but not sufficient to give voiding difficulty. In other words one is attempting to produce a controlled degree of outflow obstruction. Insufficient obstruction will give stress incontinence; excessive obstruction will cause retention. Getting the balance right and predictably so is almost impossible. The tendency should therefore be to err on the side of the

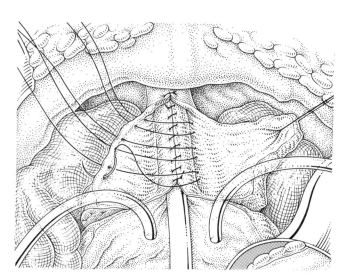

Fig. 14.8

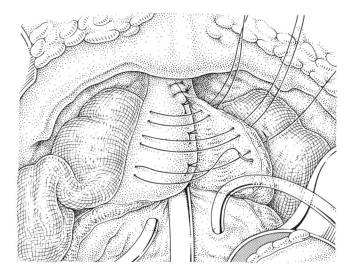

Fig. 14.9

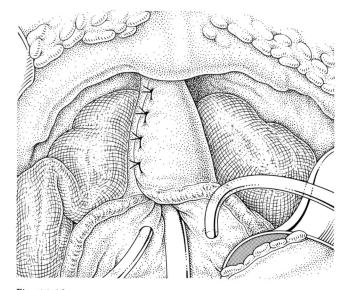

Fig. 14.10

obstruction as the female urethra is short and straight (hopefully) making intermittent self catheterisation an easy option if the patient develops a voiding imbalance. For this reason it is important to ensure that the neourethra is easily catheterisable before closing the wound. Any surgical imperfections that make catheterisation difficult are easier to correct at this stage than at a later date. (It also stops you feeling a fool if the neourethra proves to be uncatheterisable when the patient has only just recovered from the operation.)

The unpredictability of a surgeon's ability to create a competent neourethra inclines me to adopt a different approach in those children who present for treatment at or after puberty. Implantation of an artificial sphincter seems a better proposition in these patients, despite the greater than usual problems, because of the thinness of the epispadiac bladder, in getting into the plane between the bladder neck area and the vagina to place the AUS cuff.

Postoperative management

The drain is removed when it stops draining. The urethral catheter is removed after 12–14 days and the suprapubic catheter is clamped for a trial of voiding the day after. It is removed the next day assuming that the child is voiding satisfactorily without a large residual urine.

It is reassuring to have radiological evidence of satisfactory healing of the neourethra before removing the catheters and getting the child to attempt to void. For this reason I like the urethral catheter to be removed under radiological control, instilling contrast medium in the catheter as it is withdrawn. If there is extravasation of the contrast, suggesting that healing is incomplete, the catheter is pushed back into the bladder. If the neourethra appears satisfactory the catheter is removed.

The child and/or parents should be warned (if she is voiding spontaneously) that she will have frequency and urge incontinence for at least the first three months as the bladder has to have time to expand to a reasonable capacity. Likewise, if she is self catheterising, the frequency of catheterisation will have to take account of the initially reduced bladder capacity.

UROGENITAL SINUS AND CLOACAL ABNORMALITIES

There are no specific types of urogenital sinus or cloacal abnormality that can be clearly distinguished. They form a spectrum of conditions in which the perineal openings of the urethra, the vagina and, in the case of cloaca, the rectum are confluent. Some instances of urogenital sinus are due to virilisation of the female fetus caused by congenital adrenal hyperplasia or associated with other rarer congenital abnormalities. In the remainder no specific endocrine or chromosomal abnormality is found but in all patients such abnormalities should be considered as should associated abnormalities of the upper urinary tract or other organ systems.

In cloaca particularly, as with all anorectal anomalies in either sex, there is a high incidence of associated abnormalities in other organ systems, especially in the lumbosacral spine but also the heart, the central nervous system and the alimentary canal. The commonest skeletal deformities in cloaca are total or partial sacral agenesis which may be a cause of neuropathic bladder dysfunction. This may be present irrespective of the state of the sacrum but is more commonly associated with sacral malformation, the severity of which in turn correlates roughly with the level of the recto-cloacal confluence. This is only a rough correlation however. Low confluences may still have sacral malformations or neuropathic dysfunction.

The main variable factors in this spectrum of anomalies are the calibre of the confluent single channel, its length, and whether the anorectum and its musculature is involved (cloaca) or not (urogenital sinus). Occasionally the anal canal is anteriorly transposed in patients with a urogenital sinus, even if a cloaca is not present, further strengthening the concept of a spectrum. For descriptive purposes the spectrum can be illustrated

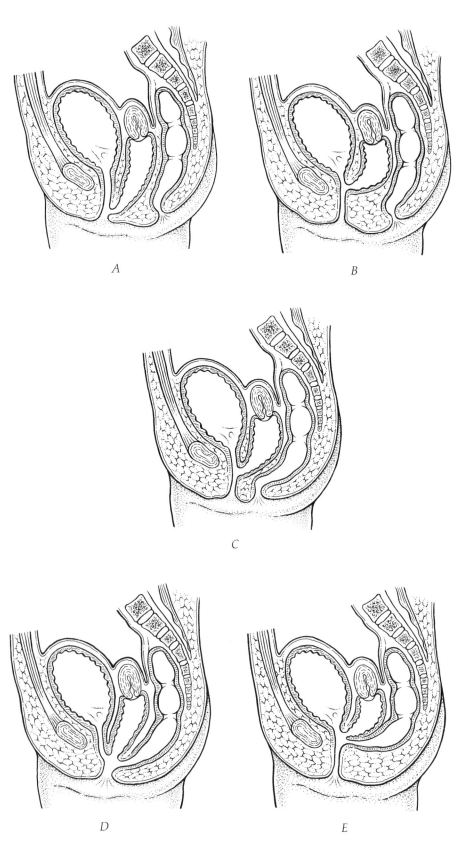

A

B

C

D

E

Fig. 14.11

in five stages of severity (Fig. 14.11):

1.   Urogenital sinus; low confluence of vagina and urethra; normal anus (Fig. 14.11a).
2.   Urogenital sinus; high confluence of vagina and urethra; normal anus (Fig. 14.11b).
3.   Urogenital sinus; low or high confluence; anterior transposition of the anus (Fig. 14.11c).
4.   Cloaca; low confluence of vagina, urethra and rectum. The pelvic floor and perianal musculature is usually well preserved (Fig. 14.11d).
5.   Cloaca; high confluence. The pelvic floor and perianal musculature is usually deficient, sometimes markedly so (Fig. 14.11e).

In all of these the impression is that the genital tract (and rectum) are draining into a confluence which is of fairly narrow calibre and which therefore appears essentially 'urethral' rather than 'vaginal' in nature. Indeed there may be a functioning distal sphincter mechanism in the expected position. The bladder neck is usually competent and the child may be continent as a result. The diagnosis of bladder neck competence or otherwise is usually obvious clinically and endoscopically, but it is best confirmed urodynamically, if possible, before any surgical treatment is planned. This is because bladder neck competence does not mean that the child will be continent. Indeed she will often be incontinent because of pooling of urine in the vagina causing urinary dribbling from the vagina between voids, a bit like the situation with a vaginal ectopic ureter and a normally sited contralateral ureter.

Two other conditions, female hypospadias (a common and relatively trivial condition in which the bladder neck is competent) and urovaginal confluence (a very much more serious condition in which the bladder neck is totally incompetent) give the impression that the urinary tract is draining into a confluence which is of rather larger calibre than in the last group and therefore 'vaginal' in nature (Fig. 14.12). Some instances of low cloaca are also in this category.

Additionally the problem in any of these situations may be compounded by urethral, vaginal or rectal stenosis at the site of confluence, by bladder neck incompetence, by vaginal duplication or hypoplasia or other gynaecological abnormalities, by vesico-ureteric reflux and/or renal dysplasia or, in cloaca, by neuropathic problems associated with sacrococcygeal dysplasia.

Of all the variables affecting the urogenital sinus or cloaca itself, the calibre of the confluent channel is the most important clinically (and when it comes to definitive treatment), because a narrow channel or outlet may cause outflow obstruction. Urinary retention in the vagina is another common consequence leading to hydrocolpos which in turn may cause outflow obstruction by compression of the bladder neck area. Obstruction may then lead to infection, impaired renal function or both. If the rectum is also involved then the problem will obviously be compounded.

Before considering treatment, another condition should be mentioned which may be confused with a urogenital sinus. This is the condition of vulval obstruction due to fused labia minora. This resembles a urogenital sinus with a low confluence but is easily treated by simple separation.

PRIMARY TREATMENT IN NEONATES

In the first instance, neonatal treatment, when indicated, is directed towards decompression of the urinary tract and, in a cloaca, the bowel. If the bladder needs to be decompressed (uncommonly, and usually because of

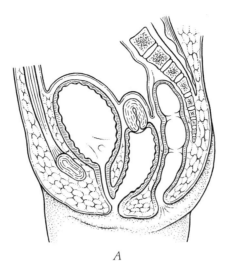
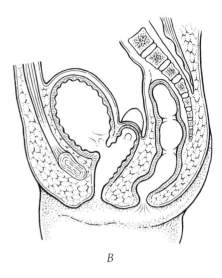

Fig. 14.12
Female hypospadias.   Urovaginal confluence

hydrocolpos) this should be achieved by catheterisation, repeated as required. If a catheter cannot be passed through the confluent channel/urogenital sinus into the bladder, usually because of a curve in the distal urethra, it may be necessary to cut back into the sinus so that the track up to the bladder is straight and a catheter can be passed but it is important only to cut back this much. Cutting back any further may damage the distal sphincter mechanism, such as there is, which may be crucially important later on. This may be sufficient treatment on its own if vaginal pooling is the main problem or to allow intermittent catheterisation if further decompression of the bladder (or vagina) is necessary. If this is insufficient on either count then suprapubic catheterisation or a cutaneous vesicostomy is indicated. If the child voids spontaneously or if CISC is necessary but easy, but recurrent hydrocolpos is a problem then suprapubic cutaneous vaginostomy is indicated but this is rarely required.

In cloacal abnormalities the bowel is best decompressed by a loop sigmoid colostomy, as a loop decompresses both sides of the colon and therefore acts as a vent for urine that collects in the distal

colon as well as a faecal channel for the proximal colon. It is perhaps worth noting that of all the spectrum of abnormalities described it is only a cloaca that will definitely be noted in neonatal life because of the anorectal abnormality and that it is only the anorectal abnormality that routinely needs prompt and early treatment.

DEFINITIVE TREATMENT

In the more minor cases of urogenital sinus, with a low confluence and a competent bladder neck, a simple, posteriorly based, skin flap vaginoplasty may be all that is required to deal with the problem, although when associated with virilisation in the adrenogenital syndrome a reduction clitoroplasty will also be necessary. Indeed it is usually only those cases with congenital adrenal hyperplasia that present in the very young because it is the clitoromegaly, not the urogenital sinus that is the obvious abnormality. In general, the more severe the degree of virilisation, the higher the vaginal opening into the UG sinus; and the higher the confluence the more extensive (and more difficult) the rotation of skin flap or flaps in order to exteriorise it.

Female hypospadias can also be treated early in life should it present that early. In fact, a urethral meatus a centimetre or so up the anterior vaginal wall is not that uncommon and is usually asymptomatic. When associated with meatal stenosis, or vaginal stenosis leading to hydrocolpos, recurrent urinary tract infection may result and this is the usual reason why the condition is brought to light. Meatal stenosis is treated by dilatation or urethrotomy and vaginal stenosis by posterior skinflap vaginoplasty.

Urovaginal confluence with absence of the bladder neck and urogenital sinus with sphincteric incompetence, because they less commonly cause recurrent urinary infection, usually present later on, at or after 3 or 4 years of age when continence is obviously abnormal. Again it should be emphasised that associated upper tract abnormalities and gynaecological problems may be present above the level of the obvious abnormality and should be looked for. They may require treatment in their own right and upper urinary tract surgery will usually take priority over correction of the local abnormality. Urogenital sinus with a competent bladder neck may not present till later still in life unless there are associated abnormalities or vaginal pooling causes problems of infection, obstruction or dribbling incontinence. In the absence of any of these to a significant degree, most girls present at puberty with gynaecological problems. These comments assume that there is no neuropathic element to affect bladder and urethral function. If there is, urological symptoms will bring the child for medical attention at an earlier age.

The urogenital sinus abnormality itself may be dealt with in one of two ways:

— If its situation and calibre are urethral in type (Fig. 14.13) then it is kept as such and the vaginal element is disconnected and brought through to the perineum. This is the most common of the more severe forms of urogenital sinus and the form commonly seen in cloaca (Fig. 14.14).
— If its situation and calibre are vaginal in type (Fig. 14.15) then it is kept as a vagina and where necessary its opening is augmented by a posterior skin flap vaginoplasty. The urethra is then constructed by means of either a vaginal neourethroplasty or a bladder flap neourethroplasty depending on the competence of the bladder neck and the calibre of the vagina.

Given the wide spectrum of abnormalities that may be found, it is only possible to generalise about treatment, particularly if there are also the effects of previous surgery to be dealt with. The procedures that will be described are:

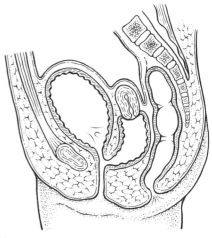

Fig. 14.13

1. The techniques for vaginoplasty for a urogenital sinus.
2. The techniques for neourethroplasty for a urogenital sinus.
3. The surgical approach to a cloacal repair.

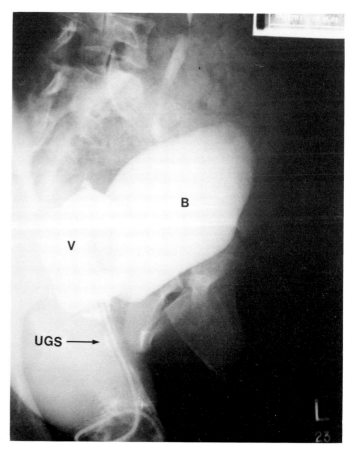

Fig. 14.14

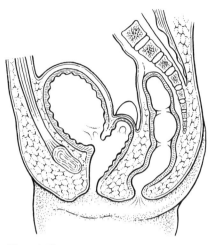

Fig. 14.15

VAGINOPLASTY FOR A UROGENITAL SINUS

When the abnormality is little more than an introital or labial fusion all that is required is a Heineke–Mikulicz type of cutback procedure with a vertical midline incision to open the introitus with closure of the wound edges to fashion the margin of the introitus.

More commonly something more than a simple cutback is required because of the greater depth of the vagina from the perineum in most instances of urogenital sinus. The crucial factor is the level of the confluence and thus the length of the vagina and its distance from the perineum. If there is a low confluence, which is more common, then a posterior flap vaginoplasty can be performed. If there is a high confluence, a simple flap vaginoplasty will not be enough; the

vagina must be dissected off the urethra and either pulled through to the perineum or have an interposition procedure to bridge the gap to the perineum.

POSTERIOR SKIN FLAP VAGINOPLASTY

When appropriate the posterior skin flap vaginoplasty is performed by making a widely based inverted-U incision with its base just in front of the anus and its apex at the posterior margin of the opening of the urogenital sinus (Fig. 14.16). This incision extends through the skin and subcutaneous tissue but no deeper and not into the sinus or the vagina. The flap is then dissected off the deeper tissues, the sinus and the vagina, and allowed to drop back (Fig. 14.17). No matter how thin the tissue block

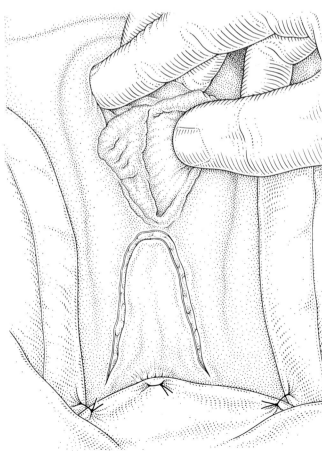

Fig. 14.16

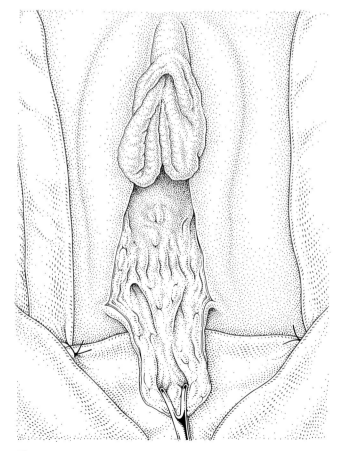

Fig. 14.17

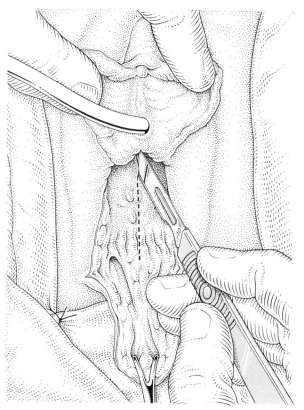

Fig. 14.18

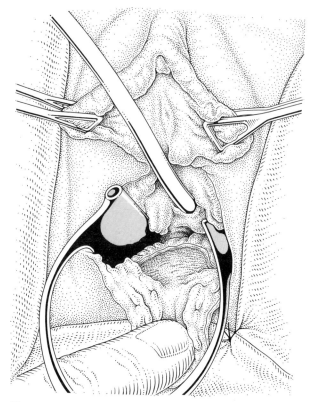

Fig. 14.19

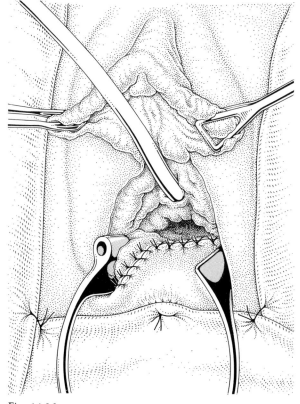

Fig. 14.20

between the skin and the sinus appears to be you should never cut straight down on to it with a simple vertical incision. A flap will always be necessary for a satisfactory cosmetic result.

The posterior sinus/vaginal wall is then exposed on its posterior aspect by dissecting through the overlying tissue in the midline (Fig. 14.18). The posterior midline of the sinus and vagina are then incised from the opening back up to a suitable point for the skin flap to be laid into the posterior vaginal wall (Fig. 14.19). This is much higher up than you might initially think, which is why it is important to make the initial incision in the form of a flap, so that you can be sure that it will reach high enough. The flap is then sewn in place with interrupted 3/0 Vicryl sutures (Fig.

14.20). If the labia minora are abnormally high riding, as they usually are, they can be dropped back to a more normal situation (Fig. 14.21).

EXTERIORISATION OF A HIGH VAGINA

For a high vagina a double skin flap variation of the posterior skin flap vaginoplasty technique performed transperineally may be adequate if the vagina is not too high and if it is fairly mobile. For a truly high vagina a combined abdomino-perineal approach will be necessary.

Preparation
No special preparation is required but there is some fairly extensive perineo-pelvic dissection so blood should

be cross matched. The urine should be sterile.

Position
Low lithotomy position is required.

Technique
To begin with, if it has not already been done the urogenital sinus is cut back, just enough to give a straight 'urethral' channel into the bladder. A Foley catheter is then passed up the sinus and into the vagina where the balloon is inflated. This aids identification by palpation during the ensuing dissection. Then, as for a simple flap vaginoplasty, a posterior inverted-U incision is made through the skin and subcutaneous tissue, but with its apex halfway between the sinus opening and the anus. A similarly orientated anteriorly based flap is then fashioned (Fig. 14.22 — the

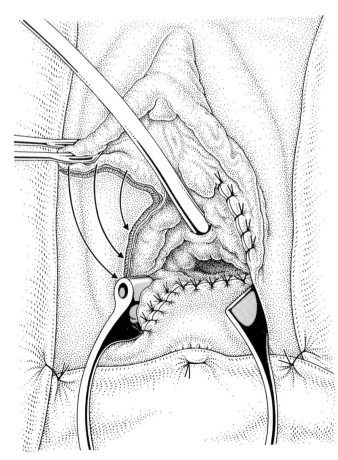

Fig. 14.21

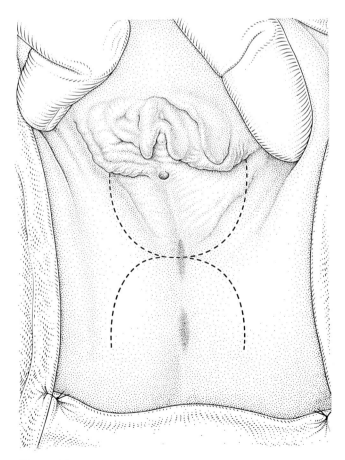

Fig. 14.22

catheter has been omitted for clarity. Note incidentally that nature shows, by areas of pigmentation (and, in adults by hair distribution), where the vagina and anus ought to be even when she places them ectopically. These landmarks are invaluable for a satisfactory cosmetic result). The flaps are then dropped back and the incision is then deepened in the midline until the vagina, urogenital sinus and confluence are exposed. A clear exposure of the lower end of the urethra is unnecessary and undesirable as the sphincter mechanism or its innervation (such as they are) may be damaged. The surgeon should stick to the midline and aim for the vagina first and then work down to the confluence.

The vagina is then disconnected from the 'urethra' leaving a sufficient margin

to close the urethra with interrupted inverting 4/0 Vicryl sutures without narrowing it (Fig. 14.23). The margins of the vagina are then mobilised to gain as much downward mobility as possible, to ensure an adequate vaginal calibre and to get good clean edges for the anastomosis to the perineal skin flaps. Quite a lot of downward mobility is possible in a toddler but this gets less with advancing age. It is important during this mobilisation to ensure that the vaginal margin to be exteriorised is of normal calibre. It is a mistake to keep as much as possible of the vagina, right up to the confluence, to facilitate the exteriorisation. If the confluence is not excised back to normal vagina of normal calibre, the patient will end up with a mid-vaginal stenosis at the site of the exteriorisation–anastomosis. This may

be a very difficult problem to resolve with a secondary procedure.

The two previously prepared skin flaps are then pushed in to reach and to be sutured to the vagina, and the lateral perineal skin margins are then undermined and advanced to complete the closure (Fig. 14.24). Again interrupted Vicryl sutures are used. This is easier to say than to do because although it is usual for the apex of both flaps to reach easily up to the vagina, it is also usual to find that there is an undesirable gap between the side edges of the two flaps along the lateral vaginal walls. Hence the need for broad flaps if a tight vagina is to be avoided.

If this mobilisation and reconstruction is not proceeding satisfactorily then the

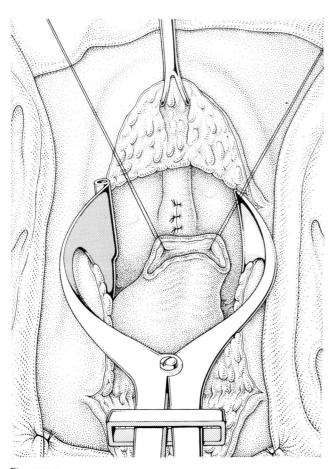

Fig. 14.23

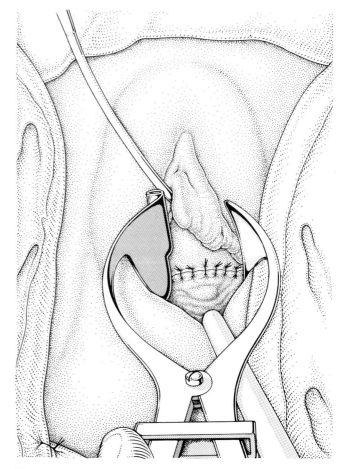

Fig. 14.24

uterus and vagina should be exposed and mobilised from above, transperitoneally (or even transvesically) to allow them to drop down more readily to the perineum.

Through a lower abdominal incision the peritoneal aspects of the bladder and uterus are exposed and an incision is made along the posterior border of the bladder to separate the bladder base from the anterior vaginal wall. The anterior vaginal wall is then followed down to the confluence with the urethra where it is (or already has been) disconnected. If access is difficult the posterior bladder wall and trigone are simply split as for a difficult fistula repair (Ch. 12).

Mobilisation of the vagina from above in this way gives considerably more downward mobility for the anastomosis to the perineal skin flaps. It also allows a cleaner delineation of the margins of the vaginal wall and, when the vagina is distended or duplicated, a greater ability to perform intravaginal corrective surgery than is possible by the transperineal route alone.

If the vagina cannot otherwise be exteriorised in either of these ways or if it is congenitally or iatrogenically rudimentary or absent then a segment of sigmoid colon can be used to bridge the gap to the perineum or to replace it. Substitution vaginoplasty is described for the Mayer–Rokitansky syndrome at the end of this chapter.

One third to one half of girls have vaginal duplication and one of the two upper vaginas is usually much more distended. When this is the case the simplest solution is to divide the bridge between the two and exteriorise the more capacious viscus. There is never any point in trying to excise the more rudimentary system.

Follow up after vaginoplasty

After all types of vaginoplasty the main problem is stenosis at the suture lines. Whatever technique is used this usually ends up as mid-vaginal stenosis as even those suture lines that seem fairly external at the end of the operation seem to retract inwards postoperatively. Mid-vaginal stenosis is difficult to treat satisfactorily and so it is wise to advise periodic passage of a vaginal dilator to try to prevent this occurrence. Many people, doctors and patients, find this rather distasteful in a young girl, perhaps not surprisingly, but it is difficult to imagine that this is as much of a problem when performed by a loving mum as multiple revision procedures later in life.

Stenosis aside, the results of vaginoplasty for low confluences are good. By contrast, a good functional result for a high vagina is unusual.

SUBSTITUTION URETHROPLASTY FOR A UROGENITAL SINUS

When the urogenital sinus is essentially a urethra into which the vagina enters, as it usually is, it is sensible to keep the sinus as a urethra and to exteriorise or reconstruct the vagina with one of the methods described in the last section. On the other hand when the sinus is essentially a vagina into which the bladder opens, either directly through an incompetent bladder neck as in urovaginal confluences or indirectly through a short length of urethra, then substitution urethroplasty is necessary.

This is best achieved with a bladder flap neourethroplasty if there is no functioning bladder neck and no urethra, and with a vaginal neourethroplasty if the bladder neck is competent, particularly if there is even a short length of urethra below it.

Bladder neck competence is the crucial factor. If present it is a much better

continence mechanism than any surgical procedure is likely to achieve. All steps should therefore be taken to preserve it.

BLADDER FLAP NEOURETHROPLASTY

This is the preferred technique of neourethroplasty in any female patient, whatever the cause of an absent urethra, when the bladder neck is incompetent.

Preparation

The urine should be sterile. One unit of blood should be cross matched for a small child, two for a teenager. Any skin problems due to incontinence with superadded fungal infections should be controlled.

Position

The patient should be in the low lithotomy position. The first part of the procedure is performed through a lower midline incision as an omental wrap is an essential part of the procedure and if omental mobilisation is necessary it will not be possible through a Pfannenstiel type of incision. The final stages of the operation are performed transperineally.

Technique

The retropubic space is widely opened to expose the bladder, bladder neck and pelvic floor fascia as clearly as possible. The pubourethral ligaments (which are present) are divided and any loose fatty tissue between them is removed. Any bleeding points are controlled. This is important because the neourethra will need to run in this area, down the front of the vagina to a meatus fashioned between the introitus and the clitoris.

The point of the confluence is then defined and the bladder neck is dissected off the vagina. The opening in the vagina is closed obliquely or horizontally with two layers of interrupted 3/0 or 4/0 Vicryl sutures, inverting the edges into the vagina.

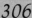

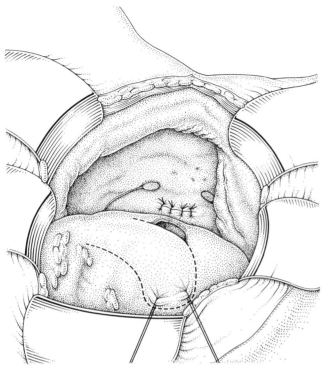

Fig. 14.25

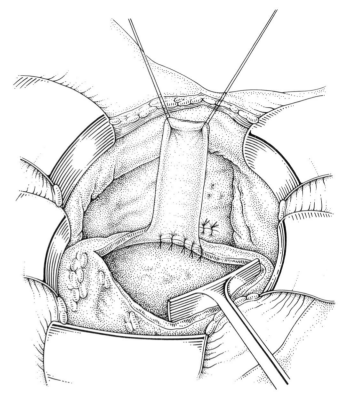

Fig. 14.26

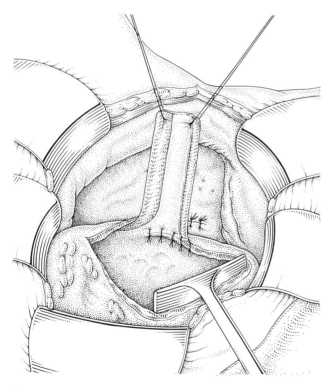

Fig. 14.27

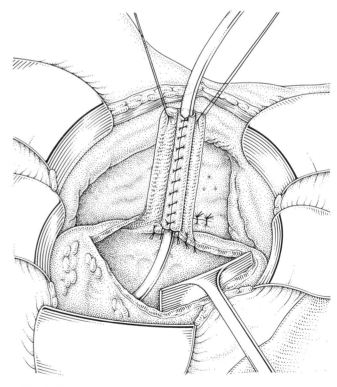

Fig. 14.28

A long, curved, oblique flap is then raised from the anterior aspect of the bladder with its base at one lateral pedicle and curving up at the bladder neck towards the dome. It should be 3–3.5 cm wide and at least 7–8 cm long (Fig. 14.25). The inferior margin of the flap, which was the anterior margin of the bladder neck and which becomes the posterior margin when the flap is viewed from its urothelial aspect, is then sutured with interrupted sutures to the posterior bladder margin to recreate the bladder neck and so that the flap can then be laid along the anterior vaginal wall as though it was an opened-out natural urethra (Fig. 14.26).

The urothelium from the side of the flap is then trimmed to leave about 1 cm bare and about 1.2 cm still epithelialised

(Fig. 14.27). The flap is then rolled in to form a tube around a 10 or 12 F Foley catheter depending on the size of the patient and closed with three layers of inverting 4/0 Vicryl sutures. The first layer closes the urothelium (Fig. 14.28). The second layer closes the muscle layer immediately adjacent to the margin of the urothelial closure (Fig. 14.29) and the third layer closes the flap of denuded detrusor muscle over the previous suture lines to make the neourethra thick and watertight (Fig. 14.30). The bladder is closed around a suprapubic catheter to ensure urine drainage.

The omentum is then brought down and wrapped around the neourethra and sutured in place to hold it there and separate the neourethra from the vaginal closure.

Next an artificial sphincter cuff of an appropriate size is wrapped around the omentum and enclosed urethra. A further layer of omentum is then wrapped around the cuff and the cuff tubing is brought out into the inguinal canal where it is left plugged off so that it can be easily found and connected to the rest of the artificial sphincter components should that subsequently prove to be necessary. (When it is routinely unnecessary, implantation of the AUS cuff can be omitted. Until you can predictably ensure continence by neourethroplasty alone an AUS cuff is a safe fallback. After about 30 of these operations I think I am beginning to get to that stage.)

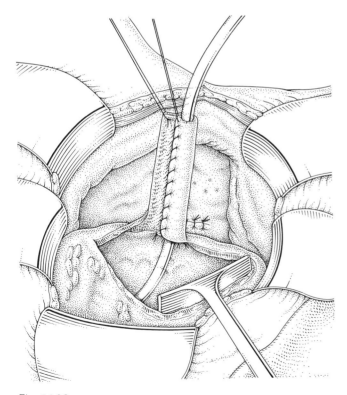

Fig. 14.29

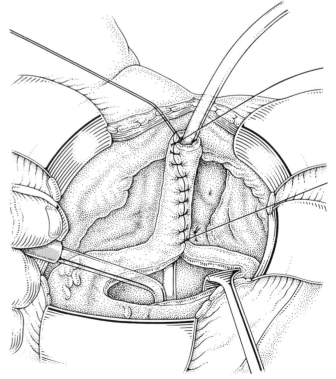

Fig. 14.30

Finally a meatus is created transperineally at an appropriate point just in front of/above the introitus and the neourethra is brought through and sutured in place (Fig. 14.31). When the neourethroplasty is complete and before the wound is closed the urethral catheter is removed and replaced to ensure that the neourethra is easily catheterisable in case CISC is required postoperatively.

Follow up

As with all instances of this type of surgery the urethral catheter is removed under radiological control after about two weeks. The suprapubic catheter is clamped off after a cystogram through it shows no extravasation (Fig. 14.32) and the catheter is then removed after a satisfactory 24-hour trial of voiding or after intermittent self catheterisation has been instituted if the child is unable to void spontaneously. Three months are then allowed to elapse to allow the bladder capacity to recover before assessing continence subjectively, urodynamically and, if necessary, endoscopically.

Note in Figure 14.32 the distance between the urethra and the vagina, which has been outlined with contrast material for this purpose. This is due to the omental wrap, in this case an omentum–AUS cuff sandwich.

Most children end up voiding spontaneously even if it takes some time to achieve it. Of those that void spontaneously about 50% will be continent without the need to implant the rest of the AUS and the rest will need the remainder of the AUS implanted, until experience gives better results without the need for an AUS. In all operations of this type, when the aim is to produce sufficient outflow resistance by virtue of a narrow calibre in a thick-walled neourethra, it is very difficult to get it just right so that there is continence but complete bladder emptying on voiding. Indeed, having tried it many times, I still regard myself

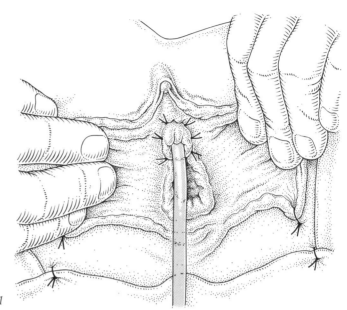

Fig. 14.31

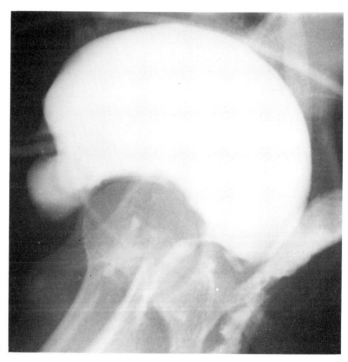

Fig. 14.32

(and the patient) lucky if it works out that way. The best it seems that the surgeon can regularly expect to achieve is a competent but obstructive neourethra that the patient can then self catheterise through. Hence the importance of ensuring peroperatively that the neourethra is easily catheterisable.

ANTERIOR VAGINAL/UG SINUS WALL URETHROPLASTY

This is not always possible because of the small vaginal calibre if the problem presents early in childhood. In older girls the vaginal calibre is usually sufficient to allow exposure unless there is scarring due to failed previous surgery. Other situations in which this approach is sometimes indicated include severe obstetric urethro-vaginal fistula, postsurgical urethral damage or after a long-term indwelling urethral catheter has 'kippered' the urethra open.

Preparation

There is no specific preparation and blood loss is not usually sufficient to warrant cross matching. The urine should be sterile and any skin problems due to incontinence with superadded fungal infection should be controlled.

Position

The patient is placed in the low lithotomy position.

Technique

Before starting the neourethroplasty a suprapubic Foley catheter is passed percutaneously. It is easier at this stage rather than later.

A strip of anterior vaginal sinus wall about 1.5 cm wide is outlined with stay-stitches from the bladder neck to the undersurface of the clitoris (Fig. 14.33). An incision is then made on one side, usually the right side by a right-handed surgeon, from the lateral aspect of the base of the clitoris to the bladder neck. This must be a full thickness incision and to get into the right plane for the vagina/sinus part of this incision it is helpful to concentrate on the more distal part of the incision initially. Here the plane between the subclitoral skin/subcutaneous tissue and the pubis is very obvious. Having defined the plane, the incision can be extended up the vagina/sinus to the bladder neck and around it. This, in turn,

makes it easier to define the plane between the vagina/sinus and the bladder, making damage to the bladder neck less likely.

When one side has been incised an incision is made on the other side in the same way (Fig. 14.34). These incisions and the subsequent neourethroplasty are facilitated by using a Turner Warwick posterior urethral speculum-retractor or a Parks anal retractor to hold the vagina open.

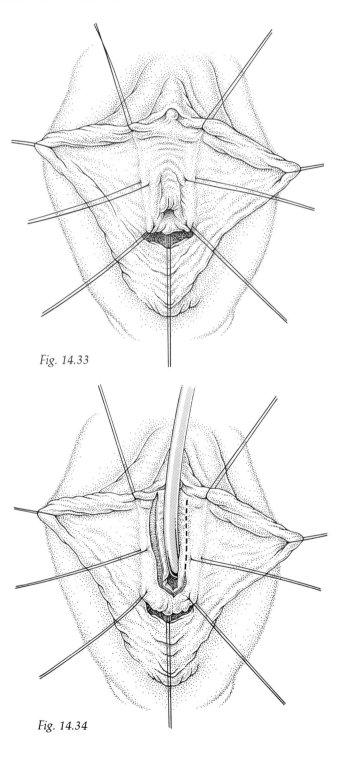

Fig. 14.33

Fig. 14.34

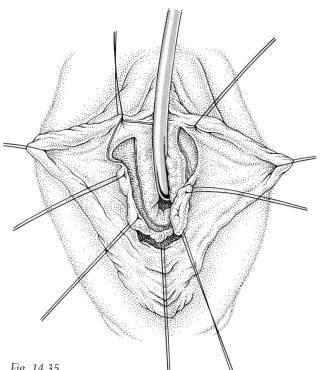

Fig. 14.35

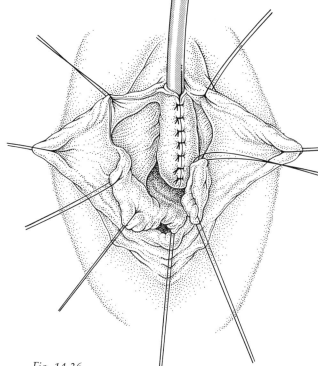

Fig. 14.36

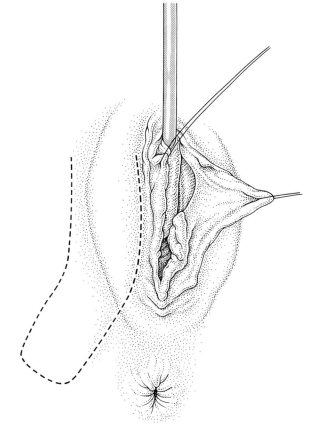

Fig. 14.37

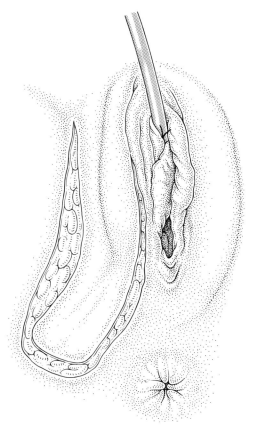

Fig. 14.38

At the upper end the incisions are extended around the bladder neck to circumcise it (Fig. 14.35) making sure that the incision above the bladder neck gives complete separation of the bladder from the vagina. If not the vaginal edge will not be good enough to give adequate closure of the vagina (either directly or with a skin flap — see below) nor will there be adequate space for a labial fat pad interposition. As a result there will be a high incidence of urethro-vaginal fistula. Distally the strip is extended as far as the clitoris to get the maximum possible length for the urethra. It should be stressed that a full thickness incision is needed all round the margins of the neourethral strip to allow it to be rolled in and closed with two layers of 4/0 Vicryl, around a 12 F catheter (Fig. 14.36). When this has been done the catheter is removed and replaced to check that the neourethra is easily catheterisable for reasons discussed in the last section.

When the neourethra has been completed there will be a defect left in the anterior vaginal wall. It is sometimes possible to close this defect directly but this is not usually possible without excessive tension. Even if it is possible a labial fat pad (see Ch. 6) should be mobilised to lie between the suture lines to prevent subsequent fistula formation.

More commonly, direct closure of the anterior vaginal wall will not be possible and a skin flap will have to be rotated in to close the defect. Anteriorly or posteriorly based labial flaps are possible and I have used both according to the circumstances but a posteriorly based flap brings hair-bearing labial skin into the anterior vaginal wall and this is obviously best avoided if possible. An anteriorly based flap of labial and buttock skin is therefore preferred as this will leave relatively hairless buttock skin on the anterior vaginal wall when the procedure has been completed.

A flap of appropriate length is raised, essentially following the margins of the labium majus and continuing posteriorly onto the buttock, curving away from the anus (Fig. 14.37). This is a full thickness flap, down to the inferior pubic ramus anteriorly, where it is composed of labium with its fat pad, and of equal depth more posteriorly where the subcutaneous tissue is ordinary fat (Fig. 14.38). To avoid subsequent ischaemic necrosis of the distal end of this flap the usual criteria for a skin flap — a length to base ratio of about 4 to 1 — should be borne in mind.

When the flap has been raised, the labium minus and vaginal margin are incised at an appropriate point to allow the flap to be rotated into the vaginal defect (Fig. 14.39). This is then held in place with interrupted 3/0 Vicryl mattress sutures (Fig. 14.40) and the

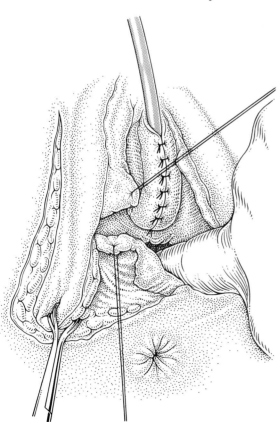

Fig. 14.39

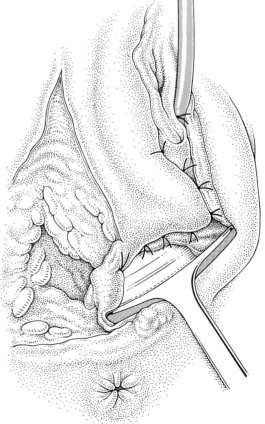

Fig. 14.40

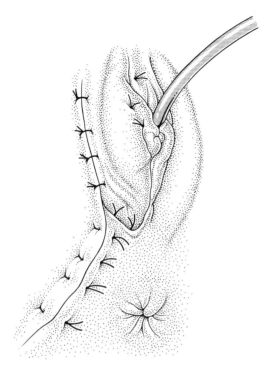

Fig. 14.41

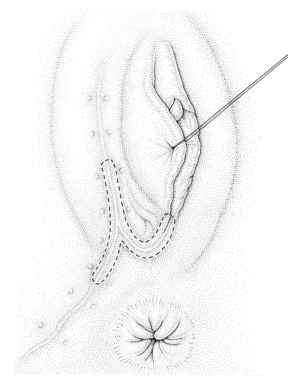

Fig. 14.42

donor defect is closed directly with interrupted 2/0 or 3/0 mattress sutures (Fig. 14.41).

Follow up

The early postoperative management and removal of the urethral and suprapubic catheters is the same as for a bladder flap neourethroplasty.

In the long term the child will be left with a rather distorted vulva, because of the buttock flap, unless something further is done. To return the vulva to a normal appearance the base of the flap is divided at some appropriate time. This should be at least two months later and preferably longer to allow time for the flap to develop a good blood supply from the vagina as a result of healing. In a young girl there is no need to do this until puberty when either she wishes to use tampons or she wishes to become sexually active. The technique is a simple Y-V plasty as illustrated in Figure 14.42. The medial curved limb of the inverted Y, which extends also up the inner aspect of the labium minus, divides

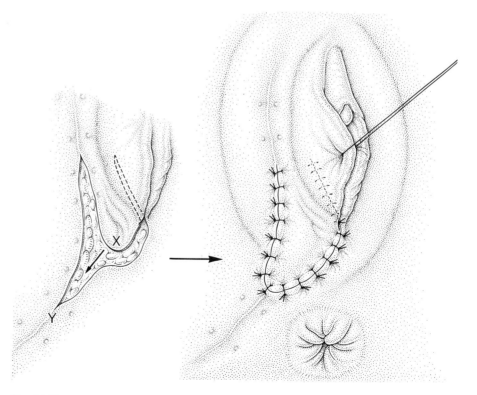

Fig. 14.43

the base of the flap and a Y-V advancement (of point X to point Y in Fig. 14.43) will restore a normal appearance.

The main determinant of continence after this operation is bladder neck competence. If it is competent (and the bladder is stable) the child will be dry. If it is incompetent (or the bladder is unstable) there is only the inherent resistance afforded by the neourethra to produce continence. This may be adequate or alternatively obstructive in which case CISC will be required. Either way the child will be continent. If the neourethra is not adequate to maintain continence in the face of an incompetent bladder neck there is little that can be done to improve matters other than to implant an AUS—omental sandwich, as described for bladder flap neourethroplasty.

CLOACAL REPAIR

In 1980 Peña described his posterior sagittal approach to anorectoplasty for anorectal atresia and since then there has been great enthusiasm for this approach, not only for anorectal atresia but for cloacal problems as well.

Preparation
This is a major surgical procedure particularly if there has been previous abdominal surgery, of which the commonest to cause difficulties is multiple colostomy revisions. The child should be fit and well with sterile urine and 2—4 units of blood cross matched depending on her age.

Position
This is essentially a perineal procedure but abdominal access is often necessary to deal with associated problems, particularly in patients who have had previous surgery. The perineal approach is best conducted with the child in a lithotomy position with the hips well flexed and the sacrum well supported,

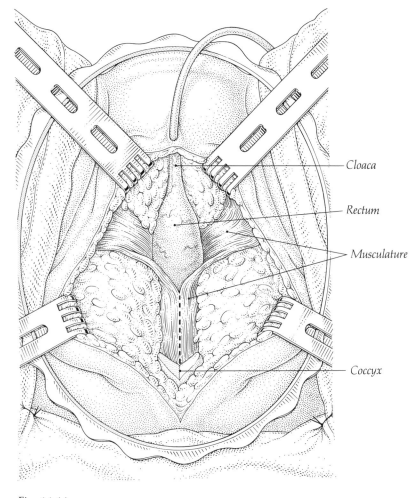

Fig. 14.44

Cloaca
Rectum
Musculature
Coccyx

but with the facility to straighten out the hips for a laparotomy without the need to re-'prep' and redrape. This may require a bit of thought during the positioning and draping (see below — next section). This is not the position that Peña himself describes; he describes the use of the jack-knife position and so presumably moves the patient's position peroperatively as indicated.

Technique
The initial steps of the Peña approach are to expose firstly the anal sphincteric and pelvic floor musculature and then the confluence through a midline incision from the tip of the spine, be it malformed sacrum or normal coccyx, to

the opening of the urogenital sinus (Fig. 14.44). To help identify the confluence within the perineum during the course of the dissection a Foley catheter should be passed through the common channel and into the rectum (as this is the most superficial viscus) where the balloon is inflated. This is not always easy: the simplest thing to do is to identify the rectal opening at the confluence endoscopically and pass a guide-wire into the rectum. A Foley catheter with the tip cut off can then be slid over the guidewire into the correct position.

The anal sphincter and pelvic floor musculature are identified most accurately by means of a stimulator but visual identification is usually adequate if a reasonable amount of muscle is present. Indeed, in my view, if the muscle is not readily identified visually then searching for it electronically is probably a waste of time as the 'muscle' will be of no functional value. The aim is to work through the centre of the muscle complex so that when the viscera are subsequently exteriorised the musculature can be closed around them to restore the anatomy as closely to normal as possible. To aid identification at the later stages of the procedure the muscle elements should be tagged with stay-stitches. In many instances it will be possible to dissect through the muscle complex without having to divide it (and then restore it later on). It is obviously preferable to divide and resuture it as little as possible. The aim

should always be to find the centre of the muscle complex — first the external anal sphincter and then the puborectal sling — and spread it open, so that there is the least disruption of continuity and thus the least disturbance of residual muscle function. This ideal is not always achievable.

Having worked through the musculture to the site of the confluence the rectum is carefully separated from the vagina and the vagina from the urogenital sinus. In both instances this is achieved by defining the margins of the communication from the posterior aspect through the opened cloaca (Fig. 14.45). This opens the inferior margin of each communication in turn. With the inferior margin open to expose the

communication, sutures are placed around the superior margin of the communication to tent the mucosa off the common wall between the two visci (Fig. 14.46). The mucosa can then be dissected off the common wall of the conjoined visci up to the point where the walls of the two visci separate. At this point the full thickness of the wall of each viscus can be defined and transected (Fig. 14.47). Each viscus can then be mobilised to allow it to be brought down to the perineum and exteriorised (Fig. 14.48). Separation and mobilisation of rectum is usually much easier than separation and mobilisation of the vagina.

The urogenital sinus is preserved as the urethra (usually — as discussed above)

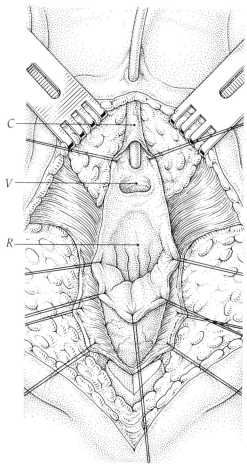

Fig. 14.45
R, Rectum; V, vagina; C, confluent channel = cloaca.

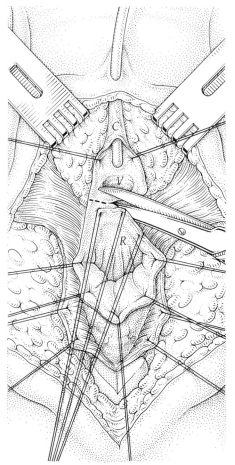

Fig. 14.46

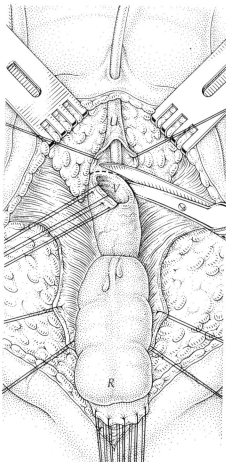

Fig. 14.47
The common channel becomes the urethra, U.

closing the defect at the site of the confluence with interrupted mattress sutures. The vagina is pulled through for a direct anastomosis, unless it is too high or too short or, on the other hand, is too rudimentary, in which case either something has to be done to bridge the gap between the perineum and the vagina or the vagina must be replaced. The younger the child, the easier it is to mobilise the vagina downwards for a direct anastomosis. If a direct transperineal anastomosis proves to be impossible, one of the techniques described above for exteriorisation of a high vagina is used to bridge the gap. I dislike using extensive local skin flaps because they tend to produce a rather untidy perineum and therefore prefer to expose the pelvis from above through a

lower midline incision and continue as a synchronous abdomino-perineal procedure.

When the vaginal anastomosis is complete the perineal body is reconstructed behind it, preferably using muscle but failing that using any available tissue. This is an important step as it strengthens the perineum and helps to form a good ano-rectal angle.

The colon is then pulled through and tapered as necessary to form an anal canal and the anal sphincter complex is reconstructed around it carefully to get the best possible functional result. The anastomosis of the colon to the perineal skin should be at the normal site as indicated by skin pigmentation where

the anus ought to be; and it should be under a bit of tension so that it tends to retract into the perineum to reduce the risk of postoperative prolapse (Fig. 14.49).

If the preformed colostomy or related scarring (or any other factor) prevents adequate mobilisation of the distal colon down to the perineum then the colostomy will have to be revised, or resited, mobilising the left side of the colon as necessary.

At the end of the procedure the child is left, besides the colostomy, with a urethral catheter, a suprapubic catheter and paraffin gauze 'wicks' across the vaginal and anal suture lines.

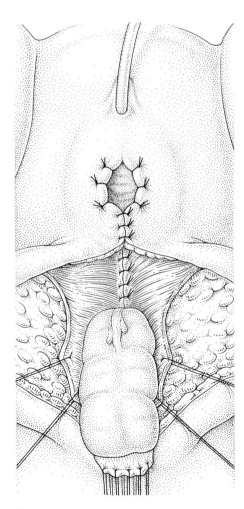

Fig. 14.48

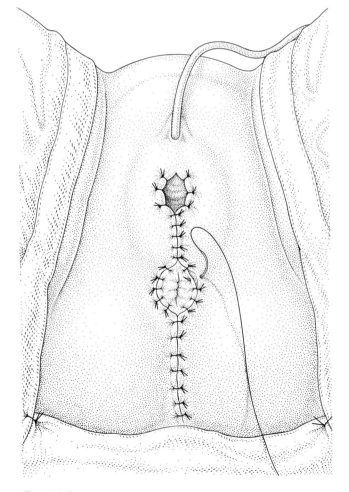

Fig. 14.49

Postoperative management

The wicks are removed after 48 hours.
Thereafter, cross adhesions of the
vaginal and anal suture lines are
prevented by passing small calibre
dilators until the wounds are well
healed. The urethral catheter and
subsequently the suprapubic catheter are
removed after three weeks under
radiological control in the usual way.
The colostomy is closed three months
later, or thereabouts, after a descending
barium study shows satisfactory healing.

Follow up

The most annoying complication is a
urethro-vaginal fistula between the point
where the confluence was closed and the
anastomosis to exteriorise the high
vagina if a direct exteriorisation to the
perineum proved impossible. This is best
prevented by omental interposition if a
peroperative laparotomy and
abdomino-perineal approach proves
necessary and is best treated in the same
way.

The most common complications are
rectal or vaginal stenosis. These are best
prevented by the use of a dilator.
Established rectal stenosis usually
requires revision using the same
technique as in the original operation.
Vaginal stenosis can usually be treated
by rotating in a labial or buttock skin
flap — another reason for avoiding the
excessive use of skin flaps during the
original procedure.

Urinary continence is primarily
dependent on bladder neck function and
every care should be taken not to
disturb this peroperatively. Persistent
incontinence is treated on its merits on
the basis of urodynamic investigation.
Urinary incontinence is not an indication
for a revision Peña procedure if the
remainder of the repair has proved to be
satisfactory. Any subsequent surgical
procedure for incontinence should be
retropubic.

Faecal incontinence is primarily related
to the level of the confluence and the
degree of preservation of the pelvic and
perianal musculature. The higher the
confluence and the less the bulk of
muscle remaining, the worse the result.
Borderline continence or even quite
marked incontinence can usually be
improved in time as the child gets older,
by attention to diet to produce
controlled constipation.

It has to be said that the Peña procedure
is not a universal panacea for all
anorectal atresias as faecal continence is
by no means always achieved. Equally
there is no doubt that it is far and away
the best available procedure and that the
standard 'pull through' procedures
hitherto used in such situations should
be abandoned.

REVISION OF A CLOACAL REPAIR IN FEMALES OR OF A 'PULL THROUGH' PROCEDURE IN EITHER SEX

The Peña approach has only recently
been introduced into paediatric surgical
practice. Most patients with anorectal
atresia and cloacal problems will
therefore have had the rectal problem
treated by a 'pull through' procedure.
Although many patients have
undoubtedly had a satisfactory result
from such a procedure it is usual to find
that bowel control is poor and that the
anal margin is not where it should be. In
simple anorectal atresia, cutaneous
pigmentation and a dimple are usually
present where the anus should be and in
adults there is the characteristic perianal
hair distribution as well. After a 'pull

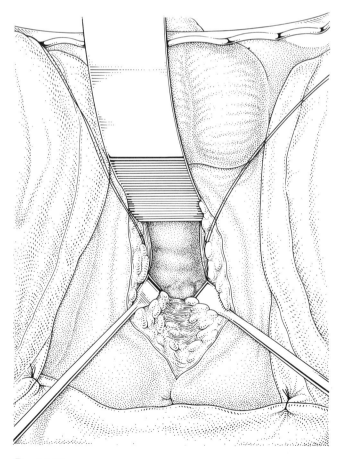

Fig. 14.50

through' the anus is usually found to be too far anterior and to one side of the midline. Furthermore, digital examination reveals that the 'rectum' runs straight through to the perineum with no attempt at formation of an ano-rectal angle and that it runs to one side or other of the pelvic musculature (when this is palpable, as it often is) rather than through it. Finally, in males, the recto-urethral fistula, usually to the prostatic urethra just below the verumontanum but sometimes to the bulbar urethra in low lesions, was often simply transected at the rectal end rather than excised, presumably to avoid damage to the membranous urethra and its innervation. This fistulous remnant is often a cause of trouble in its own right

leading to recurrent infection and stone formation.

If a patient has had an unsatisfactory result, particularly, in women, if the vagina is also unsatisfactory it is always worthwhile revising it using a Peña approach. In this type of patient a synchronous laparotomy will always be required because of adhesions and other effects of the previous surgery. In fact the exposure of the pelvic floor musculature from above gives this position a distinct advantage as the two approaches synchronously make the identification of the correct path for the colon (and vagina) to the perineum much easier. As with the Peña approach in young children careful positioning is

necessary to arrange the patient in a lithotomy position that will give adequate perineal access, and will allow adjustment to the leg supports to give differing degrees of hip flexion during the course of the procedure.

The aims of a revision procedure are the same as for a primary repair: to define the pelvic and perianal musculature as in Figure 14.50 — retracted here with stay-sutures and retractors to show the channel for the colon; to mobilise the colon and bring it through to the perineum; to reconstruct a perineal body anteriorly to the proposed anal canal (Fig. 14.51) thereby creating a good ano-rectal angle (Fig. 14.52); to reconstruct the residual perianal

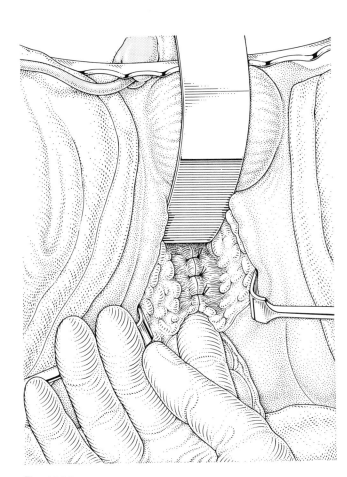

Fig. 14.51

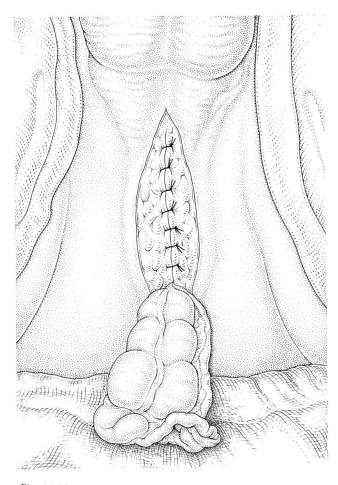

Fig. 14.52

musculature posteriorly and then put the anal margin in the spot where it should be, dividing the colon and suturing it to the skin with a little bit of tension so that it tends to retract inwards with healing rather than prolapse (Fig. 14.53). The pattern of reconstruction of the musculature, and particularly of the perineal body, as in first-time procedures, is the factor that gives an adequate ano-rectal angle and therefore the best chance of a satisfactory result. A covering colostomy is desirable.

It should be remembered that there are several causes of persistent urological problems in patients with anorectal malformations of which cloaca is but one type. This has already been mentioned but it is worth restating. Coincidental urinary tract anomalies of both the upper and the lower urinary tracts are common, particularly affecting the ureter, and so are sacral spinal anomalies and associated or unassociated anomalies of the spinal cord and its nerve roots. The peripheral innervation of the bladder may have been damaged by previous anorectal surgery, particularly in male patients. The space-occupying effect of the vagina seems to protect the pelvic plexuses in girls to some extent. Persistent infection, stone formation and even persistence of the fistula as a result of failure to deal adequately with the urethral end of a high fistula in males has been alluded to above. The alternative of an overzealous attack on the posterior urethra may of course cause a stricture. All of these are common problems, particularly ureteric problems and neuropathic bladder dysfunction, and should be considered in all patients who have had an unsatisfactory result from previous treatment, either as a consequence of that treatment or as primary abnormalities.

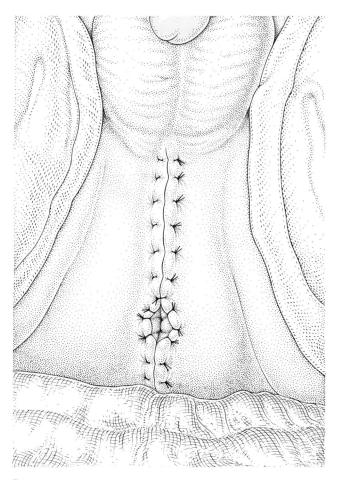

Fig. 14.53

THE FAILED EXSTROPHY/EPISPADIAS REPAIR

One of the great things about paediatric urology is that when the patient reaches the age of 16 or thereabouts he or she automatically becomes somebody else's problem — later if the procedure has been a success, earlier if it has not. In the late teens all types of urological recidivists begin to emerge from the woodwork. This process is magnified by the desire of the teenager to be as normal as possible, particularly when sexual function or performance are in any way threatened and when body image is involved.

The exstrophy/epispadias cripple in his or her late teens is therefore a recurring challenge in reconstructive surgery particularly as many of them are overweight from years of being dietetically pampered by protective parents who have attempted to compensate them for their deformities in the only way they seem to know how — overfeeding. Many are also emotionally bitter and twisted following multiple surgical procedures that have failed to produce the pelvis of their dreams.

The first thing to be impressed on these patients (gently and tactfully) is that they will never be normal. It may well be possible to give them a functioning urinary tract and genital tract but it will be functional, not normal. The urinary tract may depend on CISC or an artificial sphincter. The penis will be short and stumpy, the vagina short and prone to prolapse and neither a thing of beauty. In addition the abdominal scarring will not go away. All this is important to discuss because many patients, whether they say so or not, are hoping to be normal.

The uncertainties of further surgery need to be discussed, particularly with women with a urinary diversion because minor degrees of incontinence after an otherwise successful undiversion may be more of a problem than the diversion they have become accustomed to and that has given them total perineal dryness. This is particularly important in women because further pelvic surgery may compromise fertility (which may otherwise be entirely normal) by producing adhesions. Indeed, in my opinion, women who have established a sex life despite the psychological problems of their deformity and diversion should be positively advised not to have any further surgery until they have had any children they may wish to have. Obviously this question is more of a problem in those women who regard their deformity/diversion as a barrier to establishing a sexual relationship in the first place.

In some patients alternatives to reconstruction should be discussed. In male patients with failed exstrophy closure and no urethra or tissue with which to make a urethra, a continent diversion or conduit diversion should be considered, if they are not already diverted, because of the problems of neourethroplasty in such a situation.

General considerations

Because of the range of problems that may be encountered it is impossible to do other than generalise but certain reconstructive principles can be stated:

1. Never throw away bladder.
2. It is easier to make a bladder than a urethra.
3. It is safer to make an incontinent bladder outflow in males because of the uncertainties of catheterisability of a surgically constructed (long, curved) male neourethra. Females are more reliably catheterisable.
4. Always aim to deal with the whole pelvis. Don't leave different organ systems to different subspecialists, because one procedure may compromise others.
5. Never tamper with a functioning genital tract, no matter how unappealing it looks, for fear of disturbing that function.
6. Always expect to have to go back so leave the pelvis as you would hope to find it and don't burn your boats as far as any possible back-up salvage procedures are concerned.

From these general principles the following surgical practicalities follow:

1. If there is a small bladder remnant and a urethra of satisfactory length and calibre albeit with an incompetent sphincter mechanism, keep the remnant as a bladder base onto which a substitution cystoplasty can be anastomosed.

2. If there is a small bladder remnant and no urethra or an unsatisfactory urethra then tubularise the bladder remnant to form a urethra in females or as much of a urethra as possible in males. It may be possible to create a continence mechanism in this way but even if it is not this may be the only tissue that is sufficiently thick and sufficiently vascularised to be capable of withstanding a pressurised artificial sphincter cuff.

3. If there is a good-sized bladder and no urethra then a bladder flap urethroplasty is the best form of neourethroplasty, retaining the rest of the bladder as a base to which a substitution cystoplasty can be anastomosed. This particularly applies to females but can be used in either sex.

4. Always wrap a bladder neck reconstruction or neourethroplasty with omentum and consider the use of an AUS cuff as a back-up.

5. If no other tissue is available then, in females, some other catheterisable tube should be used as a urethra with a flap valve or tunnelled anastomosis to the inevitable substitution cystoplasty to give a continence mechanism. Suitable catheterisable tubes include the ureter if

one or other is sufficiently long, the gut (especially the colon — the most generally useful) and a labial skin tube as a last resort. The appendix could also be used but has usually been removed.

6.   In male patients there is often usable penile skin and if there is then it should be used for neourethroplasty — the help of a Michaelangelo may be necessary for its construction.

7.   A urothelial or buccal mucosa tube, if available, is another option for neuroethroplasty but if the bladder is a good enough size for this then a pedicled bladder flap will probably be possible in which case it can often replace most of the urethra as far as the glans and is preferable to a urothelial free graft — another reason for not throwing the bladder away.

8.   Female exstrophy patients have a short horizontally running vagina and a cervix more on the anterior wall of the vagina than in its vault and often require introitoplasty. An over-enthusiastic posterior flap vaginoplasty to enlarge the introitus may end up giving a major degree of prolapse, so proceed cautiously.

9.   Male exstrophy/epispadias patients have a short stubby penis with a marked dorsal chordee in addition to the obvious urethral, meatal and glanular abnormality. It is tempting to correct this chordee surgically because of its appearance but this temptation should be resisted if the patient is able to have intercourse without much difficulty (assuming the patient is of an appropriate age) for fear of interfering with potency. Don't be too bashful (or inconsiderate) to ask the relevant questions.

10.   As always suture lines should be kept apart and wrapped with omentum (or labial fat pads) as far as possible.

EXSTROPHY/EPISPADIAS IN THE MALE

The vesicourethral problem

There are three aspects to this — the bladder, the urethra and the continence mechanism. For sexual reasons — to preserve ejaculation — whatever urinary tract there was is likely to have been preserved even if there is a urinary diversion, so there is at least something to work with. A 'cystectomy' in males is rare, unlike in females.

Previous surgery will have attempted to produce a closed urinary tract, an obstructive prostatic urethra and a urethra on the dorsum of the penis down to the glans. The most likely problems to be encountered when primary reconstruction as a neonate has failed to give a satisfactory result are a small bladder, an incompetent bladder neck and a urethra that is too short (because of the coexisting dorsal chordee), too irregular (so that it cannot easily be catheterised) and ending on the dorsum of the glans rather than the tip, often with multiple fistulae along its length.

The small bladder is easily corrected by augmentation cystoplasty if its current capacity is 200 ml or more, or by substitution cystoplasty if it is less than 200 ml, bearing in mind that capacity will be reduced if bladder tissue is used for urethroplasty. If the bladder capacity is 200 ml or more, the bladder itself is supple and of normal compliance, there is no significant outflow resistance and bladder is not going to be used for a urethroplasty, then simply producing an adequate outflow resistance may cause the bladder to expand to a sufficient capacity, making augmentation unnecessary. Unfortunately I have seen this happy combination only once — all that was required was an artificial sphincter.

Adequate outflow resistance can be produced in two ways: either by a bladder neck/prostatic urethral reconstruction or by implantation of an artificial sphincter at that site. If the bladder neck is grossly patulous then a reconstruction combined with an omental and AUS cuff wrap procedure is probably the best bet so that, if this in itself does not give continence, the remainder of the AUS can be implanted at a later date without having to reopen the pelvis. Obviously it is best if an AUS can be avoided but until you are regularly achieving good results with bladder neck reconstruction alone it is safer to add an AUS cuff as a back-up to avoid the need to reopen the pelvis to implant it at a later date if it proves necessary.

Achieving a urethra of even calibre and adequate length that opens at the tip of the glans is more of a problem. The two ends are not usually difficult to deal with because there is usually sufficient epithelial tissue in the prostatic urethra and in the glans to roll in to form a tube, and sufficient prostatic and glanular tissue to overclose. The difficulty lies in between. Even if there is an even calibred urethra between, this may not be of sufficient length when the dorsal chordee has been corrected.

There are four sources of tissue for a urethroplasty which are, in order of preference: penile skin, bladder in the form of a pedicled tube, scrotal skin, and free grafts of urothelium if present or buccal mucosa or non-genital skin if it is not. All of these except buccal mucosa and non-genital skin are likely to be in short supply, particularly penile skin. Even if penile skin looks like a viable option at the start of the operation, there may not be enough to go round at the end when all the available skin of the penis and scrotum may be needed to close the various incisions without tension (see below). For this reason a bladder tube neourethra may be preferable if there is a relatively well preserved bladder but if the bladder is totally inadequate then penile skin may have to be used and some alternative found for penile wound closure—usually a scrotal flap. In fact in many situations some of the existing urethra can be retained and then revised or supplemented with penile skin or (less frequently) urothelium or buccal mucosa as it seems most appropriate. There is rarely a need to use free grafts other than urothelium or buccal mucosa, and all free grafts should be avoided if possible.

The genital problem

There are three aspects to this as well—the cosmetic problem of the appearance of the glans and the mons pubis, the length of the penis and the dorsal chordee. There is usually an epispadiac, splayed open glans, dense suprapubic scarring with separation of the hairbearing areas of the prepubic skin, a short stubby penis and marked dorsal chordee on erection that may be so severe that intercourse is impossible.

It is relatively easy to correct the deformity of the glans and the dorsal chordee, and it is usually possible to excise the scarring and approximate the hairbearing skin of the mons. Improving the length of the penis beyond the apparent increase in length achieved by correcting the chordee cannot be safely or reliably produced, although various manoeuvres to achieve this have been described. For these reasons and because it would be a catastrophe if a previously potent male was rendered impotent as a complication of surgery for chordee, genital surgery should not be undertaken in potent males except to correct the cosmetic defects.

The deformity of the glans is corrected by a variation of John Duckett's MAGPI procedure which Philip Ransley has described and called an IPGAM. The tip of the splayed open glans is incised along its length and closed transversely which has the double effect of putting the meatus more ventrally, to the tip of the glans, when it is subsequently closed, and simultaneously of advancing the intraglanular urethral epithelium at the proximal end of the incision to the tip of the penis. (It is easier to do than to describe.) The epithelium is then mobilised from the underlying spongy tissue of the glans and rolled in to form the distal end of the urethra; spongy tissue of the glans is then approximated to overclose the urethra; and the glanular skin is then closed to produce a near-normal appearance.

The defect between each half of the hairbearing skin of the mons is closed by a W-shaped incision that excises the midline scarring between the long central limbs of the W and raises the hairbearing skin as widely mobilised flaps on either side. Wide mobilisation and undermining of the surrounding skin is necessary to allow closure of the mons in the midline without tension (which would reproduce the defect).

The chordee is corrected, when necessary, by incision and division of the fibrous tissue on the dorsum of the corpora cavernosa deformity. With the corpora exposed and the neurovascular bundles on their dorsolateral aspects safely retracted or otherwise observed to be out of the way, an artificial erection is produced. As there is no communication between the corpora in exstrophy/epispadias a butterfly needle must be inserted into each of the corpora. Saline is then injected on each side to produce the chordee so that the exact point of the restriction can be defined. This is then incised transversely on each side, through the fibrosis but not into the cavernous tissue, until repeat saline infusion shows a straight erection. These incisions leave elliptical defects on the dorsum of each corpus cavernosum which can be dealt with in one of two ways. Either the two defects can be sutured together, which has the effect of rolling the corpora inwards towards each other, or, if this is not possible or causes an unacceptable degree of buckling on the lateral aspect of each corpus, the defects can be closed individually with a patch of suitable tissue. Various types of tissue have been used for this purpose—I prefer to use a free graft of dermis.

A 'typical' procedure

Having described the various possibilities in outline, a 'typical' procedure will now be described giving details of the various techniques that may be required that have not been described elsewhere in this volume. For details of the techniques of cystoplasty or undiversion the reader is referred to the appropriate chapters.

The best results are obtained when the pelvic ring is closed anteriorly by means of bilateral pelvic osteotomies as described by Salter, a Canadian orthopaedic surgeon. With this technique a transverse osteotomy is made on each side of the pelvis just above the acetabulum which allows medial rotation of the anterior pelvic ring which in turn allows closure of the pubic symphysis. This is performed as a preliminary to the procedure through separate bilateral supratrochanteric incisions before the urologist begins. Then at the end of the reconstruction the orthopaedic surgeon reappears and puts the patient in plaster. This is a recent introduction in the treatment of exstrophy and it certainly helps in younger children, particularly in gaining the maximum available length of the penis in boys. It also obviously helps in wound closure. Whether or not it gives much advantage in older children and adolescents remains to be seen as nobody (that I know of) has had much experience with it. It certainly has a place—time will tell exactly what that place will be.

Preparation

As with all major reconstructive procedures the urine should be sterile and the bowel prepared. Blood loss can be considerable, particularly during the phalloplasty, so 4 units of blood should be cross matched (for an adult-sized adolescent).

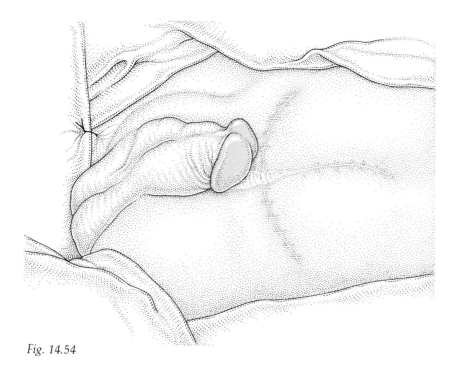

Fig. 14.54

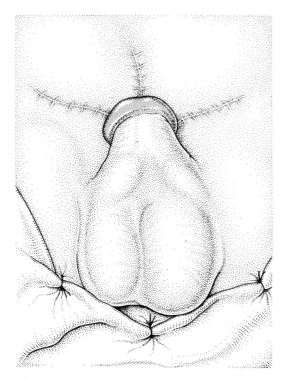

Fig. 14.55

Position

The patient should be in the low lithotomy position with drapes placed for a full length midline incision (Figs 14.54, 14.55).

Procedure

The midline abdominal scarring from the central abdomen (there is no umbilicus) down to the base of the penis is excised. At the end of the operation, when it is time to close the skin, the incision will need to be converted to a 'W' with extensive undermining of the skin to allow closure without tension. The full 'W' incision is unnecessary at this early stage. If necessary, as in this illustrative case, the lower end of the incision is extended along the dorsum of the shaft of the penis to excise the scarring there as well (Figs 14.56, 14.57).

The incision is then deepened carefully to expose the bladder, prostate and urethra bearing in mind that these are all very superficial. A urethral catheter aids identification if one can be passed.

A decision then has to be made as to how much of the urethra can be preserved. There is usually at least a short length proximally, below the verumontanum and the previously closed prostatic urethra that is smooth and regular albeit patulous. As much as can be preserved, should be preserved. Any unsatisfactory urethra is excised.

The epithelium that covers the dorsal surface of the glans, if the glans has not been closed previously, or the ventral aspect of the glanular urethra, if it has, is usually in good condition and should also be preserved so that it can subsequently be fashioned to form the distal urethra.

Sometimes the ventral wall of the urethra is satisfactory throughout its length and all the irregularities and false passages are on its dorsal aspect. In these instances the urethra is opened dorsally throughout its length, excising

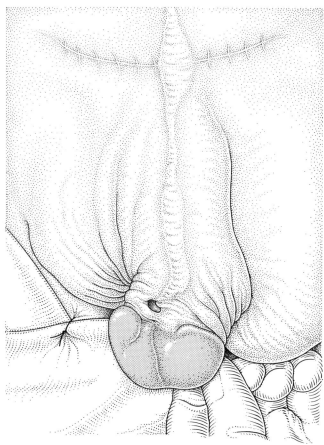

Fig. 14.56

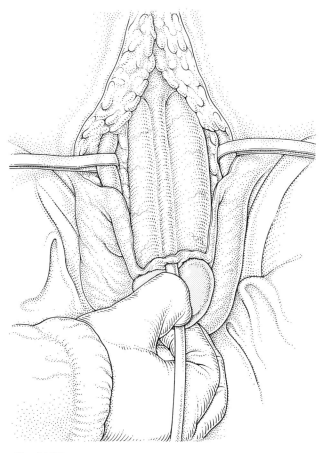

Fig. 14.57

the irregularities, leaving an epithelial strip from the prostate to the glans which can later be closed to give a regular neourethra. Occasionally the urethra is entirely satisfactory and does not need to be opened up at all. Nonetheless, it may still be too short once the dorsal chordee has been corrected in which case the urethra will need to be divided at the site of maximum curvature (Fig. 14.58) to allow correction of the chordee. The gap will then be filled with a tube graft of the appropriate length. If the urethra is hopelessly inadequate it will need to be excised.

The next step is to demonstrate and, if necessary, correct the chordee. This is demonstrated by producing an artificial erection. A butterfly needle is pushed into each corpus cavernosum and sterile saline is infused. This produces an

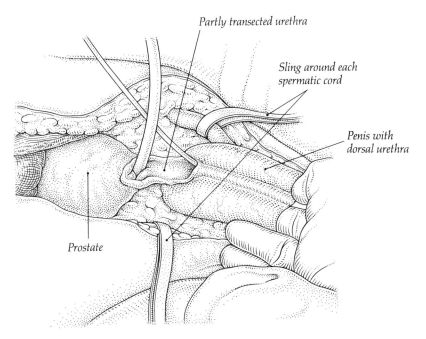

Partly transected urethra

Sling around each
spermatic cord

Penis with
dorsal urethra

Prostate

Fig. 14.58

erection and demonstrates the chordee in general and the site of maximum curvature in particular (Fig. 14.59). This site is usually 1–2 cm below the verumontanum at the point where the corpora diverge towards their bony attachments. Between the corpora at this point and immediately deep to the urethral epithelium (if it has been preserved) is the spongy tissue that represents all that remains in exstrophy of the bulb of the corpus spongiosum.

Before incising the fibrosed dorsal walls of the corpora to release the chordee, assuming this proves to be necessary, all the superficial subcutaneous tissue is reflected laterally. This exposes the neurovascular bundles to the glans on the dorsolateral aspect of each corpus which must be positively identified and if necessary retracted out of the way to reduce the risk of damage. When this has been done, the wall of the corpus cavernosum is incised on each side around the dorsal half of the circumference of each, taking care not to enter the erectile tissue any more than is absolutely necessary (Fig. 14.60). Even with all due care there can be a considerable amount of bleeding during this manoeuvre. This usually stops when

the defects are closed although more substantial bleeders may need to be stitched. Diathermy should not be used — it never works and does more harm than good. The adequacy of these releasing incisions in the corporal walls is checked by a repeat artificial erection dividing more tissue if necessary until the erection is straight.

The defects in the walls of the corpora can be closed in one of two ways. If the corpora are fairly slim and of equal size, and when the corporotomy incisions are mainly medial then they can be separated and rolled in so that the defects can be sutured together with interrupted 3/0 Vicryl sutures (Figs 14.61, 14.62). This tends to cause buckling of the lateral aspects of the corpora if the corporotomy incisions

extend more laterally so care must be taken to ensure that this is not excessive. If there is excessive buckling, or if the corpora are more substantial, or if there is considerable disproportion in size between the two corpora, then the defects must be closed with a patch. My preference for this is a free graft of dermis.

The preferred donor sites for a dermal graft are from the skin of the femoral triangle, the inner aspect of the upper arm or the flexor aspect of the forearm. A patch is outlined that will give two generous patches for the corporal defects. The word generous should be emphasised. The patch is incised down to the dermal layer of the skin but not through it (Fig. 14.63) and the epidermis is removed with a scalpel (Fig. 14.64).

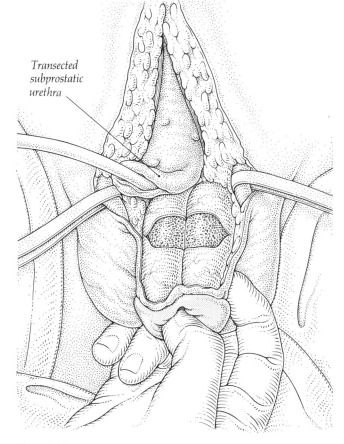

Transected subprostatic urethra

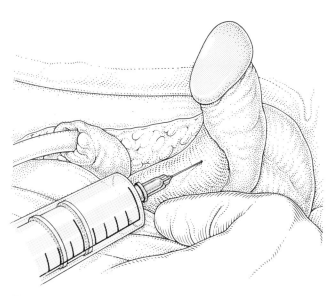

Fig. 14.59

Fig. 14.60

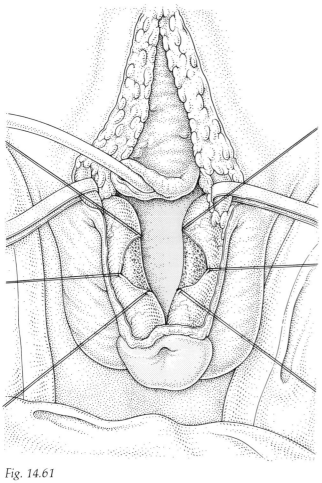

Fig. 14.61

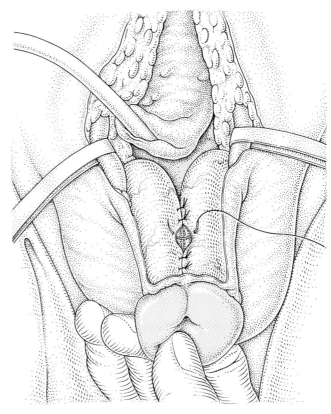

Fig. 14.62

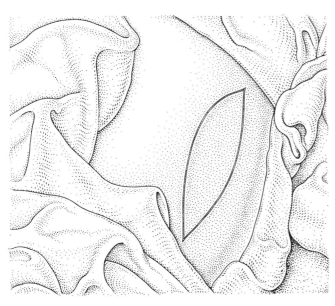

Fig. 14.63

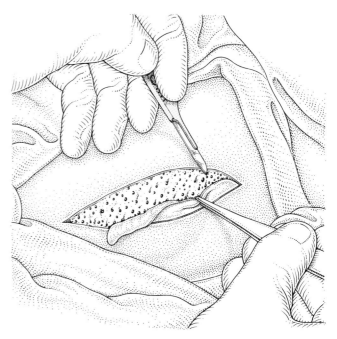

Fig. 14.64

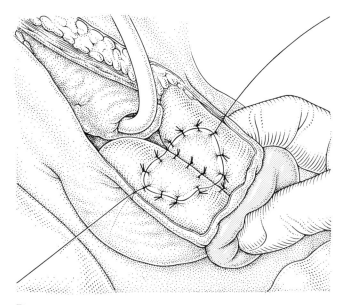

Fig. 14.65

The plane (although it is not a true tissue plane) between the epidermis and the dermis is fairly easy to define, but it usually takes three or four changes of the scalpel blade to dissect the epidermis off. When the epidermis has been removed the dermal patch is dissected away from the subcutaneous fat and pinned out on a board with the epidermal aspect face-down so that any subdermal connective tissue can be trimmed off. The graft is then divided in two and fashioned into two generous oval patches, one for each corporal defect, which are then sewn in place with closely spaced interrupted sutures (Fig. 14.65).

The next step is to reconstruct the bladder neck and the prostatic and proximal urethra using the technique

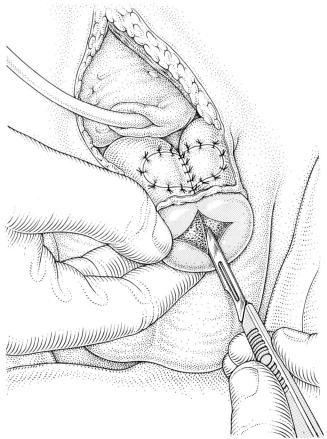

Fig. 14.66

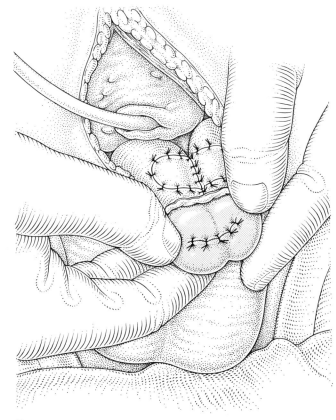

Fig. 14.67

described on pages 244—246 for adult males and on pages 295—296 for young females. This, in an adult-sized patient, should snugly accept a 16 F catheter or bougie (12 F in a smaller child). Any more patulous and it should be trimmed and reconstructed in two layers around a catheter of that size and the reconstruction should be tested by catheterisation to ensure its regularity. It is usual to find that at the original closure operation in early life the prostate and bladder neck were not properly mobilised and dropped back into the pelvis. As a result, not only is the whole urinary tract very superficial with an irregular lumen, but the anterior wall of the bladder neck and prostatic urethra are very thin as a result of being pulled together for closure without adequate mobilisation laterally. If this is the case the bladder neck and prostate should be opened and mobilised on their lateral aspects so that they can be closed to give an adequate bulk of tissue anteriorly.

The glans is then refashioned to give a distal urethral segment, a normally sited meatus and a normal appearance to the glans itself. The first step is to site the meatus. The tip of the flattened epispadiac glans is incised down into the underlying spongy tissue until the distal and ventral extent of the incision corresponds to a normal site for the meatus (Fig. 14.66). This vertical incision is then closed horizontally with three interrupted 4/0 or 5/0 sutures to restore epithelial continuity (Fig. 14.67). Two vertical incisions are then made through the skin on the dorsal aspect of the glans to outline a midline strip slightly more than 1.5 cm wide which when rolled inwards will form a glanular urethra which will accept a 16 or 18 F catheter snugly. Before it is closed in this way, the skin of the rest of the dorsum of the glans is excised so that the spongy tissue of the glans can be closed over the distal neourethra to give a normal appearance (Fig. 14.68). The skin of the glans is closed with fine mattress sutures or preferably a subcuticular suture to ensure eversion of the skin edges.

The gap between the two ends of the urethra must now be bridged using either a pedicled penile skin flap, a broad-based pedicled bladder tube graft or some type of free graft (preferably urothelial). The problems of each have been mentioned already. If there is enough penile skin both for the urethroplasty and for skin closure this is the easiest and best tissue to use for the urethroplasty. A skin strip is usually taken from the lateral edge of the penile

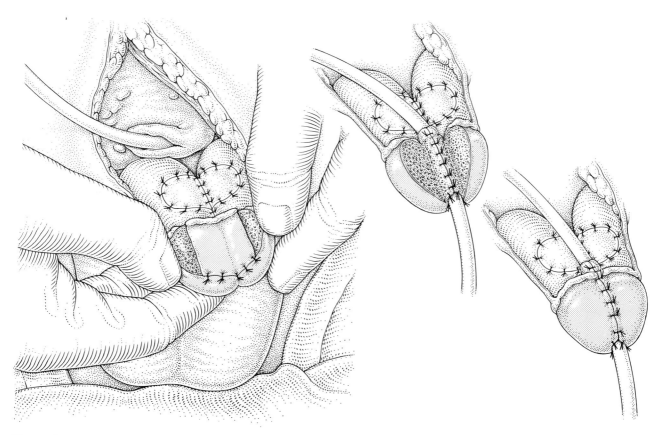

Fig. 14.68

skin incision using the dartos layer as the vascular pedicle (Fig. 14.69). If there is not enough skin then a bladder flap is the most expendable tissue. If a bladder flap of sufficient length is not possible then a urothelial free graft may still be possible. If none of these alone will bridge the gap then the skin of the hitherto undisturbed ventral aspect of the penis will be necessary.

To put these comments into persepective: if the previous urethral closure in early childhood has given a smooth regular lumen, and the only gap is that produced by division of the urethra to correct the chordee, then the gap between the two ends will be about 2−3 cm. If, on the other hand, the entire urethra from the verumontanum to the glans is unsatisfactory and needs to be completely replaced the gap will usually be 5−8 cm. Given that the proximal urethra down to the verumontanum is about 3 cm long, a bladder flap neourethroplasty will require a bladder flap which is at least 6−7 cm long (with the epithelium preserved on the distal 2−3 cm of the flap) to bridge a short gap, or 10−12 cm to bridge a long gap. This requires a fair-sized bladder although it is quite often feasible. Alternatively, if penile skin is to be used the requirement is for a strip 2−8 cm long and a little over 1.5 cm wide to give a neourethra of 16 F calibre. The width is the problem. Although there is easily enough skin on the ventral aspect of the penis for this, using this skin makes subsequent skin closure much more difficult and may also jeopardise the vascularity of the whole block of penile skin, bearing in mind the dissection so far and the mobilisation that will be necessary in addition to close the existing skin incisions.

If a bladder flap is chosen for a full length urethroplasty, this must be broad-based and laterally-based on one of the two lateral pedicles to get the best possible vascularity. The bladder is easily augmented or substituted with

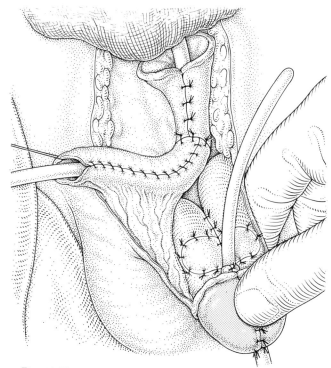

Fig. 14.69

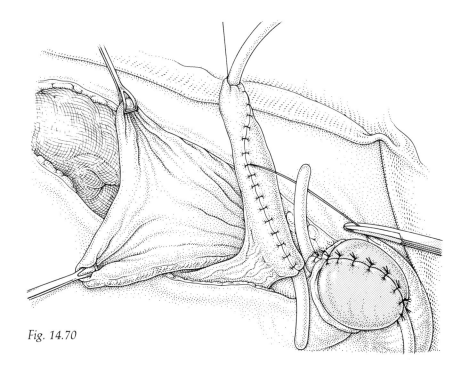

Fig. 14.70

bowel so there is no need to save bladder as bladder — all efforts should be made to get a good wide flap of adequate length to make a satisfactory urethra. When the flap has been mobilised on one of the lateral pedicles the urothelium is trimmed to size and rolled into a tube around a 16 F catheter in the usual way. The tube is closed in two layers, an inner urothelial layer and an outer detrusor layer (Fig. 14.70).

A gap of suitable size to accept the flap is then created between the corpora at the point where they diverge, proximal to the site of correction of the chordee at the apex of the proximal urethra (Fig. 14.71) if such a gap is not already present as a result of separating the corpora to correct the chordee. This, as was noted earlier, is where the spongy tissue of the bulb lies and this may bleed to an annoying degree. When a gap of suitable size has been created there a similar sized gap is made between the corpora just proximal to the glans of sufficient size for the anastomosis of the distal end of the bladder tube to the distal urethra. The proximal anastomosis is performed first, the flap is then pulled through to the ventral aspect of the penis (Fig. 14.72), and distal anastomosis of the bladder urothelial tube to the glanular urethra completes the urethroplasty (Fig. 14.73). Obviously this is all much easier if the corpora have previously been separated as part of the procedure to correct the chordee but it does not necessarily follow that it is best to separate the corpora in all instances as this may cause unnecessary disturbance to the subcutaneous supporting tissue of the ventral penile skin and unfortunate consequences. Each case must be decided on its merits.

If adequate skin is available on the dorsal aspect of the penis then it is fashioned into a tube in the usual way as described above but with this technique the neourethra will often have to be on the dorsal aspect of the penis if

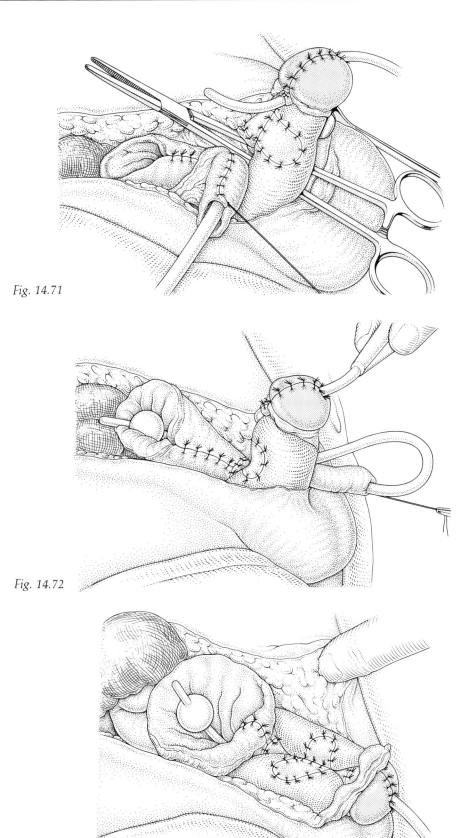

Fig. 14.71

Fig. 14.72

Fig. 14.73

the disposition of the vascular pedicle of the skin prevents placement of the urethra ventrally. For the same reason, and also to avoid excessive mobilisation of the distal urethra, simply bridging a short gap will leave the urethra on the dorsal aspect of the penis. Where possible, however, the urethra should be sited ventrally — a ventral urethra gives a better cosmetic appearance and helps to maintain chordee correction.

I have only once used a urothelial free graft in exstrophy revision as in all the other instances when there was sufficient bladder for a urothelial graft, there was sufficient for a pedicled bladder tube. On that one occasion there was excessive perivesical scarring but the posterior bladder wall was not involved. The urothelium was harvested from the posterior bladder wall. A 16 F urethral catheter was passed up the glans and out onto the dorsal aspect of the penis; the urothelial graft was rolled around the catheter and sutured with a running stitch; the distal anastomosis was performed; the catheter with the graft was then re-routed to the ventral aspect of the penis into a prepared tunnel and then brought up to the proximal urethra for the proximal anastomosis between the diverging corpora.

When the ventral penile skin has to be used, usually because of severe scarring on the dorsum of the penis, a midline strip of adequate length and a little over 1.5 cm wide is incised through skin alone, rolled into a tube and closed with a running stitch over a 16 F catheter (Fig. 14.74). The two ends are anastomosed to each end of the urethra between the corpora as described above. To avoid further dissection involving the penile subcutaneous tissue and the risks of both excessive tension and fistula formation by attempting to close the penile skin directly over the neourethra it is safest to extend the skin incisions at the base of the penis as a single incision down the scrotal raphe and then stitch the penile skin to the scrotal skin (Fig. 14.75) or alternatively to rotate a scrotal skin flap upwards to close the defect. It is then a simple matter at a later date to free the penis

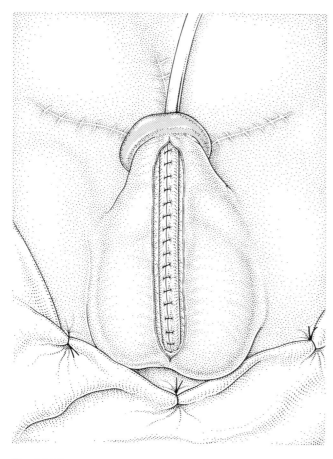

Fig. 14.74

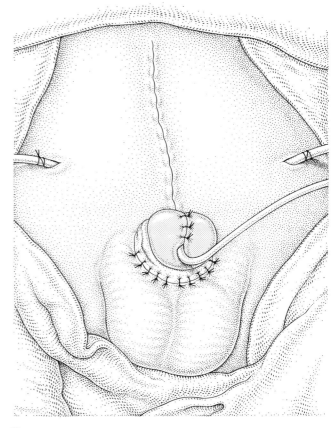

Fig. 14.75

from its scrotal bed and close the skin, either directly if there is enough penile skin or incorporating scrotal skin onto the ventral aspect of the shaft of the penis, if there is not sufficient. The advantages of this are that ventral penile skin is usually readily available and that the incision to create the neourethra acts effectively as a relieving incision to facilitate skin closure on the dorsum of the penis. The disadvantage is that the neourethra is rather mobile which makes self catheterisation difficult if it proves to be necessary.

With the chordee corrected, a normal glans fashioned and the urethroplasty performed, three manoeuvres remain to be done before the skin can be closed: the bladder is augmented or substituted as necessary, the omentum is mobilised to wrap the bladder and proximal urethral closures, and for security an artificial sphincter cuff is wrapped around the bladder neck (with the tubing plugged off and buried subcutaneously in the groin) to augment the bladder neck/prostatic urethral reconstruction and to be connected to the rest of the AUS components if they subsequently prove to be necessary.

To close the skin and approximate the hairbearing areas of the skin of the mons the long inverted V of the original skin incision is converted into a W by extending the lower end of the incision under the hairbearing area, up towards the anterior superior iliac spin on each side. The skin flaps on each side are then undermined (Fig. 14.76 — in this example an untidy lower transverse incision has also been excised). This undermining should be extensive on the abdominal wall centrally, less so in the groin in an attempt to preserve the ascending subcutaneous branches of the femoral artery. With this undermining it is relatively easy to close the abdominal skin in the midline (Fig. 14.77). Closing the medial aspects of the groin incision often requires upward mobilisation of the scrotal skin on either side of the

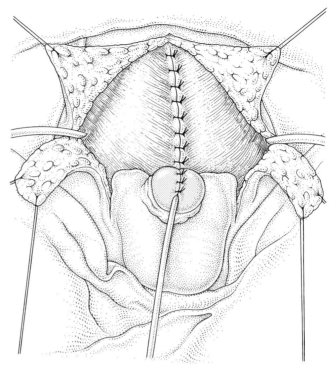

Fig. 14.76

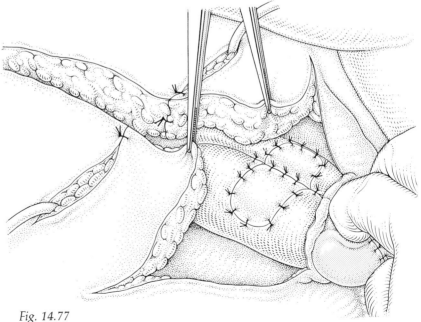

Fig. 14.77

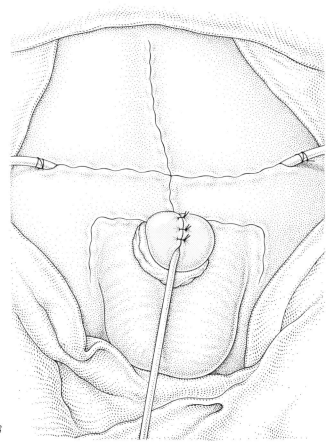

Fig. 14.78

base of the penis (Fig. 14.78). The penis itself should be closed in two layers, the first layer closing the subcutaneous tissue carefully, particularly over the two urethroplasty anastomoses (the distal anastomosis to the glandular urethra is especially vulnerable to fistula formation otherwise), the second layer closing the skin.

Further management
At the end of the procedure the patient is left with a urethral and a suprapubic catheter. As after all urethroplasties, the urethral catheter is removed after about three weeks when there is radiological demonstration of satisfactory healing. The suprapubic catheter is removed after a satisfactory trial of voiding.

For the first week or so there is usually a considerable amount of oedema. Indeed, the penis looks ghastly. This settles quite quickly.

The main problems are urethral fistula formation, particularly on the dorsal aspect of the corona down to the distal urethral anastomosis to the glanular urethra, urethral stricture and incontinence. Urethral stricture formation is not as common as might be expected given the problems of reconstruction. If follow-up radiological studies show a stricture, urethral dilatation followed by a period of self catheterisation (i.e. self dilatation) daily then weekly then monthly will usually control the problem. If not a revision procedure will be necessary — another reason for trying to preserve the ventral penile skin intact.

Incontinence is usually shown urodynamically to be stress incontinence which is treated by implantation of the remainder of the artificial sphincter. Occasionally one sees outflow obstruction with overflow incontinence

which is treated by intermittent self catheterisation.

Recurrent chordee and impotence are potential problems but — fortunately — I have not yet encountered either.

EXSTROPHY IN THE FEMALE

The problem of failed neonatal exstrophy closure in females is more straightforward, if not simpler, than in males — firstly because the genital problem is less complicated and secondly because the vesicourethral problem is easier to treat (because the urethra is shorter). Female patients are also more likely to have had their residual incontinence treated by urinary diversion. Whereas it is common to find semi-continent males, or males with a diversion but with the non-functioning lower urinary tract left in situ to preserve genital function, and very few who have had a cystectomy, this is not the case in females. If closure has not given a good functional result it is common for girls to have had the exstrophic bladder excised at the time of diversion or subsequently for pyocystis or simply for cosmetic reasons.

The vesicourethral problem
In the unusual circumstance of an exstrophic girl who has had a partially successful closure but who has a significant degree of sphincter weakness incontinence the vesicourethral problem may most easily be treated by implantation of an artificial sphincter with or without an augmentation cystoplasty to improve bladder capacity. That aside, the usual situation is of a girl with a diversion and a vesicourethral pit or cavity of variable but not very substantial size. Thus although in theory there are three aspects to the lower urinary tract problem in girls, as in boys — the bladder, the urethra and the continence mechanism — in practice there is usually little to find anatomically that can be defined as such.

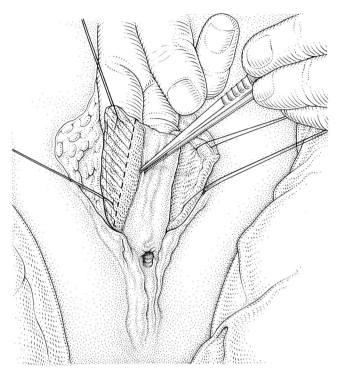

Fig. 14.79

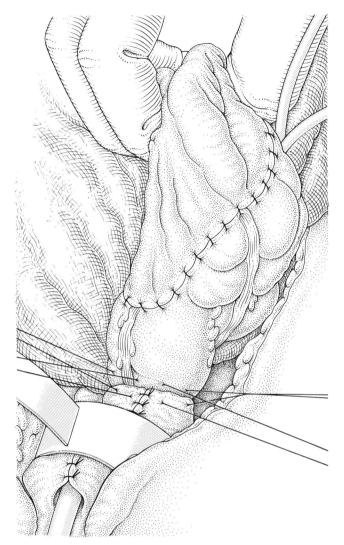

Fig. 14.81

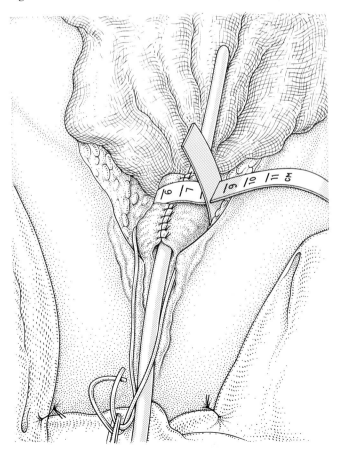

Fig. 14.80

What urothelially lined remnant there is is usually only sufficient for urethral reconstruction, if that. When possible the 'bladder' should be opened up and trimmed to form a base plate that can be rolled to form a urethra. A 1.2 cm strip of urothelium is preserved, stripping the remainder off the muscle on either side (Fig. 14.79). This is then rolled to form a tube in three layers as described above for bladder flap neourethroplasty (Fig. 14.80). A pouch type of substitution cystoplasty can then be anastomosed to the neourethra (Fig. 14.81) and a continence mechanism is usually best achieved with an

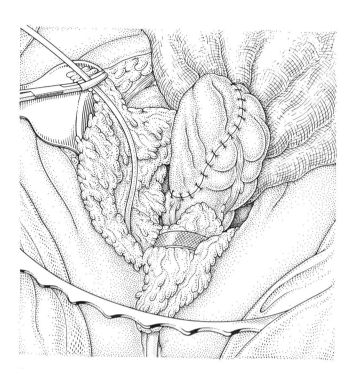

Fig. 14.82

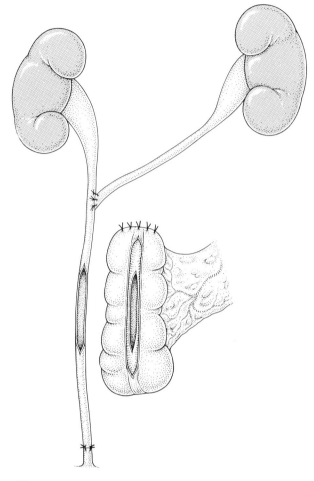

Fig. 14.84

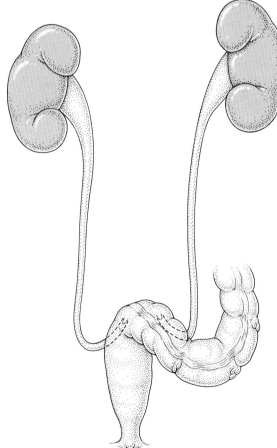

Fig. 14.83

omental/artificial sphincter wrap (Fig. 14.82), with the option of implanting the remainder of the AUS at a later date if the 'wrap' alone is insufficient. (As I have said several times already, the AUS can be omitted when you are sufficiently experienced to make your patients continent routinely without it.) As always it is important to ensure that the urethra is easily catheterisable.

If there is no bladder remnant and the patient wishes to be undiverted then suitable material will have to be found with which to make a urethra. The options that are available depend as much as anything on previous surgery. If the patient has had a ureterosigmoidostomy the ureters are often long and looped down into the

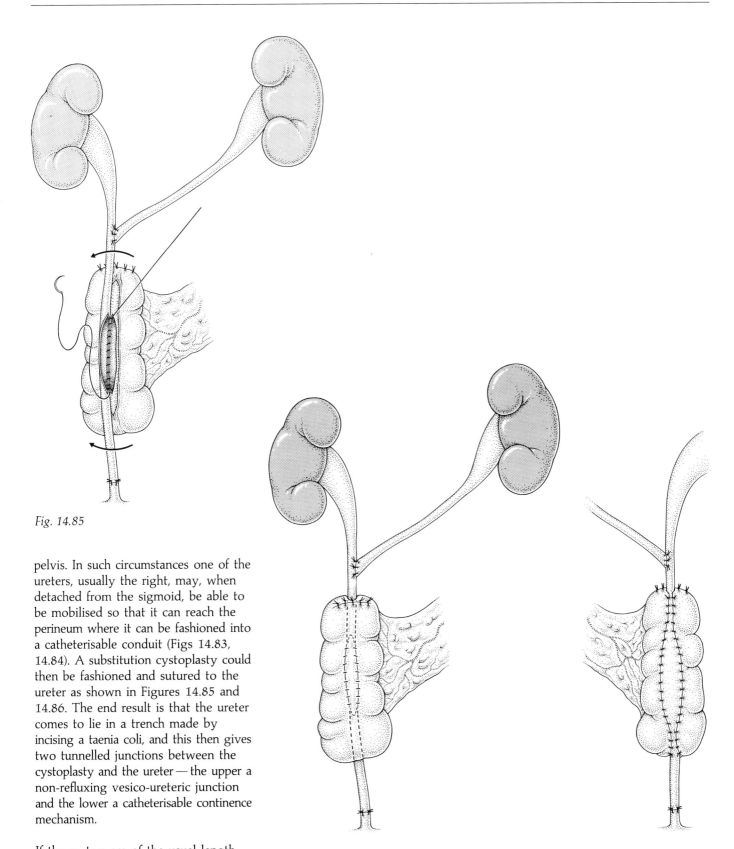

Fig. 14.85

pelvis. In such circumstances one of the ureters, usually the right, may, when detached from the sigmoid, be able to be mobilised so that it can reach the perineum where it can be fashioned into a catheterisable conduit (Figs 14.83, 14.84). A substitution cystoplasty could then be fashioned and sutured to the ureter as shown in Figures 14.85 and 14.86. The end result is that the ureter comes to lie in a trench made by incising a taenia coli, and this then gives two tunnelled junctions between the cystoplasty and the ureter — the upper a non-refluxing vesico-ureteric junction and the lower a catheterisable continence mechanism.

If the ureters are of the usual length, irrespective of the type of diversion, the

Fig. 14.86

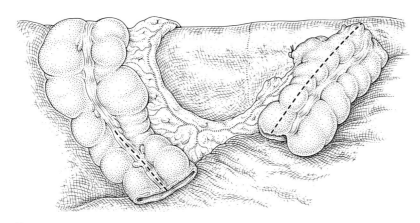

Fig. 14.87

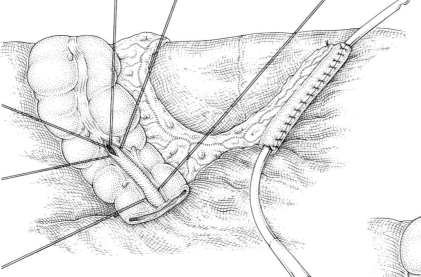

Fig. 14.88

As when described in Chapter 8, the cystourethroplasty technique illustrated on this page shows the colon un-detubularised for clarity. In fact one of the 'posterior' taeniae coli would be detubularised and patched either with adjacent ileum or the ileal conduit if there was one.

ureters could be disconnected and reimplanted into a right colonic substitution cystourethroplasty as previously described in Chapter 8. The distal end of the colonic segment is trimmed and fashioned into a tube which can then be tunnelled into the distal end of a taenia coli of the cystoplasty to form a continence mechanism (Figs 14.87–14.89).

Alternatively, if none of these choices were available in a patient diverted by means of an ileal conduit, the ileal conduit could be disconnected and rotated down to the perineum capitalising on the (usual) ease with which this can be done in a female patient with exstrophy. Similarly the transverse colon is often pendulous and, if so, the pendulous 'U' can be sutured side-to-side to form a substitution cystoplasty (Fig. 14.90). The ileal conduit

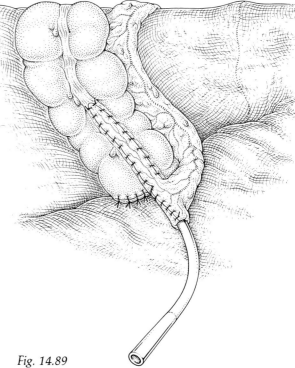

Fig. 14.89

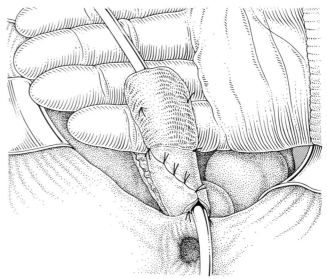

Fig. 14.91

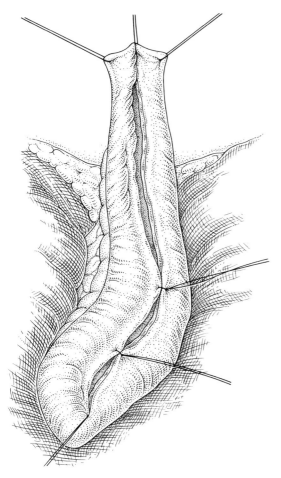

Fig. 14.90
The transverse colon is tacked together as a 'u'. The upper part will later be folded down to form a patch.

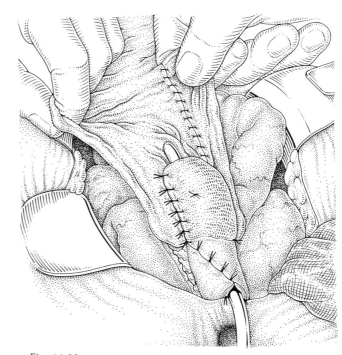

Fig. 14.92

is then trimmed to a urethra (Fig. 14.91) which can be intussuscepted into the substitution cystoplasty giving a continence mechanism (Fig. 14.92). In all of these options CISC obviously will be necessary.

The genital problem
This is less dramatic than in male patients because the genitalia are mainly internal and therefore less obvious but there may be considerable problems nonetheless.

The clitoris is bifid as in simple epispadias and the vagina is anteriorly placed, with a narrowed introitus, and lies more horizontally than normal. The cervix lies more on the anterior vaginal wall than in the vault. In addition, the entire internal female genitalia and the anorectum lack the normal support from the endopelvic fascia and the pelvic floor musculature. Thus vaginal and rectal prolapse are more common than usual.

These anatomical factors have important therapeutic implications. Bearing in mind the propensity for prolapse, reference to Figure 14.93 demonstrates how easily an over-enthusiastic cut-back introitoplasty or posterior skin flap vaginoplasty can lead to a serious degree of prolapse (Fig. 14.94). If this prolapse is then treated by some form of retropubic colposuspension procedure which pulls the uterus and vagina upwards and forwards then the deficiency of the posterior and paravaginal endopelvic fascial support thereby exposed will in turn predispose to a major degree of

rectocoele or enterocoele. Thus any narrowing of the introitus should be treated cautiously to prevent this 'vicious circle' developing. Should prolapse, particularly a severe enterocoele, require surgical intervention then it is better to hitch the vagina posteriorly up to the sacrum rather than anterolaterally to the pubic bones. In addition such a procedure will usually need to be combined with either a sigmoid colectomy or a rectopexy (or both) to reduce the risk of major rectal prolapse or enterocoele/rectocoele.

SUBSTITUTION VAGINOPLASTY IN THE MAYER–ROKITANSKY SYNDROME

This is a rare congential syndrome characterised by absence of the vagina. The ovaries and distal fallopian tubes are usually perfectly normal but the proximal tubes and the uterus are usually rudimentary. In essence you have a normal female until the labia are parted or until amenorrhoea, which is the usual presenting symptom, leads to investigation. Associated congenital anomalies of the urinary tract are not uncommon and should be looked for.

Vaginal reconstruction in these girls is best achieved by sigmoid vaginoplasty as suggested by Goligher. Some surgeons have suggested using the right colon with a technique like that of a

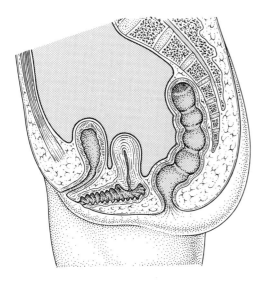

Fig. 14.93

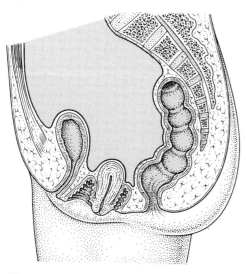

Fig. 14.94

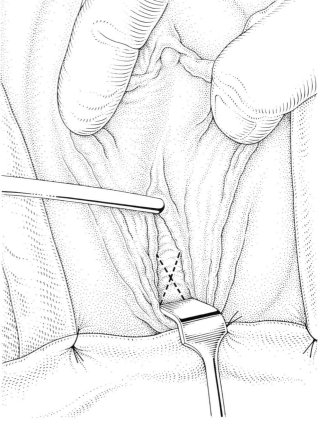

Fig. 14.95

caecocystoplasty but that generally requires a gut segment that is longer than necessary and the caecum has two additional disadvantages — it has a wider calibre and produces a more watery mucus in greater quantity than sigmoid colon therefore I prefer to use a short segment of sigmoid colon.

Generally speaking the problems with substitution vaginoplasty using gut arise because the gut segment is too long. It only needs to be 7–10 cm long bearing in mind the capacity for longitudinal stretch. Any longer and problems of excessive mucus or intra-vaginal retention of mucus (and therefore smell) arise.

Preparation
These are almost invariably fit young ladies. All that is required is adequate bowel preparation. Blood loss during the pelvic dissection may be significant so 2 units of blood should be cross matched (for an adolescent).

Position
Low lithotomy with draping for a lower midline incision and vulval incision.

Procedure
Externally the site of the introitus is usually obvious, there being a shallow pit covered by the posterior fourchette. The introitus is incised with an H-shaped or cruciate incision to open the plane between the urethra and the rectum (Figs 14.95, 14.96). The fascia that normally surrounds the vagina is present in these girls as a sheet. For obvious reasons it is safer to stay anterior to it to reduce the risk of damage to the rectum. Equally the dissection should stay in the midline to avoid damage to the pelvic plexuses.

Then, through a lower midline incision, the rudimentary uterus is mobilised and excised, opening up the plane between the bladder and rectum from above. This plane is developed to allow communication with the perineal dissection and an adequate space for the sigmoid vaginoplasty segment.

The sigmoid mesocolon is carefully inspected to identify the vascular pattern which is normally 3 or 4 loops (Fig. 14.97). The aim is to mobilise on the 1st or 2nd loop a segment of colon which is 8–10 cm long in its resting state, using the vessels of the 3rd and 4th vascular loops as an (ascending and retrograde) vascular pedicle. This will then easily rotate down into the pelvis

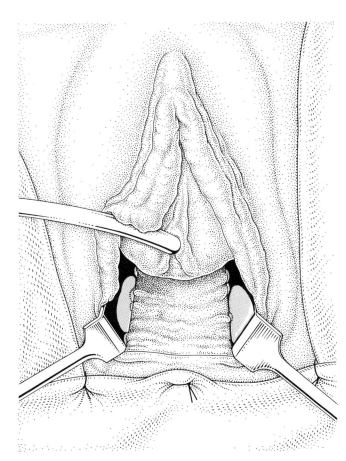

Fig. 14.96

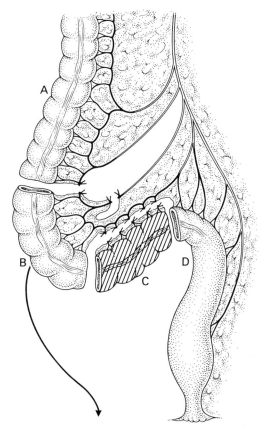

Fig. 14.97

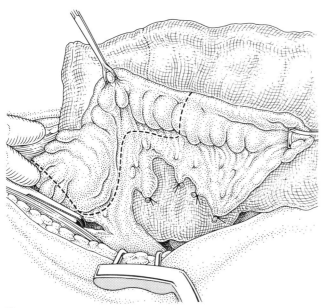

Fig. 14.98

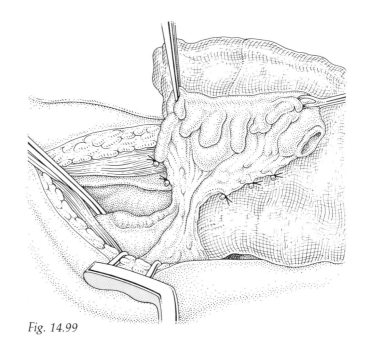

Fig. 14.99

for anastomosis to the introitus without tension. Initially the whole sigmoid colon is mobilised (Fig. 14.98). The distal half to three quarters (C in Fig. 14.97) of the bowel itself is then excised, carefully preserving the vessels (Fig. 14.99). These vessels then become the pedicle for the colovaginoplasty segment (B in Fig. 14.97). Bowel continuity is then restored by anastomosing the descending colon (A) to the rectum (D).

In a slim girl this is usually easy. In a chubby young lady with a fat sigmoid mesocolon it may be difficult to identify and mobilise the vessels. To be on the safe side, an excessive length of bowel should be mobilised and only trimmed when the bowel has been fully mobilised to the vulva.

The distal end of the sigmoid segment is anastomosed to the introitus with interrupted Vicryl sutures (Fig. 14.100) and the proximal end is closed off. The proximal end should then be tacked to adjacent structures. This helps to fix it in position, to reduce the risk of subsequent prolapse and also to help to cause retraction of the suture line into the perineum so that it is invisible and the 'vagina' is to all appearances normal.

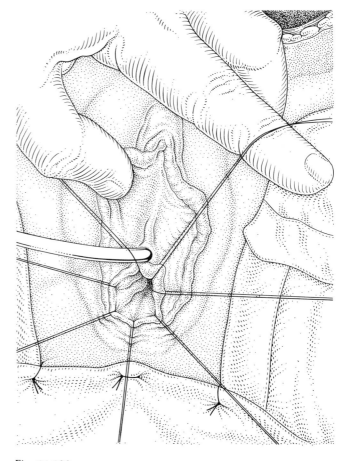

Fig. 14.100

Because there is a circumferential suture line at the introitus it is wise to let in a couple of darts of skin to prevent stenosis and for the same reason a thin paraffin gauze pack is left across the anastomosis for a few days. When that is removed a dilator is gently passed once or twice a day until healing is complete. This serves the dual purpose of preventing cross-adhesion of the suture line and psychologically accustoming the patient to vaginal penetration. More realistic activities should be deferred for about 2 months, assuming that the patient is of an appropriate age.

If the result is satisfactory at 3 months then it is most unlikely that there will be further problems thereafter so further follow up is unnecessary.

REFERENCES

Hendren's work is the prime source for urogenital sinus and cloaca problems and to a lesser extent for female epispadias. At the time of writing he has no other publications that I know of since the introduction of the Peña approach (posterior sagittal anorectoplasty), an approach that I know from conversation he has adopted. This is unlikely to have altered his views on general principles (I think).

Innes Williams' reviews are good basic reading.

Christopher Woodhouse's review is a well illustrated chapter on phalloplasty and related matters in male exstrophy/epispadias describing his technique using lyophilised dura rather than dermis for the correction of the chordee.

Revision surgery for exstrophy is not described anywhere but Howard Snyder has recently reviewed exstrophy surgery in a very well illustrated and readable fashion and this is well worth reading. He has also written a good review of paediatric reconstructive surgery in general which is also recommended.

Hendren W H 1980 Construction of female urethra from vaginal wall and perineal flap. Journal of Urology 123: 657–664

Hendren W H 1981 Congenital female epispadias with incontinence. Journal of Urology 125: 558–564

Hendren W H 1982 Further experience in reconstructive surgery for cloacal anomalies. Journal of Pediatric Surgery 17: 695–717

Hendren W H, Donahoe P K 1980 Correction of congenital abnormalities of the vagina and perineum. Journal of Pediatric Surgery 15: 751–763

Peña A, Devries P A 1982 Posterior sagittal anorectoplasty: important technical considerations and new applications. Journal of Paediatric Surgery 17: 796–811

Snyder H M 1987 Principles of pediatric urinary reconstruction: a synthesis. In: Gillenwater J Y, Grayhack J T, Howards S S, Duckett J W (eds) Adult and pediatric urology. Year Book Medical Publishers, Chicago, pp 1726–1781

Snyder H M 1990 The surgery of bladder exstrophy and epispadias. In: Frank J D, Johnston J H (eds) Operative paediatric urology. Churchill Livingstone, Edinburgh, pp 153–186

Williams D I 1982 Female urethral anomalies and obstructions — Chapter 23. Urinary tract complications of imperforate anus — Chapter 22. In: Williams D I, Johnston J H (eds) Paediatric urology, 2nd edn. Butterworths, London, pp 271–287

Woodhouse C R J 1988 Dural phalloplasty in exstrophy and epispadias. In: Mundy A R (ed) Current operative surgery: Urology. Balliere Tindall, London, pp 106–118

Chapter 15

Undiversion

Between the years 1955 and 1975 a large number of patients, including many children, underwent urinary diversion. There were several reasons for this. The first was the general popularity of the ileal conduit urinary diversion procedure. The second was the vogue at that time for an aggressive surgical approach to the management of children with spina bifida that allowed many of them to survive the early months of life (when many of them previously had died of infection of the central nervous system), to develop incontinence and impaired renal function subsequently; and thirdly there was the widespread adoption of the ileal conduit procedure for any child with bilateral hydroureteronephrosis. At that time the causes of bilateral hydroureteronephrosis in young children were poorly understood and we now recognise that many children in fact had vesico-ureteric reflux or urethral valves, conditions which nowadays would not be treated in that way.

For many years urinary diversion appeared to be a perfectly satisfactory procedure with no significant adverse long-term sequelae. Undoubtedly this was in large part due to the high percentage of patients with abnormal upper urinary tracts preoperatively and a consequent failure to notice any change or progression in the upper tracts postoperatively. Another element was the dispersal of patients over the course of their adolescent and early adult life away from the centre where the operation was originally performed, thereby being lost to follow up. Finally there were the adult patients having an ileal conduit in association with a cystectomy for bladder cancer who, in general, had a limited life expectancy and in whom long-term complications were not really an important consideration. Eventually, when long-term follow-up studies of patients diverted in early life were published, it was realised that there were problems associated with urinary diversion, both with the stoma and the conduit itself on the one hand, and with the incidence of deterioration of renal structure and sometimes function in the longer term on the other.

At about the time that reports began to appear in print about the long-term sequelae of urinary diversion, there was also a surge in the development of paediatric urology as a whole, especially in relation to vesico-ureteric reflux, posterior urethral valves, the prune belly syndrome and other conditions in which diversion had hitherto featured as an option in treatment, and a similar surge of interest in the investigation of lower urinary tract function by urodynamic studies. Together these led to a change in policy of treatment for many patients, causing a sudden decline in the number of urinary diversions performed. Finally, largely under the influence of Hendren in Boston, the concept and techniques of undiversion were developed so that this subsequently became a fairly commonplace procedure. Nowadays undiversion if anything is on the decline as most of the pool of 'undivertable' patients have already been undiverted and fewer patients are being diverted.

When considering undiversion it is important to remember that there are essentially two types of candidate for undiversion. The first is the type of patient whose underlying problem would not nowadays be treated by urinary diversion in the first place. Probably the best examples in this category are severe vesico-ureteric reflux and posterior urethral valves. In such patients with a diversion all that is required is a simple restoration of urinary tract continuity, possibly combined with a relatively minor local procedure to correct the underlying problem (i.e. by ureteric implantation or valve resection), if still necessary. This is obviously a relatively simple procedure, the only problem being to bridge any possible gap between the ureter above the level of the diversion and the ureter or more commonly bladder below the level of the diversion.

On the other hand there are patients for whom urinary diversion would still be a valid treatment, of which the largest single category will be children with neuropathic bladder dysfunction due to spina bifida. In these children a restoration of urinary tract continuity would simply recreate their initial problem and so, in addition to restoring continuity, something must be done to the urinary tract at the same time to ensure continence and adequate bladder emptying.

In other patients there is often a third factor that has to be considered and that is the presence of any complications of their disease or of their diversion. Thus:

— Patients with associated anorectal or genital abnormalities may need to have these corrected. These are usually best dealt with simultaneously with the undiversion procedure.
— Patients with non-functioning kidneys or renal calculi may need to have these dealt with. Stones are best dealt with percutaneously or by extracorporeal shock wave lithotripsy as a separate procedure.
— Patients (girls) who have had a Spence procedure (creation of a urethro-vesico-vaginal fistula) for pyocystitis will need to have the urethra and a sphincter mechanism reconstructed or alternatively, be considered for a continent diversion.

Candidates for undiversion must have all of these factors taken into consideration. The questions that therefore need to be answered are:

1. What is the nature of the underlying disease, bearing in mind that this may not be clear from the patient's original records?
2. Is the lower urinary tract capable of normal function with continence, complete bladder emptying and an

adequate time interval between voids? If not, what needs to be done to achieve these goals?

3. Is bladder function going to interfere with upper urinary tract function? Usually this resolves to two questions — is there evidence of persistent bladder outflow obstruction and is there a high-pressure bladder?

4. Are there any associated abnormalities that need to be corrected, either beforehand or at the same time as the undiversion procedure?

5. Is this patient in all ways a suitable candidate for undiversion? In this respect it is important to consider the patient's general health, intelligence and motivation and, in some instances, also their manipulative skills, mobility and general life style.

Finally in assessment it is important to remember that the effect of prolonged defunctioning of the urinary tract means that one can only estimate how the bladder is likely to behave after undiversion and that any assessment of future function of the urinary tract after undiversion is therefore only a guess, albeit, hopefully, an educated guess. It is important that the patient realises this also and thereby the possible need for secondary procedures after the original undiversion procedure, to correct any urodynamic abnormalities that remain.

ASSESSMENT

The best initial screening procedure is an IVU. This shows the general state of the kidneys, the degree of dilatation, if any, of the renal pelves and ureters, the length of the ureters above the conduit (assuming the patient has a conduit diversion), the site of anastomosis of the ureters to the conduit and the length of the conduit itself. All of these are important factors. For example, a long redundant loop that the diverting surgeon would be disappointed with is a large potential cystoplasty segment that the undiverting surgeon would be

delighted to see. If there is no clear view of the anastomosis between the ureters and the conduit, or poor visualisation for any reason, then a retrograde loopogram should supply the required information. If there is a suggestion of obstruction to the upper urinary tract then a DTPA renal scan should be ordered to confirm or refute this, and if there is any suggestion of impairment of renal function then a DMSA renal scan will show differential renal function and isolated areas of poor function in each kidney.

The next step is a cystourethroscopy and EUA. At the same time ureteric catheters can be passed up the ureters to measure the distal length of the ureters, or alternatively to get a ureterogram, just in case it proves possible to perform a direct ureteric anastomosis. This is rarely the case, so much so that I hardly ever bother to do it except occasionally in patients diverted in early childhood for reflux or some other non-neuropathic problem. Such children had big, baggy tortuous ureters initially and this superfluity of length sometimes persists, allowing a direct end-to-end upper-to-lower ureteric anastomosis — either ipsilateral or across to the ureter on the other side. At the end of the cystoscopy the bladder capacity is noted and a suprapubic catheter is left in place. Over the next few days this catheter is connected to a drip-set running in water or saline at a rate of 1 or 2 ml/min to simulate normal bladder filling. This allows an assessment of the function of the lower urinary tract and any change in its function over the next few days. If it is quite obvious that lower urinary tract function is disastrously poor because the patient is hopelessly incontinent (as, in fact, usually happens) then there is no point in continuing this beyond a couple of days as it upsets the patient and the nursing staff. But if bladder function is improving then this should be continued for a few days longer and followed by a video-urodynamic study. This period of

'bladder cycling' before urodynamic investigation allows a better assessment of bladder function. Most bladders, after they have been defunctioned for even a short period of time, tend to be poorly compliant and of low capacity. By allowing some usage compliance sometimes returns towards normal, and bladder capacity improves. Improvement in these two factors makes assessment of any urodynamic abnormality easier and in particular the larger bladder volume allows a better radiological assessment of sphincter function. A larger bladder volume also makes the undiversion procedure itself easier as explained below.

It should not be expected however that both these parameters will have returned to normal after only a few days of cycling, only towards normal. Minor degrees of abnormality are acceptable after a few days of cycling, in the expectation that further improvement will occur.

It is usually possible to predict at cystoscopy whether cycling is likely to lead to any improvement in bladder behaviour — if the capacity is less than 50 ml and particularly if the patient has a neuropathic problem it is not likely to improve. If it is 50–100 ml and repeated filling and emptying gives progressively larger volumes, then cycling is usually worthwhile as some improvement is possible particularly if the patient does not have a neuropathic problem. If the capacity is over 100 ml (or an equivalent volume in children) then improvement is likely. If the capacity is over 200 ml (or an equivalent volume in children) then you might just as well go straight on to urodynamics. Unfortunately this is unusual.

The most important role of urodynamic investigation is to identify or exclude sphincter dysfunction because of its relevance to postoperative continence and emptying. In neuropathic disease this may either be obstruction or incompetence of the urethral sphincter mechanism or more commonly a combination of the two. In the absence of neuropathy, sphincter weakness is unusual and outflow obstruction should not be present. However, some children, for example those with urethral valves, have had urinary diversions with no attempt at dealing with the local problem or may have strictures as a result of previous treatment and so it is important to be sure that the outflow tract is normal.

Although all urodynamic abnormalities are obviously important and all should be looked for, the factor of fundamental importance for the undiversion procedure itself is the bladder capacity. This is because manipulation of the bladder, by psoas hitch or Boari flap or a combination of the two, is the main way of restoring lower to upper urinary tract continuity, and because the measurement of bladder capacity is the best preoperative guide to the state of the bladder. The smaller the bladder capacity, the more difficult it is likely to be to bridge the ureteric gap by these manoeuvres.

Apart from restoring continuity the aim of undiversion is obviously to provide a low-pressure bladder of good capacity and continence. If the underlying problem is one that precludes normal continence and voiding then an alternative must be considered. There are two options — either intermittent self catheterisation through an obstructive sphincter mechanism or supplementation of a weak sphincter mechanism with an artificial sphincter. There are two general rules in this respect that I think are important. The first is that a naturally obstructive sphincter can usually be relied on to continue to be obstructive but that a surgically created 'obstructive' bladder outflow is not so reliable. It is therefore safest to supplement a 'bladder neck reconstruction' in some way, usually by placement of an artificial sphincter cuff around it, so that if

necessary the remainder of the artificial sphincter can be implanted at a later date. The second general rule is that decisions about the use of clean intermittent self catheterisation should be made well in advance of the procedure so that the patient can then start practising the technique and be shown to be capable of doing it properly and be willing to use it properly before committing him or her to using it, possibly for the rest of their lives. It is a disaster to plan on intermittent self catheterisation and then to find afterwards that the patient cannot or will not do it. As a general rule I also find that girls will accept intermittent catheterisation much more readily than boys and that complications of intermittent catheterisation are rare in girls, but much more common in boys. For this reason I would tend to use an obstructive bladder outflow and intermittent catheterisation in girls but be more inclined towards implantation of an artificial sphincter in boys.

A SUMMARY OF SURGICAL OPTIONS IN UNDIVERSION

The choice for restoring upper-to-lower urinary tract continuity is either to reconnect the upper ureter to the lower ureter or, as this is rarely possible, to manipulate the bladder in some way to bridge the gap.

The choice for the bladder is either to retain it and use it to restore continuity between the upper and lower urinary tracts with bladder augmentation to provide an adequate capacity if necessary, or, if the bladder is too thick-walled or otherwise diseased, to remove it by subureteric subtotal cystectomy and then use substitution cystoplasty to replace it. Restoration of continuity between the ureters and the lower urinary tract is very much simpler with a substitution cystoplasty as this will easily bridge any gap but the complication rate is higher than when

continuity is restored by a direct anastomosis between natural ureter and natural bladder.

The choice for the bladder outflow depends on whether it is obstructive or incompetent; it is rarely normal. If it is obstructive, which is generally only seen in neuropathy, then it is best left alone, relying on CISC postoperatively for bladder emptying. The problem is to decide preoperatively whether it is obstructive enough to give reliable continence. The best method of assessing this, if it can be assessed, is by the volume of residual urine in relation to intravesical pressure on preoperative urodynamic testing. If there is a significant residual volume despite elevated intravesical pressures then there is usually sufficient sphincteric resistance for adequate continence. If not, outflow resistance will need to be enhanced in some way. If outflow resistance is low and the patient has a neuropathic problem then an artificial sphincter is the best way of providing continence. If the patient has a non-neuropathic problem such as exstrophy then a bladder neck reconstruction may be possible but an AUS may still be a better option. In some instances sphincter function is unpredictable and definitive control of continence has to be left to a second stage. Absence of the bladder or bladder outflow are discussed later on in this chapter.

Abnormalities of the upper urinary tract discovered during assessment are usually one of two types: firstly a non-functioning kidney, which can be treated by nephrectomy or nephroureterectomy at the time of undiversion, or secondly, calculous disease. This is best treated by extracorporeal shock wave lithotripsy or by percutaneous removal of the stones before undiversion, as renal access is adequate for nephrectomy through a midline anterior abdominal incision, but not for any intricate intrarenal manipulations.

UNDIVERSION AND CONTINENT DIVERSION

Continent diversion has already been referred to several times in this book and specifically in Chapter 8 when my preferred technique was described, the indication in this instance being irradiation cystitis; in Chapter 10, various techniques of continent diversion were described for use in certain patients with spina bifida; in Chapter 12, again for irradiation cystitis; in Chapter 13 for certain patients with bladder cancer and in Chapter 14 for the reconstruction of girls with exstrophy. I have not however as yet discussed the concept of continent diversion in any depth, which some readers may find surprising given its current popularity. As undiversion and continent diversion are so regularly discussed together I have chosen to discuss it here.

It is quite common to see descriptions in the urological literature of patients being 'undiverted' from an ileal conduit to a continent diversion or otherwise 'reconstructed' by means of a continent diversion. As far as I am concerned a continent diversion is still a diversion, as a point of terminology, however much better than a conduit diversion it may be for the patient. Consequently I regard it as semantically wrong to describe the use of continent diversion for undiversion or reconstruction, the end result of which, in both cases, should be voiding through a naturally sited meatus. Some may regard this as rather a trivial point but in my opinion some of the biggest problems in communicating, discussing, understanding and describing the subject of reconstructive urology have been due to inaccuracies or vagueness in terminology. Needless to say this is an arguable point but there are however two important practical issues involved in this question of undiversion/reconstruction on the one hand as against continent diversion on the other. The first concerns the

interchangeability between the two approaches in relation to the surgical techniques used. The second concerns those situations where one or other is positively indicated.

There are many techniques that have been described for continent diversion that can often be used for (continent) undiversion as well. Typical examples are the many complicated gut pouches made from the ileum that have been described and attributed to various cities of the Northern hemisphere. Unfortunately they cannot routinely be brought down into the pelvis for anastomosis to a natural or substitute urethra because the length of the small bowel mesentery prevents this in 10% of patients (and a much higher percentage of patients with spina bifida). The mobility of these pouches is in any case reduced by folding the mesentery into an S, U, M, W, or any other shape which additionally restricts the capacity of the pouch to expand by the tethering it produces at each 360° arc of the S, U, W, M, or whatever. The end result is that however mathematically advantageous these convoluted pouches may be on paper (without a mesentery and a third dimension) they are somewhat less magical both in capacity and in range of mobility when it comes to putting theory into practice. Consequently, if the surgeon insists on using a specific technique for bladder substitution which is based wholly or substantially on ileum then a reconstruction or undiversion may prove impossible on occasions and a continent diversion will be the only option. While I recognise that all surgery has an inherent element of unpredictability I believe that it is wrong to compound this unpredictability by using a technique which, by its very nature, is unpredictable and may not therefore allow the surgeon to do what he would like to do, unless of course he always aims to give his patients a continent diversion.

On the other hand, techniques of bladder substitution based on the right colon have all the advantages of a straight marginal artery pedicle with a potentially very long arc of rotation which contrast sharply with the limitations imposed by the short looped pedicle of the small bowel mesentery. Furthermore the nature of the pedicle means that the bowel can be opened and pouched if it is so desired without the restrictions of either expansibility or mobility that the mesentery imposes on small bowel pouches. These bladder substitutes, whether straight (undetubularised) or pouched, are therefore truly interchangeable and the surgeon can choose in advance either to use his technique for either undiversion/reconstruction or continent diversion according to the nature of the patient's problem. This is the reasoning behind my preference for the colonic cystourethroplasty technique I described in Chapter 8 which can be used for continent diversion with an umbilical meatus or rotated through 180° with a perineal meatus for undiversion/reconstruction.

The second issue concerns those situations where either reconstruction or continent diversion is positively indicated. Whether or not you agree with what I have just said the crucial factor in both approaches is the competence of the continence mechanism of the outflow from the substitute bladder, and whichever approach is used the problems of creating such a mechanism are broadly similar. The complication rate of each approach — undiversion/reconstruction or continent diversion — could therefore be expected to be similar and therefore technical factors do not play or should not play much part in the decision of which to choose although obviously they sometimes do. Given a free choice most patients would obviously prefer to be as normal as possible and so they would opt in most instances for reconstruction. We are then left only with disease considerations which might dictate against reconstruction and in favour of continent diversion, and in my view there are three situations in which continent diversion is indicated with any frequency:

— male patients requiring cystourethrectomy for bladder cancer,
— spina bifida patients who would otherwise be suitable for reconstruction but who cannot self catheterise urethrally because of an associated urethral problem, because of calipers or some similar situation,
— patients with severe irradiation cystitis in whom a diversion away from the field or irradiation is obviously desirable.

In all these instances a conduit diversion would obviously be an alternative approach.

SURGICAL TECHNIQUE

All patients are explored through a long midline incision. This is the only incision that will allow extension to the required degree to allow exploration of the abdomen, pelvis and retroperitoneum.

THE DECISION AS TO HOW TO PROCEED

(In the last few chapters I have been more concise in my descriptions of surgical technique, believing that most readers will either have read through the previous chapters or already have some experience of reconstructive urology. In this chapter I have reverted to being verbose and long-winded. To the experienced urologist I apologise but as the commonest candidate for undiversion is a patient with a neuropathic bladder many readers may have skipped to this chapter without reference to the rest of the reconstructive section of the book.)

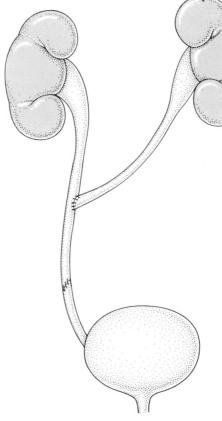

Fig. 15.1

The first steps are to open the retropubic space widely and to make a final assessment of the ureters and bladder. The state of the bladder (if it is still present) will determine whether it can be retained, as it usually can, or whether it is so badly diseased that it will need to be excised. There is rarely a sufficient length of ureter above and below the level of the diversion to allow direct anastomosis on either side, but this should be confirmed, particularly in those who are likely to have had long tortuous ureters at the time of their diversion. Upper-to-lower urinary tract continuity will usually have to be restored by either a psoas hitch or a Boari flap or, more commonly, a combination of the two. With a bladder of normal capacity it is possible to do this without the need for bladder augmentation, although augmentation

may nonetheless be necessary to correct any intrinsic urodynamic dysfunction. If, as is usually the case, the bladder is not of normal capacity but is nonetheless usable then a psoas hitch and Boari flap sufficient to allow a tunnelled ureteric reimplantation may use up so much of the bladder that all that is left of the bladder is a flat plate onto which a gut segment, usually the ileal conduit, will need to be patched to restore the bladder to a useful size. If these manoeuvres are not going to be possible, usually because the bladder is too thick-walled and trabeculated to allow it, then the bladder is excised and a substitution cystoplasty is performed. As the urethral sphincter mechanism is not normally innervated and normally functioning in the vast majority of patients having an undiversion an ileocolic pouch technique is used for the substitution cystoplasty to ensure as far as possible that the new bladder is a low-pressure system. The ureters are then plumbed directly into the cystoplasty.

In summary then the approaches to undiversion, depending on the operative findings, are as follows. If there is sufficient ureteric length above and below the level of the diversion, on one or both sides, for a direct anastomosis without tension, then this is the preferred option, but rarely possible (Fig. 15.1). If this is only possible on one side, the other ureter is mobilised for an end-to-side transureteroureterostomy (TUU) to the reconnected side at a point well above the anastomosis. The bladder is then augmented or not, depending on the urodynamic findings.

If there is not sufficient ureteric length for a direct anastomosis but the bladder has near normal capacity and wall thickness then a psoas hitch should bring the bladder up sufficiently to allow a tunnelled reimplantation of the ipsilateral ureter (Fig. 15.2). An end-to-side TUU of the contralateral ureter is then performed above the ipsilateral ureteroneocystostomy (UNC). Again the bladder is then augmented or not, depending on the urodynamic findings (usually this will be necessary).

If the bladder has a reduced capacity but is not so badly diseased that it cannot be used — which is the usual situation — then a combined Boari flap and psoas hitch will usually bridge the gap to allow a tunnelled ipsilateral UNC. A TUU is then performed to restore continuity of the contralateral ureter and the bladder is then augmented to restore capacity using the ileal conduit and a second gut segment alongside it if that alone is not big enough (Fig. 15.3). In these circumstances the deficiency of the bladder wall makes all other urodynamic considerations irrelevant because the bladder will have to be augmented anyway.

If the bladder is so bad that a combined Boari flap and psoas hitch are impossible, or if the bladder has previously been removed, then a substitution cystoplasty is used. This serves the dual purpose of providing a bladder and bridging the gap. The ileal conduit (if present) can be incorporated into the substitution cystoplasty to form a detubularised pouch (Fig. 15.4). The ureters are tunnelled into a convenient area of the cystoplasty or anastomosed to the ileal tail of the cystoplasty before it is anastomosed to the bladder base or urethra.

In all the options given so far it is assumed, as is usually the case, that the urinary diversion has left the ureters intact and more or less normal down to about the level of L4–L5, just above the common iliac vessels on one or other side of the midline. In other words the problem of restoring urinary tract continuity — of 'bridging the ureteric gap' — is entirely below the level of the diversion. This is not always the case for one of three reasons: firstly the proximal ureters may be grossly dilated as a result of longstanding obstruction or reflux, in other words not intrinsically normal; secondly they may be strictured and obstructed or otherwise intrinsically diseased proximal to the diversion, but still draining reasonably functioning kidneys; thirdly they may have been replaced by a longer than usual ileal conduit, perhaps reaching up to the

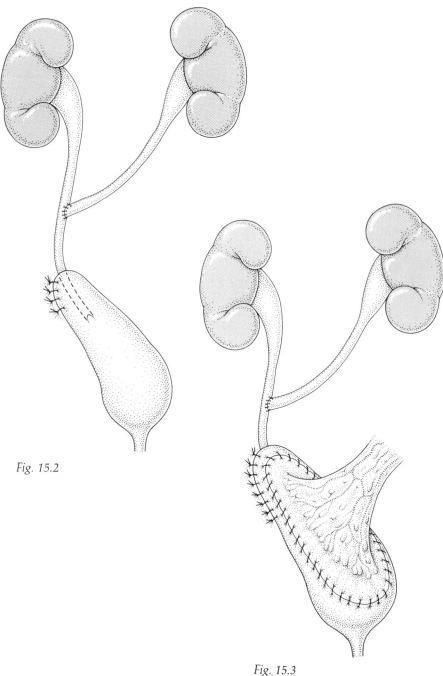

Fig. 15.2

Fig. 15.3

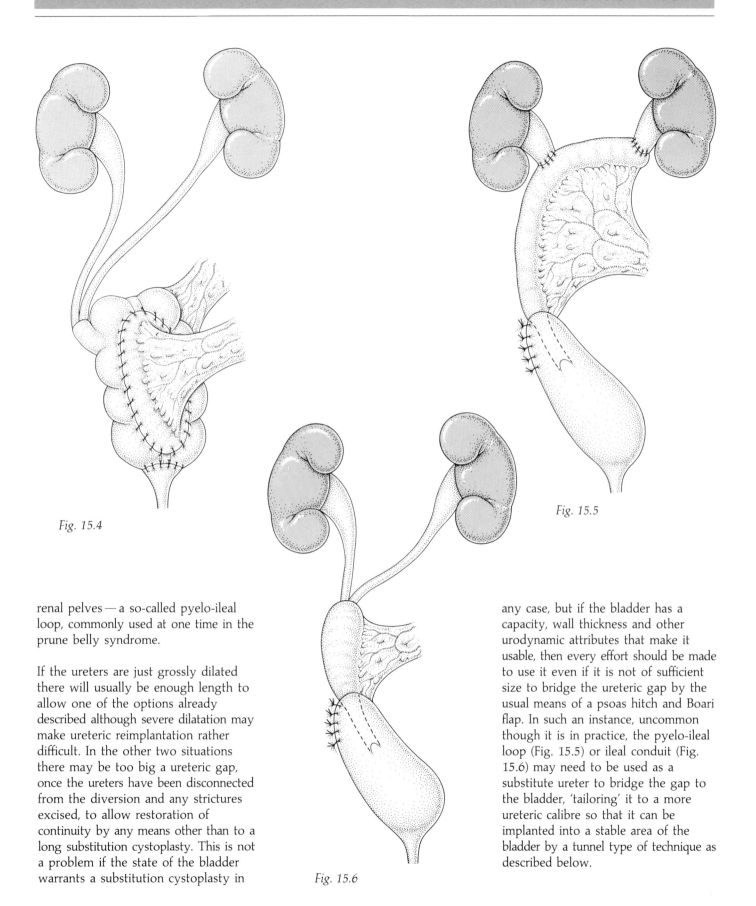

Fig. 15.4

Fig. 15.5

Fig. 15.6

renal pelves — a so-called pyelo-ileal loop, commonly used at one time in the prune belly syndrome.

If the ureters are just grossly dilated there will usually be enough length to allow one of the options already described although severe dilatation may make ureteric reimplantation rather difficult. In the other two situations there may be too big a ureteric gap, once the ureters have been disconnected from the diversion and any strictures excised, to allow restoration of continuity by any means other than to a long substitution cystoplasty. This is not a problem if the state of the bladder warrants a substitution cystoplasty in

any case, but if the bladder has a capacity, wall thickness and other urodynamic attributes that make it usable, then every effort should be made to use it even if it is not of sufficient size to bridge the ureteric gap by the usual means of a psoas hitch and Boari flap. In such an instance, uncommon though it is in practice, the pyelo-ileal loop (Fig. 15.5) or ileal conduit (Fig. 15.6) may need to be used as a substitute ureter to bridge the gap to the bladder, 'tailoring' it to a more ureteric calibre so that it can be implanted into a stable area of the bladder by a tunnel type of technique as described below.

Whatever the operative findings the guiding principle should be to bridge the ureteric gap and restore upper-to-lower urinary tract continuity by means of a urothelium-to-urothelium anastomosis wherever possible. If the bladder is grossly deficient a substitution cystoplasty will be necessary and if the ureters are grossly deficient then an ileal ureter or substitution cystoplasty will be necessary depending on the state of the bladder. In all other situations every effort should be made to bring the bladder and one ureter together (with a TUU for the other ureter) to maintain urothelial continuity. The complication rate of undiversion is much lower when urothelial continuity has been achieved than when a gut segment has been interposed.

So far I have only discussed the undiversion of patients with ileal conduits, mainly because they are by far the largest group. Patients with colon conduits, cutaneous ureterostomies and ureterosigmoidostomies are dealt with in much the same way. Colon conduits pose almost exactly the same problems as ileal conduits, but in general cutaneous ureterostomies and ureterosigmoidostomies are less of a problem because the ureters tend to be longer so there is less of a gap to bridge.

BRIDGING THE URETERIC GAP BY DIRECT UROTHELIAL CONTINUITY

On the rare occasions that it proves possible to achieve a direct anastomosis between the ureter above and below, this is the procedure of choice. When mobilising the ureters the surrounding connective tissue should be carefully preserved to preserve their vascularity as far as possible. However normal the upper ureter, the lower ureter below the diversion is likely to be thin and miserable-looking. Both ends should be mobilised along their full length and the

anastomosis between the two should be widely spatulated and splinted with an infant feeding tube of an appropriate calibre. On even rarer occasions when it is possible to do this on both sides this is done, otherwise the contralateral ureter is mobilised across the midline for a TUU well above the level of the end-to-end anastomosis.

Direct anastomosis aside, the three basic procedures for bridging the ureteric gap with direct urothelial continuity are the psoas hitch with or without a Boari flap, a transuretero-ureterostomy (TUU) and a tunnelled ureteric implantation of the one ureter thereby created into the psoas hitch/Boari flap. It is best to anastomose one ureter to the bladder

rather than both because after the psoas hitch the bladder will lie to one side of the pelvis and the contralateral ureter is likely to be too short to reach. Even if it is long enough it is likely to be kinked as it angles across the midline and then downwards into the bladder at the site of reimplantation. Hence the need for a TUU.

1. PSOAS HITCH

The aim of the psoas hitch is to hitch one side of the bladder up to the ipsilateral psoas, preferably to the psoas tendon, alternatively to the psoas fascia. In patients with big bladders this is usually a simple matter and requires no

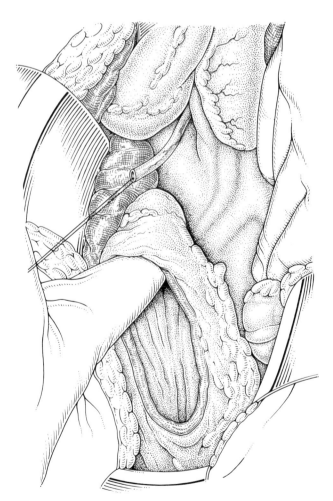

Fig. 15.7

real mobilisation of the bladder but big bladders or even normal-sized bladders are rare. The smaller the bladder the greater the degree of mobilisation required.

The first step is to open the retropubic space widely all the way around both sides and the next is to incise the peritoneum and underlying fascia on each side (the fascia being the more important) all the way along the anterolateral margins of the bladder, back to the lateral vascular pedicle of the bladder and then over the pedicle and medially along the posterior margin of the bladder to the midline. Mobilisation simply by dividing the fascia that tethers the bladder to the brim of the pelvis on one side may suffice to allow the bladder to be

hitched up to the contralateral psoas tendon (the left side of the bladder is mobilised for a right-sided psoas hitch and vice versa). If this is not enough, it will be necessary to divide the vascular pedicle as well. To do this fully would require division of the ureter on that side which would be an obvious limiting factor in any situation other than an undiversion procedure, when that ureteric stump will probably be superfluous. It may however still be a limiting factor to some degree during undiversion if a psoas hitch alone is not going to be sufficient to allow restoration of urinary tract continuity because if a Boari flap is also going to be necessary, as it usually is, then it is obviously desirable to preserve as much of the blood supply as possible. It is therefore a good idea to keep intact at

least the inferior vesical component of the contralateral vascular pedicle to maintain the blood supply of the bladder as far as possible. In practice if division of the obliterated umbilical artery, superior vesical vessels and ureter does not give sufficient contralateral mobility, further division of the inferior vesical vessels is unlikely to make much difference.

When the bladder has been mobilised sufficiently to reach comfortably to the ureter for a tunnelled reimplantation (Fig. 15.7) the peritoneum is incised to expose the underlying psoas muscle and tendon, if present (Fig. 15.8). The bladder is then fixed to the psoas with a series of interrupted 2/0 Vicryl sutures (Fig. 15.9). Each suture takes the full thickness of the bladder wall except the

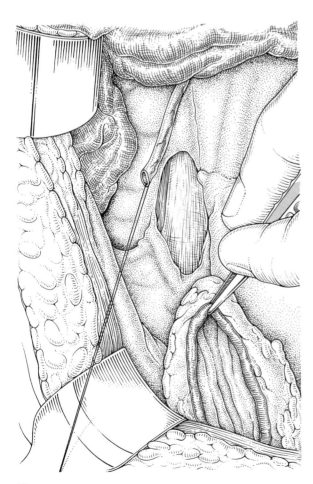

Fig. 15.8

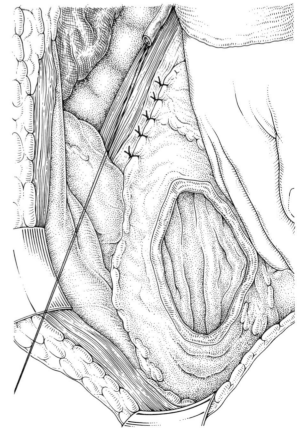

Fig. 15.9

mucosa and a good bite of the psoas tendon or fascia. Care should be taken to keep to the medial aspect of the psoas when taking a bite of the muscle itself for fear of damaging the femoral nerve which lies deep in the groove between the psoas and the iliacus muscles. Sutures are placed about a centimetre apart, aiming to get two rows of 3 or 4 sutures with each row also being about a centimetre apart. This should provide 6 or 8 anchoring sutures which is quite adequate. It should be emphasised that these sutures are not to put traction on the bladder to drag it up to the psoas, but merely to hold the adequately mobilised bladder in place without tension. A tension-free hitch is the only way that the hitch can be guaranteed to survive — otherwise the sutures will cut out. The hitching sutures should aim to give not only fixation to the psoas tendon but also lateral spread of the collapsed bladder over the area of fixation to stretch it flat and so avoid a concertina effect which may make the subsequent ureteroneocystostomy and bladder closure more difficult and less satisfactory.

2. BOARI FLAP

In general terms I prefer a psoas hitch to a Boari flap as a single procedure to overcome deficiency of ureteric length because the psoas hitch, in addition to bridging a ureteric gap, also provides a stable unmoving part of the bladder into which the upper ureter can be reimplanted. This stability means that there will be no kinking of the vesico-ureteric junction thereafter with varying degrees of bladder filling. The Boari flap is therefore complementary to the psoas hitch when a 'hitch' alone is insufficient, rather than a true alternative.

In theory, a psoas hitch of a bladder of normal capacity should get the bladder up above the pelvic brim and this point of fixation then acts as the axis of rotation for the Boari flap enabling the

technique to bridge a gap at least up to the lower pole of the kidney. Thus (in theory), any bladder that is capable of a psoas hitch will also be capable of providing a Boari flap that will bridge almost any ureteric gap. Hence the rare need for techniques involving an ileal ureter. In practice, the theory falls down because in undiversion the bladder is not usually of sufficient capacity to be hitched up to the psoas, let alone higher, except by means of a Boari flap. In other words the Boari flap is done to make the psoas hitch, and therefore a tunnelled ureteric reimplantation, possible.

In practice therefore, I begin an undiversion by mobilising the bladder as for a psoas hitch, then see whether or not it will reach up sufficiently. If it will not, as is usually the case, I then raise a bladder flap to see if that will reach up to the ipsilateral upper ureter. With very small bladders this bladder flap may represent as much as half of the bladder wall. But even with a bladder that seems at first sight to be very small it is usually possible to bridge the 'ureteric gap' for a tunnelled reimplantation above the level of the common iliac

vessels if it is mobilised and 'flapped' to this degree. A bladder that is too small for this will usually be so severely deranged that it will warrant subtotal cystectomy and substitution cystoplasty in any case.

Because the extent of the Boari flap required is an unknown quantity until after the bladder has been mobilised the bladder should not be opened for whatever reason by anything more than a short cystotomy until after it has been fully mobilised because any larger incision in the bladder may compromise the incision subsequently necessary to raise an adequate Boari flap.

When raising the flap it is important to remember that it must be wide enough to maintain an adequate blood supply, to accommodate a ureteric reimplantation and then (if a cystoplasty is not to be performed) to be rolled into a tube during closure, and this means in most instances a flap that is at least 3 or 4 cm wide. Any narrower and there is a risk of compromising the blood supply and also of being unable to close the bladder with ease, thereby possibly compromising ureteric drainage.

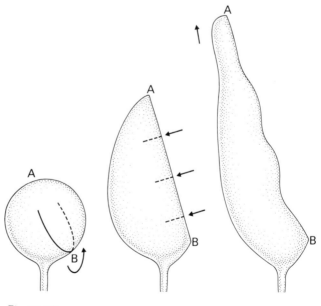

Fig. 15.10

When a flap has been mobilised (Fig. 15.10) it is common to find, because of the natural curvature of the spherical bladder wall, that the edges of the flap are rather tight by comparison with the centre of the flap. The wider the flap is in proportion to the size of the bladder as a whole the more marked this phenomenon is, particularly in small bladders. This tightness of the edges of the flap restricts the overall length of the flap and prevents it reaching as high as it otherwise might.

The solution is to make a series of 'nicks' in the margins of the flap, every 2 cm or so along each margin to allow them to expand as illustrated diagrammatically in Figure 15.10.

When the flap has been raised (Fig. 15.11) it is fixed to the psoas tendon/fascia and the retroperitoneal fascia, as with a psoas hitch, to stabilise that part of the bladder and to prevent it retracting during the course of the subsequent ureteric reimplantation (Fig. 15.12).

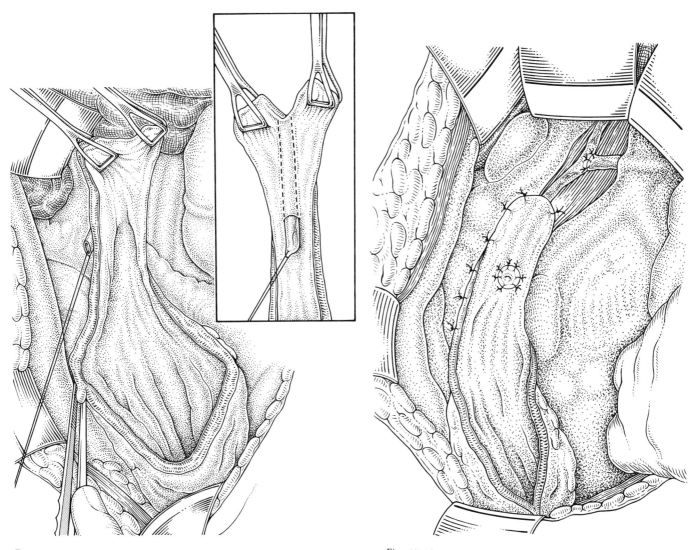

Fig. 15.11   *Fig. 15.12*

Sometimes a bladder with a sufficient capacity to allow a good psoas hitch, with or without a Boari flap, is then capable of closure without the need for bladder augmentation (Fig. 15.13), assuming that there is no other reason for augmentation, as for example poor compliance or hyperreflexic or unstable bladder activity. If a bladder augmentation is necessary, as it usually is, it is important to bear in mind the principles of the 'clam' procedure and split the bladder down to the bladder neck region if this has not previously been done in raising the bladder flap. Usually, augmentation is required as a matter of course (Fig. 15.14) and the first choice for the cystoplasty segment is the ileal conduit — mobilised and opened to form a patch — if it is long enough.

So far we have considered the psoas hitch and Boari flap techniques principally in relation to bladder size. It might therefore be useful to summarise the approach in relation to the more common clinical conditions seen in patients undergoing undiversion.

The majority of patients have neuropathic disease and therefore most bladders are small capacity, poorly compliant and hyperreflexic. For all three reasons an augmentation cystoplasty will be necessary. The small capacity will mean that both a psoas hitch and a Boari flap will be required to bridge the ureteric gap, leaving the bladder open as a flat, laterally based plate onto which the augmentation cystoplasty can be patched.

Many of the remaining patients will have small bladders even if they are not neuropathic, so the same approach will need to be adopted.

Those with normally functioning or acontractile bladders of more or less normal capacity (rare these days — most were undiverted long ago) will usually just require a psoas hitch and simple bladder closure.

Those with normal-sized bladders but with unstable or hyperreflexive detrusor activity will require a cystoplasty to correct this. They could therefore be treated by a unilateral psoas hitch, a TUU and a cystoplasty to close the bladder but an alternative to capitalising on the size of the bladder to avoid the TUU is to bivalve the bladder in the

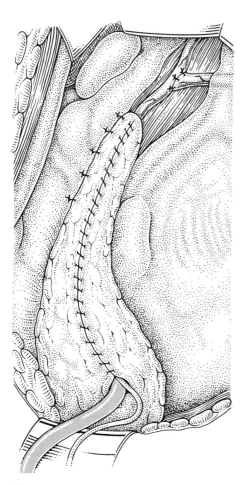

Fig. 15.13

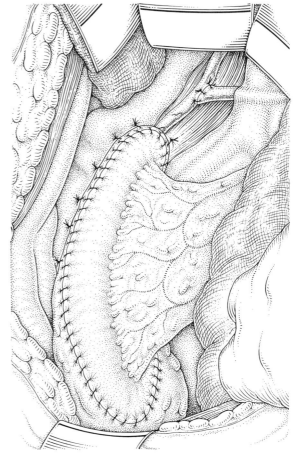

Fig. 15.14

sagittal plane, perform a psoas hitch on each side, reimplant each ureter separately and then close the sagittal central defect of the bivalved bladder with the cystoplasty.

All this assumes that the ureters are of the usual length, ending in a conduit at about the level of the aortic bifurcation, and that they are normal above that level.

3. URETERONEOCYSTOSTOMY

It might seem sensible at first thought, having mobilised the upper ureters from the diversion and checked that the ipsilateral ureter will reach the Boari flap/psoas hitch comfortably, to perform the TUU next. It is better however to

reimplant that ipsilateral ureter first to ensure that when the TUU is performed it is well away from the ureteroneocystostomy and to avoid compromising both by having them too close together when the bladder is eventually closed.

It is worth emphasising again the importance of providing a stable base for the ureteric reimplantation (by psoas hitching), particularly when it is combined with a TUU of the contralateral ureter (and even more so when an ileal segment is being used to replace the ureter as described below).

A second point is that creating a submucosal tunnel is rarely easy, particularly in a previously defunctioned bladder. The simplest way out of the

problem is to incise the urothelium along the length of the ureteroneocystostomy site and then reflect it for a few millimetres on each side (Fig. 15.15). The spatulated ureter is then stitched in place and the reflected urothelium is then tacked to the ureter so that re-epithelialisation will create a tunnel as healing takes place (Fig. 15.16). This is what one might call a 'trench' reimplantation as distinct from a true tunnel. This is particularly useful when the 'ureter' is a tailored ileal segment as it is much larger than a natural ureter making a neatly dissected tunnel of adequate size almost impossible.

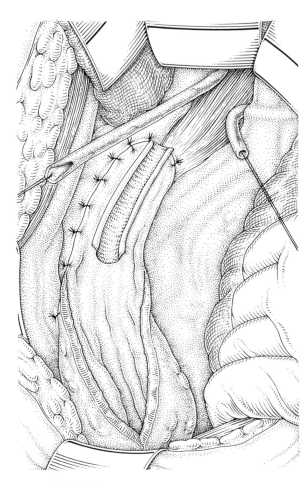

Fig. 15.15

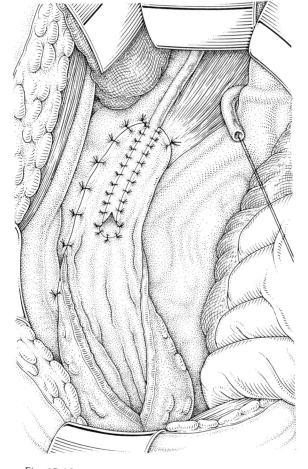

Fig. 15.16

4. TRANSURETERO-URETEROSTOMY

In many ways it was the combination of transureteroureterostomy (TUU) and psoas hitch that led to the development and widespread use of undiversion. The principle is to use the TUU to provide a single ureter to be reimplanted into a bladder that has been elevated and fixed by a psoas hitch to bridge the ureteric gap and provide a stable area for the ureteric reimplantation. This is still a very useful principle and one that should always be aimed for in order to achieve urothelial continuity.

The first important point in TUU for undiversion is that almost invariably the original diversion procedure will have involved passing one of the ureters under the inferior mesenteric artery to the other side. Most patients will have had ileal conduits and the left ureter will have been passed to the right side. When it comes to mobilise the ureters for undiversion it is important to remember this because mobilisation of the left ureter to gain any extra length will involve mobilisation back to the side on which that ureter originally lay, and the inferior mesenteric artery is therefore vulnerable during the dissection involved. The second point is that the only way that much additional length of that ureter can be gained is by rerouting it above the level of the inferior mesenteric artery unless the surgeon who performed the ileal conduit divided the ureters at an unusually low level.

If mobilisation of the ureters is necessary to gain extra length it is important to mobilise a substantial amount of periureteric tissue with them. This is easy to do if one is dissecting around part of the ureter which has not previously been operated on, but it can be rather difficult to do otherwise. To ensure that one is carrying sufficient vascularity for the ureter during the course of the dissection it is a good idea to mobilise the gonadal vessels and the ureter together. In this way adequate vascularisation of the ureter can be guaranteed. With short ureters it is also important to mobilise them as high as possible on each side to gain as much as possible elastic lengthening of the ureter. If we assume that the bladder has been hitched up onto the right psoas and a Boari flap raised as necessary, then for the TUU the right ureter should be mobilised up with its 'mesentery' to the lower pole of the kidney or higher and the left ureter should be mobilised back across to the left-hand side, rerouting it above the inferior mesenteric artery if necessary to gain extra length before bringing it back across to the right side for the TUU.

To prepare the ureters for a left-to-right TUU the left ureter is spatulated and a small window is cut in the right ureter of equal size to the spatulated end of the left ureter and safely above the UNC. The two are then anastomosed with interrupted 4/0 chromic catgut sutures (Fig. 15.17). A ureteric stent is passed up from the bladder through the single right ureteric orifice and then up across the TUU into the left kidney. A drain is left alongside the TUU and the area is wrapped in omentum. If the ureter (the right ureter in this case) that is used for uretero-vesical anastomosis is grossly dilated and capable of taking two ureteric catheters then one is passed up into each kidney, but if only one can be used it is important that it cross the

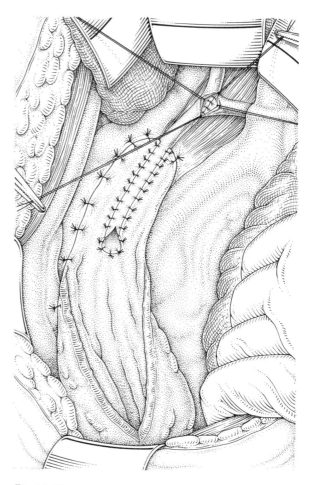

Fig. 15.17

TUU rather than pass up to the ipsilateral kidney.

During the postoperative period it is to be expected that the wound drain draining the TUU will function for at least a day or two. Indeed it is more worrying if the drain does not function (as this usually means that the drain is not working and that extravasated urine is collecting around the TUU) than if all of the urine appears to be passing out through the drain. The surgeon should be in no hurry to remove either the ureteric stent or the wound drain and should not be discouraged by having to face the possibility of keeping them there for more than the usual length of time. The risk of taking the stent or the wound drain out too early is to be left with a urinoma with a high risk of subsequent stricturing in the region of the TUU which can be extremely difficult to correct.

5. BRIDGING THE URETERIC GAP WITH AN ILEAL URETER

I have said above that if a bladder can be brought up above the common iliac vessels with just a psoas hitch then the combination of psoas hitch and Boari flap can overcome almost any ureteric gap. There are however, occasions where the bladder is inadequate, when the ureteric deficit is so long that it cannot be bridged in this way, or when the patient has already had a pyelo-ileal loop. The latter is particularly common in patients who have been diverted for prune belly syndrome. In patients like this who are being undiverted the ileal conduit or pyelo-ileal loop is converted into an ileal 'ureter'. A psoas hitch is then performed, as usual, to provide a stable base for implantation of the ileal 'ureter'. Obviously, for a reimplantation of an ileal ureter, the 'hitched' and 'flapped' part of the bladder will have to be wider than that required for a natural ureter.

To get the ileal 'ureter' to a size where it can be readily implanted into the bladder it must be tailored. The aim is to tailor it down to a calibre that will comfortably accommodate a 14 F catheter (Fig. 15.18). Even so this leaves rather a bulky ileal 'ureter' because of course the mesentery has to go through the tunnel with the 'ureter' itself. Some trimming of the mesentery may therefore be necessary in addition to trimming of the ileum itself. When both these together have been achieved, the combined ileal 'ureter' and mesentery will be about 2 cm wide. Given that a length to width ratio of 4:1 is required to prevent reflux the length of the

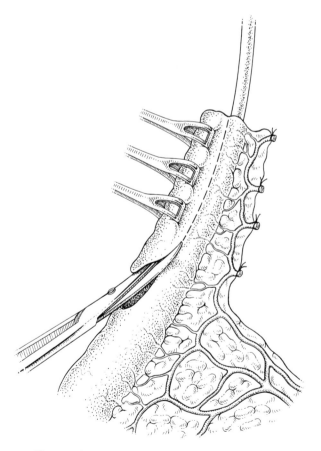

Fig. 15.18

tailored segment and the length of the trench in the bladder mucosa for the segment to lie in will both need to be about 8 cm long to allow an anti-refluxing anastomosis. Thus the aim is to trim the 'ureter' to a calibre of 14 F over a length of about 8 cm. This usually involves excising about half the thickness of the ureter on its antimesenteric side, bearing in mind that after excising this there tends to be retraction of the muscular coat of the ileal wall and a relative surfeit of mucosa. Such excision must therefore be made carefully. The closure of the serosal and muscular layer of the tapered ileum must not end up being too tight because of failure to trim the mucosa sufficiently. A 'trench' type of ureteroneocystostomy is then performed, as described above (Figs 15.19, 15.20).

6. LOWER URINARY TRACT SURGERY

Many aspects of this have already been discussed. There are occasional patients in whom nothing further will need to be done, as when the previous problem for which the patient was diverted was vesico-ureteric reflux or obstruction. This will have been corrected by the ureteroneocystostomy so, having reconnected the upper urinary tracts to the bladder, the bladder can simply be closed. There are others who have a normal bladder but sphincter weakness incontinence who require correction of this but nothing further to the bladder. Again the bladder can simply be closed. More commonly the patient will require bladder augmentation for reasons of

capacity, compliance or for detrusor instability/hyperreflexia and this is dealt with using the ileal conduit to provide the augmentation patch if it is adequate for the purpose, or a newly mobilised gut segment if it is not. Sometimes two gut segments — the conduit and a new patch — will be necessary to give a bladder of adequate capacity. Finally there are the patients in whom a direct anastomosis of the ureters to the bladder has not been possible because either the bladder is too small or too diseased for it usefully to be preserved. In such patients substitution cystoplasty will be necessary using an isolated ascending colonic segment with the conduit or a separate, freshly prepared ileal segment patched onto it to provide an ileocolonic pouch. This serves the dual purpose of

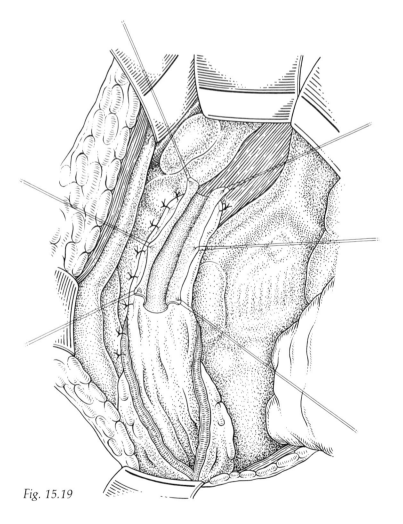

Fig. 15.19

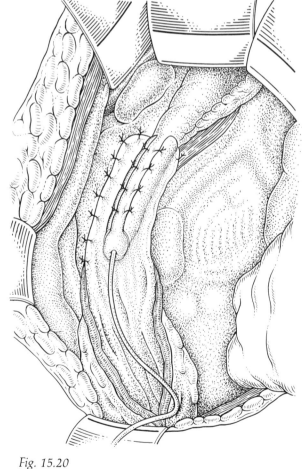

Fig. 15.20

providing a bladder and, by virtue of its length, bridging the ureteric gap. In such patients tunnelled ureteric reimplantations direct into the dome of the 'bladder' are performed having opened the colonic segment but before sewing in the ileal patch.

UNDIVERSION IN PRACTICE

Having described the principal manoeuvres involved in undiversion it may be helpful to describe the way an undiversion usually proceeds in real life with the more common variations.

Given the choice, the incision should be in the midline but one is often obliged to excise and reopen an existing paramedian scar. Adhesions will normally need to be divided before the self-retaining retractor can be placed.

If the bladder outflow requires attention it may be easiest to deal with it first as this can be the most difficult part of the procedure in more complicated cases. Even if reconstruction of the bladder outflow is not actually performed at this stage the decision as to how it will be done should be made early on.

The general rule with urethral reconstruction is that it is easier to make a bladder than a urethra so the demands of urethral reconstruction come first. In males the bladder outflow is usually present and the most common requirement is for an AUS, with either a retropubic or a bulbar urethral cuff to correct sphincteric incompetence. In the unusual event of there being no bladder outflow at all the two options are to use the bladder remnant or a pedicled skin tube (Fig. 15.21). If neither of these two options exists the patient is a candidate for a continent diversion only. Obviously there are several potential variations on these themes. A bladder tube can be anastomosed to a skin tube and the anastomosis can be along the 'traditional' perineo-pelvic route or can be transpubic through a wedge pubectomy. In practice the two most common causes of severe urethral deficiency are after cystourethrectomy for bladder cancer and after cystectomy and subtotal urethrectomy for rhabdomyosarcoma in childhood. In

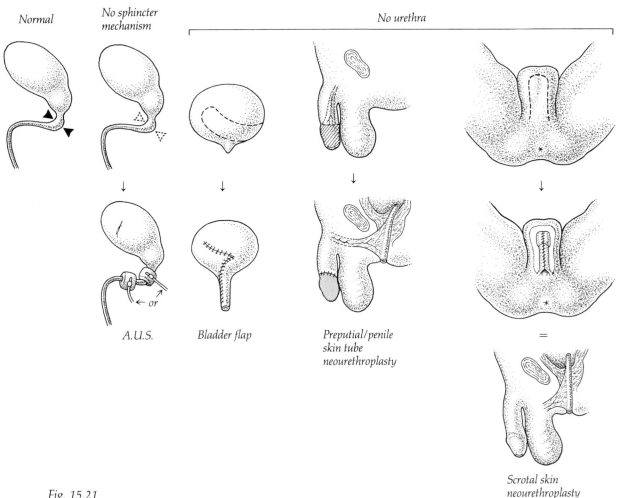

Fig. 15.21

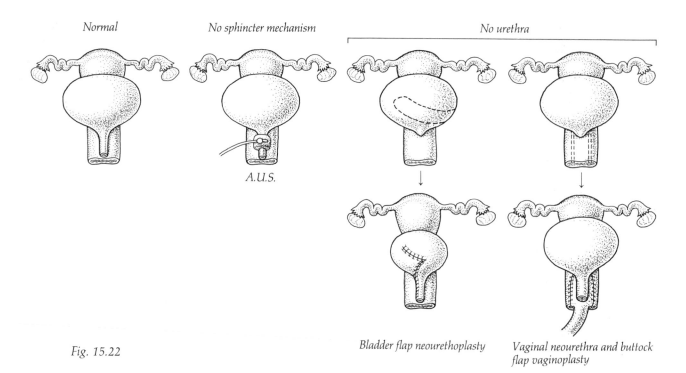

Normal   *No sphincter mechanism*   *No urethra*

A.U.S.

Fig. 15.22

Bladder flap neourethroplasty   *Vaginal neourethra and buttock flap vaginoplasty*

both instances a substitution cystoplasty will be required. With a urethral remnant there is often enough to mobilise and reroute transpubically onto the cystoplasty. The more difficult alternative is to core a channel through the pelvic floor to bring the cystoplasty through to anastomose to the bulbar urethra in situ — this is also more likely to disturb any residual potency these patients sometimes have. In bladder cancer patients who have had a total urethrectomy the only possible urethral substitute is a skin tube. If this is possible with penile skin it is worth trying. If scrotal skin is required then it is probably not worth trying as a scrotal skin tube is usually difficult to catheterise and CISC will almost certainly be required with substitution cystourethroplasty. In fact it is rare for a patient with bladder cancer to be considered for undiversion — a continent diversion, as discussed above, is usually much better.

In females also the commonest requirement is either a bladder neck suspension or an AUS for sphincter weakness. In a patient requiring urethral

substitution or reconstruction (Fig. 15.22) and in whom there is a good-sized bladder but no functional bladder neck then a bladder flap neourethroplasty is the best option. If there is a good-sized bladder and functioning bladder neck then a vaginal wall urethroplasty is

better, capitalising on bladder neck function for continence. If the bladder (and any residual outflow tract) is so small (Fig. 15.23) that as a bladder it is useless but not so badly diseased that it requires excision — common in exstrophy patients — then the remnant

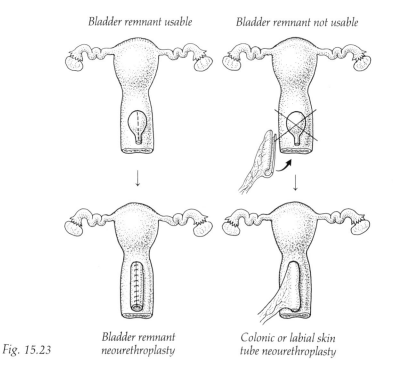

Bladder remnant usable   *Bladder remnant not usable*

Fig. 15.23

Bladder remnant neourethroplasty   *Colonic or labial skin tube neourethroplasty*

should be rolled into a tube to form a neourethra. If none of these options are available because there is no lower urinary tract at all the patient will require a substitution cystoplasty and substitution urethroplasty and the neourethra will need to be anastomosed to the substitute bladder in some way that will provide a continence mechanism — either a flap valve or a nipple valve. Of the latter two, the flap valve is more reliable. A flap valve is produced by tunnelling a tube-like neourethra into a cystoplasty to create a structure resembling the normal vesico-ureteric junction. To create such a neourethra either a colonic neourethral tube (Ch. 8) or, if that is not possible, a pedicled skin tube (Ch. 12) is fashioned. Alternatively, as a last resort and if it will reach, the ileal conduit is mobilised down to the perineum for anastomosis to a meatus with intussusception of the proximal end into a substitution cystoplasty to provide a nipple valve continence mechanism (Ch. 14).

The state of the bladder should be known from preoperative urodynamic studies and bladder cycling. It is usually one of four types — more or less normal capacity and function, with or without cycling (rare); more or less normal capacity but abnormal function (poor compliance, hyperreflexia, instability), correctable by augmentation; of reduced capacity and almost certainly abnormal in function but sufficient to serve as a base for augmentation (commonest); or a write-off requiring substitution cystoplasty. Occasionally there is no bladder at all following a previous cystectomy.

A bladder that is more or less normal both in capacity and function after cycling will require no further attention. The conduit, assuming that there is a conduit and not ureterostomies or ureterosigmoidostomies, can then be discarded. In any of the other circumstances bladder augmentation or substitution will be required in which

case the conduit will be useful and so is retained.

Thus, having dealt with the bladder outflow, attention is next directed to the conduit (Fig. 15.24). In theory the conduit will be short because that is the way it ought to be if it was constructed properly. In practice most conduits, unless they have been revised, are fairly long either because they were made that way or because of a tendency to elongate with time. For undiversion, length is a useful attribute.

Adherent loops of ileum are first dissected off so that the conduit can be

traced from one end to the other taking great care not to damage the vascular pedicle. The distal end is amputated as it passes through the abdominal wall, and the part within the abdominal wall and externally is then excised from the outside and the body wall defect is closed. Only occasionally does the need for length of the ileal conduit for the purpose of cystoplasty warrant dissection of the full length of the loop, which in any case carries a fairly high risk of damage to the vascular pedicle of that part within the abdominal wall.

Next the uretero-ileal anastomosis and the terminal segments of the ureters are

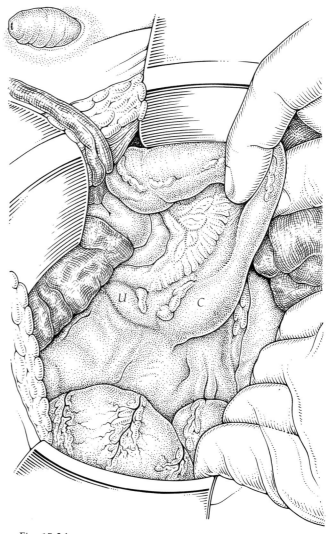

Fig. 15.24

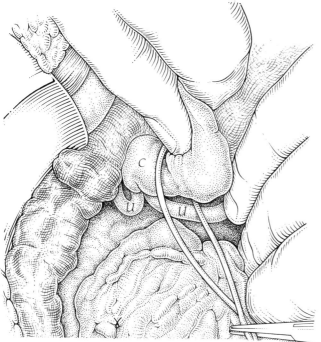

Fig. 15.25

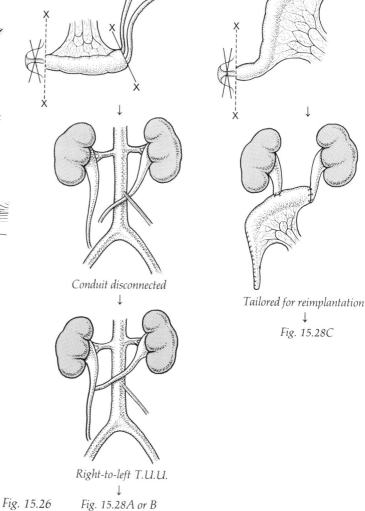

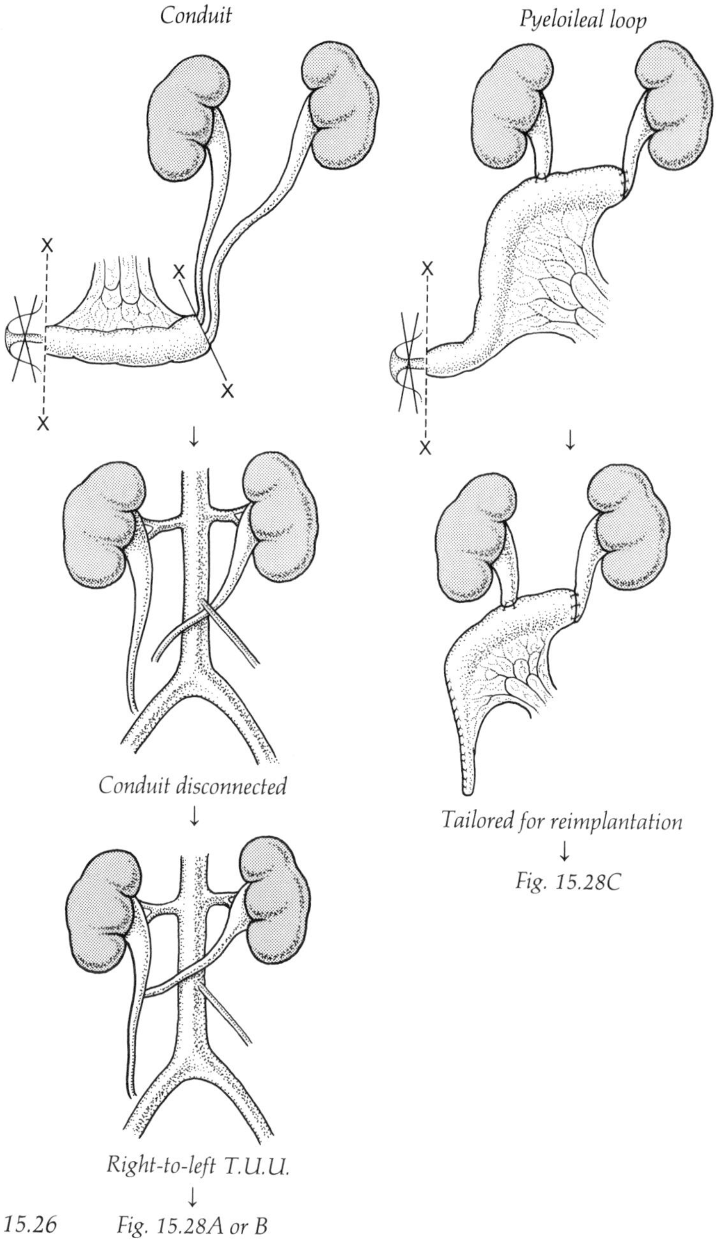

Conduit

Pyeloileal loop

Conduit disconnected
↓

Tailored for reimplantation
↓
Fig. 15.28C

Right-to-left T.U.U.
↓
Fig. 15.26   Fig. 15.28A or B

defined. Sometimes the anastomosis is adherent to the lower end of the inferior vena cava or to the right common iliac vein so care should be taken at this point. It is best to mobilise the distal ureters all the way down to their junction with the conduit before dividing them (Fig. 15.25) in order to preserve as much ureter length as possible. The ureters are then divided just proximal to the anastomosis and the anastomosis is then excised, thereby completing the mobilisation of the conduit. The ureters are then mobilised proximally (Fig. 15.26).

Colon conduits are treated in the same way as ileal conduits. In these patients the conduit is usually on the left side.

If the patient has been diverted with cutaneous ureterostomies great care has to be taken from the moment the surgeon begins the skin incision. Some ureters meander all over the abdomen and through the abdominal wall before they reach the stoma. This can sometimes be anticipated from

preoperative radiological studies, but not always.

If the patient has ureterosigmoidostomies it is important to excise both uretero-sigmoid anastomoses completely with either a cuff of surrounding colon or a short segment of colon if the anastomoses are close together. If the anastomoses are left behind then the risk of malignancy at those sites remains. If the patient has

a pyelo-ileal loop or if the ureters are so short that the conduit will be needed as an ileal ureter then mobilisation of the anastomosis is obviously unnecessary.

When mobilising the ureters, a wide margin of surrounding tissue is included to incorporate the ureteric 'mesentery' unless the mesentery itself is clearly definable. It is not usually necessary to mobilise the full length of both ureters but it may be so, particularly if the left ureter will not reach over to the right (for the TUU) in its usual situation below the inferior mesenteric artery. If so the ureter will have to be mobilised throughout its length and brought across the great vessels above the inferior mesenteric artery.

Having made the decision as to how to deal with the bladder outflow and having mobilised the ureters and the conduit, attention returns to the bladder and the question of restoration of urinary tract continuity (Figs 15.27, 15.28). It is rare to be able to do a direct anastomosis between the ureteric ends above and below the level of the previous diversion. I have only been able to do that on two occasions. The bladder, natural or substitute, will therefore be crucial for restoration of continuity in the vast majority of patients.

If a psoas hitch of a nearly normal bladder is possible then that is obviously best (Fig. 15.27) but this is rare. At the other extreme, the bladder has previously been removed or there is more commonly a grossly diseased bladder which will need to be excised

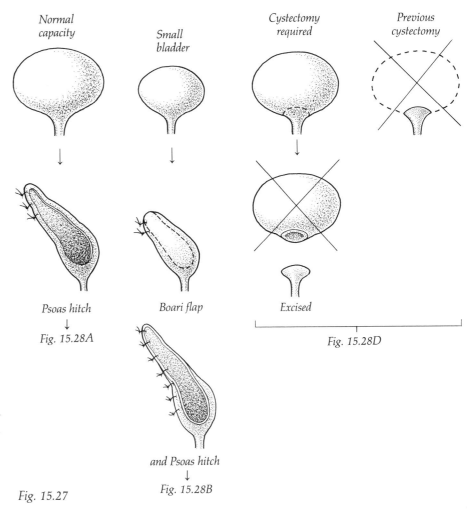

Normal capacity

Small bladder

Cystectomy required

Previous cystectomy

Psoas hitch
↓
Fig. 15.28A

Boari flap

Excised

Fig. 15.28D

and Psoas hitch
↓
Fig. 15.28B

Fig. 15.27

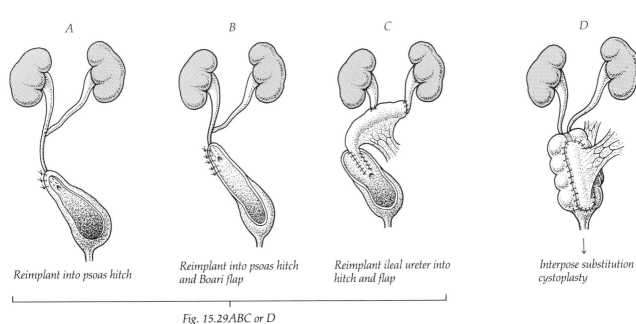

A

B

C

D

Reimplant into psoas hitch

Reimplant into psoas hitch and Boari flap

Reimplant ileal ureter into hitch and flap

Interpose substitution cystoplasty

Fig. 15.29ABC or D

Fig. 15.28

except for the bladder neck and trigone which will then act as a base for a substitution cystoplasty.

By far the most common situation is the finding that the bladder is not so diseased that it requires a substitution procedure but not so good that a simple psoas hitch is all that is required. Typically the bladder is small and thick-walled with a capacity of 50–100 ml, but even if it holds 200–300 ml it will usually require augmentation because of neuropathic or other dysfunction. Even if such a bladder is unlikely to contribute anything useful either to bladder capacity or to contractile/expulsive activity, it does provide the best material with which to restore urinary tract continuity. A bladder of this type can usually be made to reach up to the proximal ureter with a combination of a Boari flap and psoas hitch. One half of the bladder is raised as a flap which will then allow a contralateral hitch.

Having bridged the 'ureteric gap' by one or other of these methods, the ureter is reimplanted (Fig. 15.28). In most instances the right ureter is anastomosed to the hitched bladder (with or without

a flap) with a suburothelial tunnel of adequate length. Alternatively the ileal ureter or pyelo-ileal loop is reimplanted if such is the situation, and if the patient has required bladder substitution the ureters are tunnelled into the cystoplasty at an appropriate point or anastomosed to the ileal tail.

All that now remains is to close the bladder (Fig. 15.29). The (rare) normally functioning bladder is simply closed, discarding the conduit. In the most common situation of a bladder 'base plate' after a flap, a hitch and a ureteric reimplant, an augmentation is required. With a baggy conduit all that is necessary is to open the conduit up to form a patch and then to sew that on to the bladder 'base plate'. With a small or narrow base plate or a short conduit this may not be enough, in which case a second gut segment is mobilised. The two gut segments, both opened along their antimesenteric borders, are sewn together side-to-side and then together to the bladder remnant. When the ileal conduit is so small or so immobile that it cannot be used, it is discarded and the bladder base plate is augmented with a right colonic segment that has been opened along one of its taenia coli.

The key to more complicated undiversions is the ability to adapt or vary the basic techniques described here to fit the circumstances of the case in question.

A

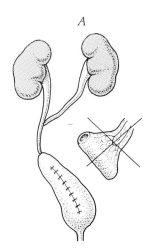

Close bladder discard conduit

B

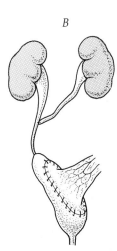

Close bladder with conduit patch

C

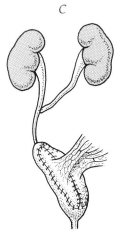

Close bladder with conduit patch and second ileal patch

D

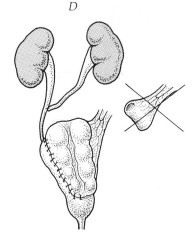

Close bladder with right colonic cystoplasty discard conduit

Fig. 15.29

POSTOPERATIVE MANAGEMENT

The postoperative management after undiversion is essentially the postoperative management of the procedures that were used to achieve it and most of these have been described elsewhere in this volume.

The average patient will have a wound drain to the retropubic space, a wound drain alongside the TUU and ureteric reimplantation, a suprapubic or urethral catheter or both and a ureteric stent running up the ureteric reimplantation and across the TUU to the contralateral kidney. The drains are removed when they stop draining. The ureteric stent (or stents if the ureters were more than usually dilated) is removed on about the 8th postoperative day after retrograde radiological studies (a 'stentogram') have shown satisfactory healing and, specifically, no extravasation at the TUU (Fig. 15.30, 15.31). If there was no urethral or bladder neck reconstruction — in which case there is only a suprapubic catheter — this is clamped on the 10th postoperative day for a trial of voiding. If spontaneous voiding does not occur the patient is started on clean intermittent self catheterisation (CISC). If a bladder neck or urethral reconstruction was performed — in which case there will be a suprapubic and a urethral catheter — both catheters are left for 3 weeks (2 weeks for healing, 1 week for paranoia!). A cystogram and urethrogram are then performed before removing the catheters to be sure that all the suture lines are well healed and the suprapubic catheter is left in (clamped) as a safety valve until a 24-hour trial of voiding or CISC has proved satisfactory.

An IVU is obtained 3 months later to assess upper tract drainage and bladder emptying before and after voiding by whatever means the patient is using to

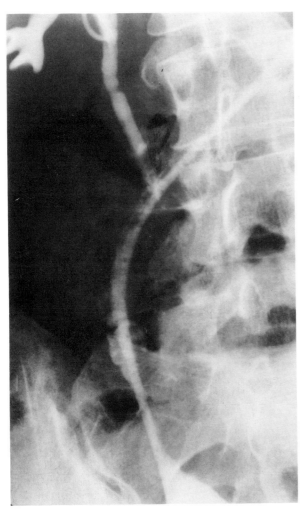

Fig. 15.30

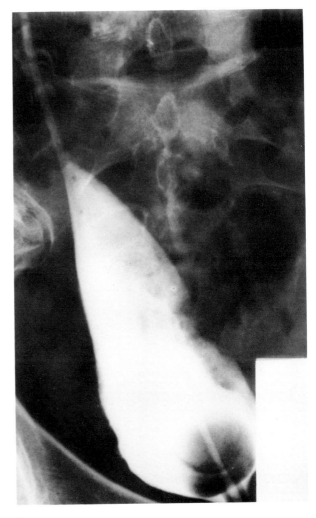

Fig. 15.31

empty. Ultrasound studies of bladder emptying and DTPA renal scanning of the upper tracts may be more appropriate studies than an IVU in some patients, but an IVU gives a good overall screening of the urinary tract after undiversion and is a useful baseline study for the future. Figure 15.32 shows the typical appearance after TUU and reimplantation of a normal ureter and Figure 15.33 shows the appearance with a tailored ileal ureter (arrowed). Note in both instances that it is almost impossible to detect the augmentation cystoplasty — this is often the case with a single view taken in one plane which is characteristic of an IVU. Figure 15.34

shows the appearance when a substitution cystoplasty has been used to serve the dual purpose of dealing with both the bladder problem and short ureters.

Video-urodynamic studies at 3 months are another important baseline for the future in patients with neuropathy or those who have abnormal upper urinary tracts.

COMPLICATIONS

The three main complications are upper tract problems, poor bladder emptying (which may be a cause of upper tract problems) and incontinence.

Poor bladder emptying is much the most common. It is treated by CISC if it is causing impaired upper tract drainage, frequency, overflow incontinence or recurrent urinary tract infections. Otherwise it can be left alone but should be followed by serial ultrasound studies of the upper and lower urinary tracts, before and after emptying, to make sure that the situation does not deteriorate.

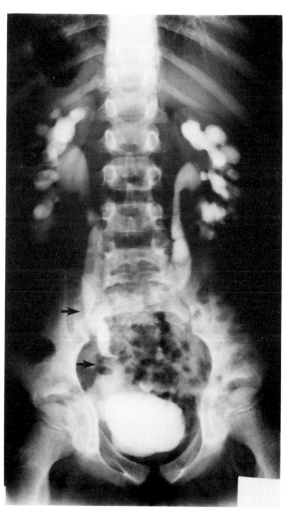

Fig. 15.32

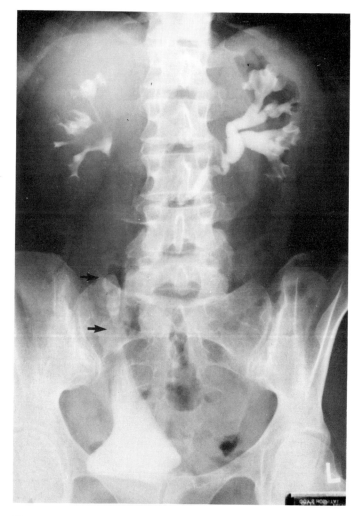

Fig. 15.33

Upper tract problems otherwise are rare. If they occur they will usually be related to ureteric obstruction at either the ureteroneocystostomy or the TUU. These will require surgical revision. Occasional patients have persistent vesico-ureteric reflux which is not likely to be a problem if the bladder is functioning satisfactorily and in the absence of recurrent urinary tract infection except that, for some unknown reason, reflux after undiversion almost always causes annoying loin pain. This may be severe enough to warrant revision of the UNC irrespective of bladder function or infection — another reason to prevent reflux if at all possible.

Another problem is ureteric failure — grossly dilated ureters, usually draining poorly functioning kidneys. When reimplanted in undiversion using an anti-reflux technique, ureters of this type tend to become obstructed. Although I believe this is rare when urothelial continuity is achieved, as hopefully it can be, it can nonetheless be a serious problem in a few patients and is often a problem when such ureters are reimplanted into gut by an anti-reflux technique. The problem can usually be resolved when it does occur by plumbing the ureters into an isolated segment of ileum which is then converted into an ileal ureter. The ileal

ureter is then reimplanted into the bladder, natural or substitute, using an anti-reflux technique. Distancing the anti-reflux mechanism from the incompetent ureters in this way seems to eliminate the obstructive element although the reason why this should help (just as why an anti-refluxing implantation of an incompetent ureter should become obstructed in the first place) is not clear.

Incontinence is usually due to sphincter weakness but may be due either to contractile activity in the bladder in patients with instability or hyperreflexia who were not treated by an adequate cystoplasty, or to poor emptying with overflow incontinence. Urodynamic investigation gives the definitive diagnosis which is then treated on its merits according to the nature of the problem.

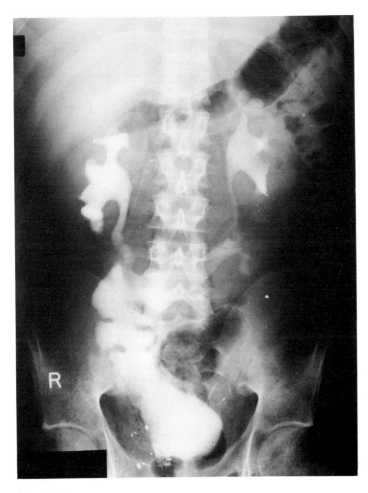

Fig. 15.34

REFERENCES

The main references on undiversion come from Hendren who has written numerous original papers and reviews on the subject. The review cited here is one of his more recent ones on the subject and refers to all his previous writings on specific aspects of the subject. My own recent review is also given.

Hendren W H 1986 Urinary tract undiversion. In: Welch K J, Randolph J G, Ravitch M M, O'Neill J A, Rowe M I (eds) Pediatric surgery, 4th edn. Year Book Medical Publishers, Chicago, pp 1264–1285

Mundy A R 1987 Refunctional urinary tract surgery with particular reference to undiversion. In: Hendry W F (ed) Recent advances in urology/andrology — 4. Churchill Livingstone, Edinburgh, pp 147–168